The following incidents of patients being harmed or killed by medical care have made the news headlines:

- A man undergoes surgery to have a gangrenous foot amputated and later finds that the doctor removed the wrong foot.
- Defective heart catheters that are used to remove blockages cause 50 patients to undergo emergency bypass surgery before the defective devices are removed from the market.
- A woman enters a top hospital to have a brain tumor operation and the doctor operates on the wrong side of her brain.
- A young woman undergoes surgery to remove her appendix and is accidentally given a hysterectomy instead.
- A nurse notices a piece of rubber sticking out of a woman's surgical wound and discovers that it is a glove left behind from surgery.
- A man undergoes surgery to have a cancerous kidney removed and the medical team removes the wrong kidney.
- A man who underwent surgery to remove a cancerous lung finds out that the wrong lung was removed .
- A young man decides to have liposuction and ends up dead from an overdose of anesthesia.
- A doctor is convicted of fondling patients while they were under anesthesia.
- A woman goes to the hospital for scar revision surgery and ends up with massive infections that require months of medical care to save her life.
- Two doctors unknowingly and separately prescribe medications that when taken together can have a fatal result, and the patient dies.
- Dozens of women who go to a doctor to be impregnated with donated sperm later find that the doctor was using his own sperm and may have fathered more than 70 children.
- A man finds out that an operation he had was done for no other reason than to help the doctor obtain her board certification.
- A doctor accidentally prescribes radiation therapy for a patient who does not have cancer.

The list goes on and on, and unfortunately all the stories are true. Millions of people undergo surgery every year. What happens to them when they enter the doors of an operating room can depend a lot on what it is they know about the surgery.

This book examines healthcare, explains how to evaluate doctors, lists what books to read, and tells you what questions to ask and what to expect before, during, and after surgery.

Also by John McCabe

Plastic Surgery Hopscotch:
A Resource Guide for Those Considering Cosmetic Surgery
Carmania Books, 1995

SURGERY ELECTIVES

What to Know Before the Doctor Operates

A·GUIDE·FOR·THOSE·CONSIDERING·ELECTIVE·SURGERY

EXPANDED AND COMPLETELY REVISED 2ND EDITION

by John McCabe
edited by Miriam Ingersoll

CARMANIA BOOKS

Surgery Electives: What to Know Before the Doctor Operates
2nd edition
by John McCabe, edited by Miriam Ingersoll

Address all letters concerning this book to:
    Carmania Books
    P.O. Box 1272
    Santa Monica, California 90406–1272

Carmania Books E-mail: CarmaniaBk@aol.com

John McCabe E-mail: TheJMcCabe@aol.com

All company names and products should be considered registered trademarks.

Printed in the United States of America

Published only in soft cover
by Carmania Books – 1994 (1st edition), 1997 (revised 2nd edition)

Health   Medicine   Self Help

Library of Congress Catalog Card Number 95-71658

ISBN   1-884702-22-8   (USA) $19.95   Soft cover   2nd Edition

The book *Plastic Surgery Hopscotch: A Resource Guide for Those Considering Cosmetic
Surgery* ($19.95), and additional copies of this book (also $19.95) are available from
Carmania Books at the address listed above. Postage of $3 must be included for the
first book and $1 for each additional book ordered. California residents must include
sales tax.

This book is available to the bookstore and library markets through the major book
wholesalers. For further information contact Carmania Books at PO Box 1272, Santa
Monica, CA 90406-1272.

Disclaimer

The information contained in this book has been compiled from thousands of sources and is subject to differences of opinion and interpretation. Every attempt was made to present accurate information as it could be gathered and cross-referenced before the publication date. This book is sold with the understanding that the publisher, author, and any related parties are not rendering medical or legal services. The opinions, suggestions, and advice given in this book are meant to inform readers and to provoke thought only, and should not be used as a substitute for needed healthcare or other professional help.

Neither the publisher, author, nor any involved and interested parties assume any liability for omissions or errors in this book, and therefore are not responsible for the interpretation or implementation of information contained in this book, and are not liable for any damages or loss caused or alleged to be caused directly or indirectly by information contained in this book including, but not limited to, legal disputes.

Because medical information is continuously being updated; many records are incomplete; new methods of treatment continue to be found; new laws are constantly being put into effect; and many scientists and others dedicated to the study of the human body have their own findings, beliefs, and opinions, no book on health is ever complete and the information contained here should not be considered the final say on any subject.

Although doctors, lawyers, editors, and others have adjusted some of the wording in this book, it was written by the author using his understanding of the issues covered. Therefore, some subjects may not be explained as fully as some readers may need for their specific health needs. As with any work this size, there is the possibility that typographical and content errors exist.

This book is focused on non-emergency health concerns. When experiencing a health emergency, a person should do what it takes to preserve his health and seek prompt medical attention. A person who is experiencing severe pain or a high fever, has suffered a broken bone, has been inflicted with an injury, such as a deep cut or burn, or any ailment that is interfering with the normal functions of his body, such as those that interfere with movement, vision, or breathing, should seek immediate medical care. Even in non-emergency situations it is important to seek the correct treatment early in the disease process or when any health concern arises, rather than to wait for the condition to worsen before finding treatment.

Each reader is encouraged to do his own research on issues that interest or concern him. For information on particular health subjects, referring to the many books and organizations listed in the *Research Resources* section of this book may prove to be helpful.

For physical and psychological issues, contact a properly licensed and certified, responsible doctor or health professional who is well trained in the area of your health concern.

Laws change as new cases are decided and new laws and regulations are enacted and interpreted. The legal information within this book is not to be used as a substitute for or in place of private legal advice. For legal matters, contact a legitimate lawyer who is familiar with the laws in your area. (Some information on seeking legal counsel is given in the *Research Resources* section of this book under the heading *Legal Assistance*. Persons interested in the legal concerns of healthcare consumers may want to read the book *The Consumer's Legal Guide to Today's Healthcare: Your Medical Rights and How to Assert Them*, by Stephen L. Isaacs, JD, & Ava C. Swartz, MPH; Houghton Mifflin Co., 1992. They may also find some help by contacting one or more of the groups listed in the *Research Resources* section of this book under the heading *Patients' and Consumers' Rights*.)

He Said/She Said about Him/Her

It is not the intent of the author to express any gender bias. Because most doctors are men, this book uses the masculine pronoun when referring to them. To make it easier on the reader (and writer), the patient is also referred to as a male. The author does not intend to offend anyone by referring to the doctors and patients as male, but he does think it is labor-intensive to constantly have to write and read "him/her," "his/her," "himself/herself," and "he/she." (The subject of women working in the male-dominated world of medicine and the role-playing, paternalistic, insensitive behavior of doctors toward women is covered in the book *Outrageous Practices: The Alarming Truth About How Medicine Mistreats Women*, by Leslie Laurence and Beth Weinhouse; Fawcett/Columbine, 1994.)

My thanks to the people and groups who supplied me with medical and legal advice, assisted in editing, sent me information, connected me with the right people, gave me support and encouragement, and helped me in their own various ways.

Some of them include Nancy S., Jonathan K., Terry M., Christina A., Marion C., Ray S., Marilyn M., Cheryl D., Lorin L., Cynthia E., Danny & Amy B.W., Rob & Bonnie B., Steven H., Hugh B., Marjorie B., Julie B., Lynda R., Dan P., Trevor E., John R., Bernard K., Brant L., Janet VW., Bill S., Bill E., Nanette J., Curt F., Bill P., Peter K., Judy S., Joyce P., Tom and Cheryl R., Patrick D., Amy C., Lee S., Margo T., Susan M., Teryl Anne N., Margaret Rita Murray C., and Miriam I.

I especially want to thank the many victims of medical negligence whom I interviewed for this book and who wish to remain anonymous. Without their input this book would not be what it is.

– John McCabe

CONTENTS

Introduction

This book may be too harsh on the good doctors but not critical enough of the bad doctors. It also may not go into as much depth about certain approaches to treating ailments as some people may need. While reading this book it may be good to remember that there is more than one side to every story, everyone seems to have an opinion, and all points of view are biased in some way. Those who are considered experts will disagree with some of the material, but other than possible errors in statistics, definitions, or facts, there is no opinion expressed in this book that is unshared.

Many volumes have been written about medicine — enough to fill large libraries. Many books written about the business of medicine raise questions concerning the necessity of surgery. Other books are based on the subject of unnecessary surgery and the reasons why it takes place. This book covers a little of everything.

The medical industry has always had its critics, including 19th-century preachers who warned that doctors were influenced by Satan. Today there are consumer awareness groups that work to empower patients and there are people inside and outside the medical community who write books like this one. Some of this input is helpful because it has been effective in stimulating change and developing better therapies and safety measures. Although some may criticize this book for mentioning so many malpractice cases and occurrences of negligence, it is through studying past mishaps with the delivery of medicine that a person can learn what can go wrong and know what to look out for when seeking healthcare.

Rather than instill fear in the minds of medical consumers, this book was written to suggest to patients what questions to ask and to direct them toward the information needed to make well-balanced, informed decisions on whether surgery will be beneficial in improving well-being and quality of life.

This second version of *Surgery Electives* not only provides information on what to know about surgery, but also considers what caused patients to experience the health problem that landed them in the doctor's office. Other than for injuries and genetic disorders, surgery is most often prescribed as a treatment for illnesses created by food choices and lack of exercise. All the information here is presented to inform patients of their healthcare rights or show them how to take charge of their health. By using the references in the *Research Resources* section of the book, a person should be able to find information on practically any health topic and come to a clearer understanding of the subjects discussed.

During the time I spent writing and rewriting this book I spoke to a wide variety of patients, medical doctors, psychologists, lawyers, nurses, holistic practitioners, physical therapists, consumer advocates, lawmakers, librarians, government workers, authors, magazine editors, and journalists. I also received boxes of letters from, and spoke on the phone with, people who have been victims or are related to victims of medical malpractice. The books, pamphlets, articles, letters, and videos these people have provided me, along with what they have told me, helped this project slowly grow into the book you now hold in your hands. Many people also read and reread the manuscript as I was writing it, and many of their comments have been written into the text.

The first version of this book was published in 1994 and was purchased by many public libraries. Although it was written for consumers, it became popular with malpractice attorneys, who seemed to be using the book to figure out what happened to their clients and to help pinpoint where malpractice may have occurred. This second version has been updated and a lot of reference material has been added to it.

Rather than provide information for malpractice lawyers, I hope this new version of the book will be used more often by medical consumers to help prevent situations in which they may be harmed and even killed at the hands of pompous, incompetent, and untrustworthy healthcare providers.

Doctors are not all-knowing and do not always possess good judgment. Their knowledge is limited and may be biased toward certain ways of treating the body based on personal beliefs and what they learned in medical school. Whenever people subject themselves to treatment by a medical professional, it should never be assumed the professional is going to do what is best. Nor should it be assumed the doctor will relay every important piece of information regarding their care.

There are many reasons why patients may not be told of optional or alternative treatments. There are also many reasons why patients may not get the treatment that is best for the condition. Although it is deplorable, much of the reasoning behind more and more medical decisions revolves around money — who is getting it and who is spending it — rather than the health needs of the patients.

Unfortunately, the medical professionals Americans rely on most often for health information — allopathic doctors — are strongly influenced by the actions of big-money medical device manufacturers and drug companies, who lobby heavily in Washington. They provide financing to medical schools; offer incentives to doctors; buy nearly all the advertising space in allopathic medical journals and magazines; and rent most, if not all, of the booth exhibition space at medical conventions. For example, even though it is well known that diet, nutrition, and exercise can play the largest role in preventing and reversing most heart disease, the doctors, cardiologists, scientists, and others who attended the American Heart Association Scientific Sessions in Anaheim, California, in November 1995 were exposed to four buildings full of booths rented by medical device and pharmaceutical companies promoting surgical and drug therapies.

Surgery and medical procedures can cause adverse consequences that are not ordinarily anticipated in advance. Some of the operations being performed may be of no benefit to the patients, and some do nothing but introduce problems into patients' lives, while some other surgeries and therapies make sick patients even sicker.

Time and again as new procedures are developed they often become overused by some segment of the medical profession. This includes many of the more common surgical procedures. Numerous expensive studies that have involved reviewing the records of hundreds of thousands of patients and that have been published in the most popular and respected allopathic medical journals have concluded that many surgeries are done too often, are of questionable value to the patients, and may cause more problems than the surgeries were meant to solve.

In addition to the problems with surgeries that harm patients is the evidence that the x-rays the patients are subjected to, the tests that are performed on them, and the drugs prescribed may also be more damaging to the patients' health than the conditions the treatments are meant to cure. In the long term, some forms of surgery and testing procedures may cause problems and diseases that will show up years later in the patient, and some drugs may cause health problems in the patient's posterity. Some people who go into the hospital with the goal of getting medical care end up getting post-mortem care as their body is prepared for its trip to the cold hospital morgue.

Because people are never more vulnerable and emotionally fragile than when ill, consumers entering the medical world need to be aware of what is and is not acceptable, and what is and is not good medicine. They need to know what to look for when they seek healthcare so they can prevent situations in which they may be taken advantage of and harmed by the negligent acts of caregivers. They should know that medical professionals vary in their knowledge, their therapeutic philosophies, their skills, and the techniques they use. They need to understand that not all patients with the same ailments respond in the same way to the same treatments. They should realize that even simple medical decisions can affect the rest of their lives.

Patients can play a large part in the success of their medical treatment. The first step to success with any choice is that of becoming informed. The less people know about a medical treatment, the more susceptible they are to mistreatment, especially when they have been misdiagnosed. Confidence can be gained from knowledge, which can help patients protect themselves from harm.

People need not figuratively wear a blindfold when first consulting the doctor, nor do they need to accept the doctor's first reflex of prescribing drugs or surgery. Many patients do not understand that they have the right to refuse any type of treatment or medication that is offered or prescribed.

In the past, doctors left the patient out of the decision-making process and often did not do much explaining about the diagnosis, treatment options, or risks involved. This caused patients to be unprepared for and frightened about undergoing surgery. Patients are now becoming more assertive. Today patients can educate themselves about their options and play a major role in deciding what treatment — if any — will be prescribed.

Open communication between a doctor and a patient is important. Patients who understand their diagnosis and prescribed treatment are more realistic about what to expect from a doctor. Doctors who take time to listen to their patients are also more likely to gather information that can be crucial to proper diagnosis and treatment.

A study published in the *Journal of the American Medical Association* (November 23, 1994) reported that patients are more likely to be satisfied with their medical care if they communicate well with doctors from the very start. Many other studies have shown that patients who are informed about their options, who know what to expect when undergoing medical care, and who become active participants in their own treatment recover faster than patients who are not informed or involved. Doctors are told by their associations and insurance carriers that open communication with patients is helpful in reducing medical malpractice suits. At least one insurance company has provided a decreased malpractice premium to doctors who complete a workshop on doctor-patient communication. Many medical schools are now offering classes in the doctor-patient relationship.

The healthcare world is changing quickly, and more forms of treatment are available now than have been available in the past. The wide variety of therapeutic options that are offered deserve to be explored by anyone who is experiencing a serious health problem. These forms of treatment are delivered by both allopathic and osteopathic medicine specialists, as well as by very knowledgeable holistic practitioners who specialize in such forms of medicine as Chinese, ayurvedic, homeopathic, and herbal.

As the holistic approaches are becoming more popular, many people are recognizing the roles nutrition and physical fitness play in bringing them to and keeping them in good health. Nutrition is important during sickness and in maintaining health because every one of the trillions of cells in the body uses nutrients to function properly. All the therapies that are delivered by the various types of doctors would be of little avail if the body were not able to heal. In addition to proper nutrition, the way people heal is often related to fitness level, state of mind, physical surroundings, and the strength of the immune system. Doctors are not magicians; they do not heal people. It is the body that heals; therapies only assist the process.

Through it all, the type and quality of medical care patients receive in large measure depend on their taking the initiative to educate themselves and on asking the right questions before deciding on a course of treatment. Information specific to each health concern can be attained through library research, consultations with health professionals, speaking with other patients, and contacting specialized health organizations.

In any situation where elective surgery is suggested, the final authority on whether the surgery takes place should be none other than a well-informed patient who knows the options, who has had more than one professional opinion, and who understands and has weighed the physical, emotional, and financial risks.

— John McCabe
c/o Carmania Books, PO Box 1272, Santa Monica, CA 90406-1272
E-mail: TheJMcCabe@aol.com

1 • THE CUTTING EDGE

Altering Procedures

There is no defined area of knowledge that can be mastered in regard to the human body and the ways to treat what goes wrong with it. Thousands of books have been written about the human body and how it works; magazines and medical journals are filled with articles and studies about it, and it is the subject of numerous television talk shows and news programs, but still there is no one who thoroughly understands it.

Probably everyone has some type of physical condition that a doctor can find some reason to alter. A bothersome toenail, a mole he does not like, a slight chip in a tooth, or a recurring soreness in a joint are some small examples. These are things a doctor can correctly or incorrectly claim need medical attention: the toenail could cause an infection; the mole could become cancerous; the chipped tooth could lead to tooth decay; the sore joint could deteriorate.

On the other hand, these might never amount to any significant problem that could interfere with the person's health and happiness, and they might be better left alone. A couple of the conditions — the toenail and the stiff joint — might even heal themselves, whereas surgical intervention might lead the person to experience more problems than the conditions otherwise would have caused. More serious conditions that are often treated with invasive surgery may not only result in a physical change but may even have a negative emotional impact on the patient.

The world of medicine is filled with these and other more serious types of decisions where a vital organ, a major function of the body, or a person's overall health might be adversely affected.

It is often hard to determine what aspects of certain procedures are most important for each patient, as what may seem unimportant at one moment may become life-altering at another time.

•

How your health condition is treated may depend on what area of the US you live. For instance, mastectomy operations for breast cancer are more commonly performed in New Mexico with 57.7% of women with breast tumors (ductal carcinoma in situ, or DCIS) being treated with mastectomy as compared to Connecticut with 28.8% (*Journal of the American Medical Association*, March 27, 1996).

•

In any situation in which a person is experiencing physical-health problems there can be many ways of treating the condition.

Perhaps the remedy may be simple, such as improving the quality of the person's food choices and fitness level, or the person may need some immediate attention where surgical intervention is the best form of treatment. It is hoped, in the case of surgery, the right diagnosis and choices will be made, and the most beneficial techniques will be used.

Healthcare Access

With all the modern developments in health science, when an individual in the US is in need of medical attention you would think that person could go to a doctor and receive the best care possible. Unfortunately, that is not true as often as it should be.

The healthcare world is not a perfect place where everyone does what is right and everyone wins. It revolves around big money and career advancements; therefore, people do not always do what they are supposed to do. Many of the actions of doctors and hospitals these days are motivated by financial gain, and they too often judge their success by it. Many surgeries and other treatments are financially driven rather than symptom-driven, and the financial and legal interests of today's medical industry are clouding over the real needs of the patients, while healthcare providers are conducting business within a system that has a flagrant disregard for consumers' right to know. It is also a healthcare system in which the accessibility to quality healthcare declines and the chances of mistreatment increase in proportion to the individual's lower financial status and the darker his skin color.

The eruption of the AIDS epidemic in the last fifteen years has helped to expose the way the medical industry delivers healthcare. As thousands of young and educated people infected with HIV have fought to find a cure for AIDS, they have revealed questionable activities in the way drugs are developed, tested, researched, and approved by the FDA, and have unveiled the way the American health insurance and medical industry misspends, mismanages, and altogether "misfunctions."

> During the Clinton healthcare campaign it was noted by White House officials that only 40% of Hispanics were covered by employer health insurance, compared with the 70% figure for all Americans.

As the talk of restructuring the healthcare industry blew through the mass media and the halls of lawmakers, many Americans were made aware of the problems facing medical consumers. Some attention was given to the abuses that occur within the medical industry and the fact that doctors do not always know or do what is best as they work in an industry in which patients and government health plans are regularly overcharged.

The healthcare industry is an industry just like any other — driven by the goal of making profits for investors. The well-financed medical trade groups at the top hire lobbyists who influence lawmakers to pass laws that protect key medical industry players and help them make more money. The result is that doctors do not live by the same standards and rules that govern the rest of Americans; some abuse the power they have been given, and at times there are those who seem literally to get away with murder.

As in every other profession, there are good people working in the medical industry who are well educated and who excel in and enjoy their work. There are those who flourish in the atmosphere where life-or-death decisions are often made, and others who do not cope well in a tense work environment. Some doctors, because of the treatment they receive from their superiors and the turf disputes and abuses that happen around them, are burned out and endure stress because they are not financially or professionally able to walk away from the bad working conditions that interfere with the high quality of care they aim to supply.

Not all doctors are alike. While there are ethical doctors who try to do what is right and give more than they receive, there are others performing life-altering procedures while strung out on drugs and alcohol, and they subject patients to gross negligence. There are also many doctors who hand out drug prescriptions too freely with no explanation of side effects and little if any follow-up, and who too quickly decide on surgery without considering other options.

As insurance companies continue gaining power, more and more healthcare decisions are being made for financial reasons rather than for reasons that would benefit the patients.

Currently, the governing bodies that are set up to enforce standards that protect medical consumers, such as state medical boards and peer review groups, do not always do their jobs properly. Very often when these governing bodies investigate bad medical care, they seem to protect the negligent practitioners more than the consumers who register the complaints. Often, boards use the term "acceptable standards of practice" to describe actions that border on malpractice, or that at least amount to treatment that is not in the best interest of the patient.

In 1994, the Illinois Department of Professional Regulations fielded 636 complaints against doctors for gross negligence; dishonorable, unethical, or unprofessional conduct inimical to the public interest;

incompetence; or immoral conduct. It issued only 21 sanctions for offenses in those categories. The year before, a similar number of complaints in those categories came in, but only a single doctor was disciplined.

— *Bad Medicine*, by Anita J. Slomski; *Chicago Magazine*, March 1996

•

Some of the medical professionals who read the manuscript of this book mentioned that doctors may not report a bad doctor to the state medical board because the medical boards, which are run by doctors, do not like tattle-tale doctors. They said the medical boards may take steps to remove the licenses of the reporting doctors in retaliation for being tattle-talers. They also mentioned that nurses who report bad doctors are not taken seriously.

•

In a way, the existing disciplinary system practically requires consumers to be the supervisors of the doctors. The information source that state medical boards rely on to learn of bad medical care usually consists of patients who recognize and report when a doctor is out of line. Among the sources that patients should be able to consult to learn about negligent doctors are state medical boards. Unfortunately, as you will learn by reading this book, lobbyists working for the medical and insurance groups have been very successful in getting laws passed that protect negligent doctors. These laws limit consumers' access to such information and help secure insurance company profits by limiting court awards.

If patients are better educated and demand more information about medical procedures, devices, and pills; ask more questions; and request better treatment, the patients themselves can raise the level of acceptable standards.

The reason many healthcare organizations are launching quality-improvement and quality-assurance programs is that healthcare consumers are asking more questions and demanding better quality.

Licensed to Perform

Anyone who has a medical license can legally perform surgery. Surgery is performed by doctors who may or may not have specialized training along with a staff who may have insufficient medical knowledge. Many of the new medical technologies, such as videoscopic surgery and improved anesthetic processes, have created less invasive, less complicated, and less expensive surgical procedures done through small incisions, and this has resulted in speedier recoveries. More than half of all surgical procedures are now performed on an outpatient basis, which has brought about greater patient responsibility. Many procedures that once required a hospital stay now allow patients to go home just hours after surgery, but they are then responsible for their own recovery.

Surgical procedures that can be performed in a doctor's office can be done to high standards by caring doctors but also attract doctors who would not be able to meet the standards of many hospital peer review committees, which limit what procedures a doctor can and cannot do in the hospital on the basis of experience. The surgeon operating outside the hospital setting can also hire surgical assistants, nurses, and anesthesiologists who might not be accepted into a hospital based on their own professional histories. Some of these physicians have not had any formal training in the area of medicine they practice. Many of them are performing newly learned procedures on patients who believe the doctors are well trained and experienced. The result is that people are sometimes left maimed, psychologically distraught, financially burdened, and sometimes even dead.

In 1984, dozens of researchers from the fields of medicine, law, economics, peer review, policy analysis, and statistics analyzed the care of patients in New York State. The study included interviewing patients, doctors, and surgeons, and reviewing insurance claims, hospital records, and malpractice suits. Out of an estimated 2.7 million patients hospitalized there were 98,609 (or 3.65 %) who suffered an injury that could be attributed to the medical care they received rather than to their ailment. More than 13,000 (about 0.5 %) of the patients' deaths were in part a result of injuries or poor care.

The advertising that the medical industry puts out, the doctors themselves and their office staff may speak of surgery too lightly. They may downplay the recovery period while overlooking the details the patient should know pertaining to the risks, the extent of the injuries inflicted by the surgery, the information needed for post-operative care, and the length of the recovery time. They may also place promises where promises cannot truthfully exist.

The American College of Surgeons *Socio-Economic Factbook for Surgery* **lists the following as the ten most frequent operative procedures performed on patients in short-stay nonfederal hospitals in 1991*:**
1. Episiotomy (almost always an unnecessary procedure) with or without forceps or vacuum extraction (during childbirth) (1,684,000 performed).
2. Cardiac catheterization (1,000,000 performed).
3. Cesarean section (933,000 performed). (The US has one of the highest rates of cesarean sections. In Japan, where the cesarean section rates are lower than that of the US, the infant survival rate is higher.)

4. Repair of current obstetric laceration (795,000 performed).
5. Artificial rupture of membranes (775,000 performed).
6. Cholecystectomy (gallstone removal) (571,000 performed).
7. Hysterectomy (removal of the female reproductive organs) (546,000 performed).
8. Oophorectomy (removal of an ovary) (458,000 performed).
9. Open reduction of fracture (418,000 performed).
10. Coronary artery bypass graft (407,000 performed).

* According to the American College of Surgeons there was a total of 22,411,000 surgical operations performed in short-stay nonfederal hospitals in 1991.

The top five procedures performed on men in nonfederal short-stay hospitals during 1991 were:
1. Cardiac catheterization (603,000 performed).
2. Prostatectomy (363,000 performed).
3. Reduction of fracture — excluding skull, nose, and jaw (337,000 performed).
4. Direct heart revascularization (coronary bypass) (296,000 performed).
5. Excision or destruction of intervertebral disc and spinal fusion (258,000 performed).

The top five procedures performed on men 65 years and over in nonfederal short-stay hospitals in 1991 were:
1. Prostatectomy (295,000 performed).
2. Cardiac catheterization (235,000 performed).
3. Direct heart revascularization (coronary bypass) (144,000 performed).
4. Pacemaker insertion or replacement (117,000 performed).
5. Biopsies on the digestive system (89,000).

The top five procedures performed on women in nonfederal short-stay hospitals in 1991 were:
1. Procedures to assist delivery (2,558,000 performed).
2. Cesarean section (933,000 performed).
3. Repair of current obstetric laceration (795,000 performed).
4. Hysterectomy (546,000 performed).
5. Oophorectomy and alspingo-oophorectomy (458,000 performed).

The top five procedures performed on women 65 years and over in nonfederal short-stay hospitals in 1991 were:
1. Cardiac catheterization (211,000 performed).
2. Reduction of fracture — excluding the skull, nose, and jaw (174,000 performed).
3. Arthroplasty and replacement of hip (124,000 performed).
4. Biopsies of the digestive system (107,000 performed).
5. Pacemaker insertion or replacement (128,000 performed).

Surgery should never be taken lightly. It inflicts trauma on the body and causes the person to become temporarily unwell. Depending on which procedure is done, surgery can involve taking drugs to prevent infection and pain. It may involve some sort of anesthesia to which the patient might have an allergic reaction, and, in the worst case, can kill the patient. It nearly always involves cutting into the flesh, where there are blood vessels and nerves to which irreversible damage can occur. It may involve breaking, cutting, chiseling, sawing, shaving or drilling of bone and cartilage. It may involve removal of part of the flesh, muscle, cartilage, bone, or part of an organ that cannot be put back once it is taken away. It usually involves blotting or suctioning blood and stitching flesh and sometimes organs and muscles, and setting bones and cartilage back into place. Whatever was removed is eventually dropped into a hazardous-waste bin.

Even after surgery, any number of known and unknown complications may arise that can endanger the patient's physical and mental health for the sake of a goal that is not always met in operations that cannot be reversed. During the recovery period that starts immediately after the surgery is completed, the patient might experience bleeding, severe swelling, intense bruising, and infections. There is always a risk of improper healing, along with the question of how the surgery site will change over the years. Depending on what procedure is done, and how it is done, the altered body part may age in undesirable ways.

•

When doctors in Israel went on strike, the mortality rate declined by 50%.

In Bogota, Colombia, when doctors struck for 52 days, the death rate decreased by 35%.

When doctors in Los Angeles County protested the rising cost of malpractice insurance by not performing non-emergency surgery for the first 35 days of 1976, the county mortality rates declined. The rates increased to their normal level soon after the doctors resumed their practices.

•

There is no accurate record of how many people have died during surgery. Unexpected deaths are not always reported to the correct authorities. Deaths in surgery centers away from hospitals, where many surgeries are performed, are not always recorded accurately. The death certificate may simply state that the person died from heart failure or respiratory failure and not list the consequences or the disease that led to the death. In his book *The Making of a Surgeon* (Random House, 1968), William Nolen tells about how patients who died on the operating tables were pronounced dead after they were taken off of the operating table so that the doctors could avoid having to fill out stacks of complicated forms that were required to explain why a patient died during surgery. Even if the patients were already dead, the anesthesiologist would continue to administer oxygen until the doctors could suture the incision and then transfer the patient to a stretcher before the patient was declared dead.

Listing the true cause of death is important for recognizing threats of contagious diseases, product fault, criminal activity, and medical malpractice. The lack of accurate death certificates causes inaccurate health statistics and makes it difficult to trace the incidence of diseases and inherited health problems.

Surgical Intent

Basically, there are two reasons why people agree to have elective surgery:
- To alter a birth or genetic defect, or to repair a body part that has been changed by an accident, wear and tear, or disease.

    — or —

- To change a body part for cosmetic/vanity reasons.

Surgery is a way of altering what nature, heredity, and life have drawn on the body. People undergo surgery for many reasons. It could be something as simple as pulling a tooth or as complex as transplanting a heart. Whatever the reason for someone's being on an operating table, there is always the chance of a complication with the operation. There could be a problem with bleeding, an adverse reaction to anesthesia, or any number of common or uncommon complications. It could be a simple problem that can be easily avoided, or it could be a complication that can result in the death of the patient.

Whereas a certain number of mistakes are to be expected in any profession, all too often it is not an injury or sickness that does the most harm to the patient, but the medical treatment the patient receives that causes injury or death. Although the number of fatalities in operating rooms has dropped dramatically over the last few decades, current estimates of the number of patients who die each year because of operations that have gone bad are still uncomfortably high. Many of these deaths are untraceable because of the way medical records are kept.

Elements that increase the chance of unexpected surgical results or injury are:
- Putting too much trust in the doctor and his staff.
- Letting the doctor and his staff's knowledge and authority intimidate you.

- Having a doctor who does not have enough training.
- Having a doctor who works too fast.
- Having a doctor who does not have enough help or is assisted by a staff who lack thorough training.
- Having a doctor who tries to cut costs in the office and the operating room by not purchasing and maintaining emergency supplies and equipment.

Whenever surgery is performed, there can be no guarantee on the results. Surgery can produce a result that is opposite to what the patient expected. It may turn out better than the patient thought it would, or it can leave the patient deformed or alter the normal function of the body. A negative result can cause a patient to fall into a mind-wrenching obsessive depression, and send him to search for another doctor who may or may not be able to fix a surgical disaster.

Surgery cannot give a patient an entirely new body. Alterations can be made to change various parts of the physical structure. Sometimes the outcome is very successful. Some surgeries are relatively simple compared with others, but surgeons have botched even the simplest operations. Even with the best medical attention there is no guarantee that the surgical goal will be obtained. The patient's health, the techniques used by surgeons and their medical team, and the patient's healing abilities all play a part in the final result of surgery.

For these and other reasons, anyone seeking medical care needs to look very closely at any physician approached for treatment. No one should ever automatically trust someone simply because that person has a doctoral degree in medicine. Those about to undergo an operation or any medical procedure deserve to know his rights and how to recognize a bad doctor and bad medical treatment.

There is always more activity behind the scenes of a hospital that the patients are not exposed to. In his book *The Making of a Surgeon* (Random House, 1968), William Nolen tells about how one particular intern he worked with made the diagnosis of a hernia on every male patient. Most of the patients accepted the diagnosis, and some underwent surgery for the conditions that didn't exist. The doctors probably made money, the hospital probably made money, and the patients probably never knew their surgeries were unnecessary.

Just because someone has an MD attached to his name does not automatically mean he is honest and caring. While some people feel cheated when they leave a doctor's office without some kind of diagnosis, drug prescription, or orders for some type of test, no one has to accept a doctor's diagnosis, judgment, or prescribed treatment.

Because a doctor agrees to operate on you does not always mean you need an operation. You may have been misdiagnosed, the doctor may not be knowledgeable of or current on alternative treatments, or the doctor may have ulterior motives.

Other than for financial reasons, treatments prescribed by doctors are often based on what has worked in the past. When a doctor prescribes a treatment it does not necessarily mean that it is the only treatment available for your condition. It may be the treatment the doctor is most familiar with. There may be newer or older procedures the doctor is unfamiliar with that can be more effective in treating your condition. There may be a less invasive procedure that is not only more effective but is also safer. Some conditions heal by themselves with no medical intervention. Other conditions improve when diet and fitness level are improved.

Questions to answer before undergoing surgery:
- What are the likely benefits of the surgery?
- What are the valid reasons that determine your need for the surgery?
- Do you know how it is done?
- What are the short- and long-term risks?
- Do you know what your body's response to the surgical wound will be?
- Do you know the length of time you will need to recover from the surgery and what type of care you will need during this time?
- How will the surgery affect all areas of your life?
- What are the educational backgrounds and professional histories of the doctor and the surgical team?
- Are the doctor and staff going to do what is best for you?

Not everyone looks or feels better after surgery. If you are considering surgery, you should not be too enthusiastic about hopping up on an operating table. You should take caution with each step toward surgery. When no immediate health threat exists, you should not let a doctor or the staff set a date for an elective surgical procedure, get you to pay for the operation, or get you anywhere near the operating room before you are able to make an informed and responsible decision as to whether the surgery is best for you.

The Hand That Holds the Scalpel

A doctor always plays God.
— Dr. Jack Kevorkian

Up until the last century those people who became doctors learned the trade by working with an established doctor in an apprentice system (this is still the practice in some parts of the world). Learning was accomplished and techniques were often developed by observation of each patient. Many of these old-time doctors never held a degree, were not supervised by anyone, were governed by few laws, and were not subject to certification boards or insurance company guidelines. Primitive treatments were practiced, surgery was performed without anesthesia by doctors who wore no special sanitary surgical clothing, and ineffective and dangerous remedies were the norm, while improvements were few and far between and opportunities for quackery were broad and common.

Even the clumsy medicine of the 18th and 19th centuries was a great improvement over treatments performed in Europe during earlier centuries. During the Dark Ages human ailments were thought to be the workings of evil spirits, medicine was more of a religious mystery, and patients were subject to exorcisms and visits by priest-doctors. By the 17th century people in England thought offensive smells would keep illnesses away, so they burned things and kept rotting animals around to drive away the diseases. People did not know about bacteria, where diseases came from, or how they were transmitted.

.

The children's singing game *ring-around-a-rosy* is actually about the spread of disease within a family at the time of the plagues. The rosy rings that showed up on the skin were the sign of disease. The *"pocket full of posies"* referred to the smelly things they kept in an ignorant attempt to keep the disease away. The *"ashes, ashes"* part actually was originally *"achoo, achoo,"* and had to do with the first person in the family sneezing. As the disease spread in the family, they would all begin to sneeze and eventually *"all fall down"* and die.

.

Luckily the early days of medicine contrast dramatically with the standards of today's medical community, which continues to experience many revolutionary changes — but unfortunately some of the quackery element still exists.

People who become doctors are not derived from some form of unique human pedigree. They are simply people who have gone through years of specific schooling and learned certain things to obtain a degree in medicine.

There are some very good doctors who seek to have an up-to-date knowledge in their area of medicine, are experienced in the treatments they prescribe, possess a keen understanding of how the body works, and always try to do what is best for their patients. Some doctors have performed medically miraculous operations. There are doctors who spend their careers in distressed areas of the world with limited medical supplies, working against the odds to try to improve the health of people who otherwise would not have had the chance to receive proper healthcare. There are doctors who form teams and fly to war-torn countries to perform free operations on people who have been injured, and doctors who remain in war zones to save the lives of innocent victims.

However, there are also some selfish, psychologically and socially immature, arrogant, and manipulative doctors who show more interest in making money than in guarding the welfare of their patients. These doctors prescribe therapies and procedures that are done for no reason other than to get money from the patients and insurance companies. Many of these doctors have been sued, many have had their licenses taken away, and some have been sent to jail for many kinds of unprofessional, deceitful, injurious, and life-threatening actions. There are also doctors performing procedures simply to gain more experience and others using unknowing patients as part of research projects. There are unskilled doctors misrepresenting their experience, doctors who do more harm than good, and doctors who perform operations that, for one reason or another, should not be done. There are doctors who have been sent to jail for raping their patients while the patients were under anesthesia. There are doctors who misuse their accessibility to drugs and regularly abuse them. Some doctors are so addicted that they perform surgery while under the influence.

Steps taken in the United States to become an allopathic medical doctor:

- Obtain Bachelor of Science degree.
- Take either the Graduate Medical Aptitude Test or the Medical College Admissions Test that is administered by the Association of American Medical Colleges.
- Attend (usually) four years of medical school. This includes classes in anatomy, biochemistry, histology, microbiology, pharmacology, and physiology.
- Two years before graduation from medical school and at the end of the fourth year, take the standardized US Medical Licensing Examination. The exam is administered by the National Board of Medical Examiners to determine placement in residencies and helps determine whether the student should remain in medical school.
- Serve (usually) one year of internship. Internships, like residencies, are coveted positions and key to allopathic medical training in the US. They also provide hospitals with a ready supply of needed healthcare workers.
- Obtain a state medical license. If practicing in a town near a state border, a license can also be obtained in the neighboring state. If working for the federal government, a medical license from any state in the nation is accepted.
- Get a Drug Enforcement Agency registration number so he can legally prescribe drugs.

- Complete a residency program. The residency system was developed several decades ago at Johns Hopkins University in Baltimore, Maryland. The Resident Matching System assigns residents to the hospital where they will serve their residency. The residency can last for two or more years depending on the specialization. During the residency program the residents work long hours and are exposed to a wide selection of cases. As the residency period is served the resident take on greater responsibility. In the last part of the residency he may perform entire operations while being supervised by a senior surgeon. Residents are paid, but the pay varies from hospital to hospital.
- Go into private practice or join an existing practice or organization.
- Apply for privileges at nearby hospitals. The hospital will ask for information about the doctor's educational and professional experience along with references, proof of state license, proof of Drug Enforcement Agency license, and malpractice insurance. The hospital is also supposed to contact the National Practitioner Data Bank to find if there are any records of the doctor being in trouble with state medical boards or having a history of malpractice, criminal behavior, or drug abuse. The hospital will grant privileges based on this information. Some hospitals are more thorough in doing background checks than others. Hospitals with rigid standards will restrict the doctor to scheduling and performing procedures on patients in the hospital based on the doctor's training. Hospitals with less rigid standards will let the doctor govern his own limitations and hope the doctor does so wisely.
- Pass specialty board exams and present a portfolio that details cases of patients that have been treated.
- Sometimes continue with fellowship training in a subspecialty area.
- Attend continuing education programs to keep updated. Continuing education class settings vary greatly. They may involve classes at a university medical school, or seminars given at a resort hotel where the doctor watches a video and listens to a speaker before heading off to snorkel in the ocean or ski on the slopes. The seminar conductors may have the doctor performing a new surgical technique on a cadaver or an animal, or learning to use a new type of medical instrument by using a medical mannequin or a computer. At the end of the seminar a class photo may be taken, and these often end up mounted on plaques hung on doctors' office walls.

According to the Association of American Medical Colleges, a record 42,500 people applied for 15,975 slots at 126 US medical schools for the 1993-94 school year.

If doctors who have been educated in another country want to practice medicine in the US, they must complete an equivalency exam in order to obtain a medical license in the US. They also may be required to complete an internship in the US.

•

In past centuries it was common for a doctor to have little, if any, formal training, and even the best doctors prescribed barbaric treatments, such as trying to bleed the sickness out of a patient. Since then the standardization of medical schools combined with the advancements seen in medical science have led to the modern-day doctor's training that is rigorous, pressured, stressful, time-consuming, expensive, and involves committing a large amount of information to memory.

However, it is hard to ignore the great financial incentive for all the time, money, and energy a person spends to become a doctor. Doctors make many times the income of an average American; currently a doctor in the US makes an average annual income of just over $170,000 (cardiosurgeons, orthopedic surgeons, cosmetic surgeons, neurosurgeons, radiologists, reproductive endocrinologists, anesthesiologists, and some other specialists make much more than this, on average).

The medical industry has hundreds of billions of dollars flowing through it every year, and doctors are at the mouth of the funnel. While many Americans struggle to make a common wage, many doctors *bring home* several thousand dollars a day. It is why some people joke that "MD" stands for "Making Dollars."

Doctors' standing in society is promoted to a high level of respect by commercials that use wording such as, "In clinical studies doctors agree that . . .," or, "Nine out of ten doctors . . ." Many people take these testimonies as truth without questioning who the doctors are, what kind of doctors they are, who paid for the studies, and what it is that is being considered "clinical." The studies may also be biased, flawed, or based on out-of-date or falsified information.

•

One early radio personality, Henry Morgan, made fun of this advertising lingo when he spoke about the fictional town of More, Utah. Morgan said the town of More had two doctors and those doctors were who the commercials were referring to when they claimed that "More doctors recommend . . ."

•

The authority figure they represent can be and is used by some doctors to their advantage. Some patients expect their doctor to wear the white "authority" jacket or they do not feel as if they are talking to a doctor.

•

Medical students and interns often wear white pants or skirts. These clothes are often supplied by the hospital. Residents and attending physicians who are working in hospitals often wear white coats. The coat of the attending physician is longer than that of the resident.

•

Some people are intimidated by any sign of authority, and many people automatically become more reverent and respectful in its presence. Within medical facilities there might be what is called "white-coat hypertension." This is when a patient becomes nervous around medical authority and experiences an elevation in blood pressure (*Journal of the American Medical Association*, January 8, 1988).

Some doctors become just like some movie stars in that they believe in their own publicity. Some doctors are so caught up in being authority figures that they use their titles everywhere they go. Some are so uptight that they are offended when anyone refers to them on a first-name basis.

Many have learned the hard way that doctors are not perfect, they sometimes make mistakes, and some have very bad judgment. There was a man in Europe who went in to have a cancerous leg removed but woke up after the operation to find the medical team had amputated the wrong leg. There was a well-known case in Florida of a man who had the wrong foot removed. A man in Illinois had the wrong knee operated on. A woman in Michigan had the wrong breast removed. A woman in New York had the wrong side of her brain operated on. There have been at least two recent incidents of patients having the wrong kidneys removed. One California woman who went in for an appendectomy (removal of the appendix) was accidentally given a hysterectomy (removal of the female reproductive organs). Another California woman had the wrong eye operated on. One woman who went in for a nose job sued her plastic surgeon after he surprised her by also giving her cheek implants. Every once in a while there is a person who is misdiagnosed with a terminal illness and, after going through the mental anguish of expecting to die, later finds that there was a misdiagnosis. Many people have gone through operations and later found that the operations were not at all necessary and sometimes were done only so the doctor could make money, practice a new technique, or become eligible for board certification.

Some doctors make a very good income by performing operations that are not necessary. Surgery rooms are where much of the money is spent in medicine and is the most expensive area of the healthcare industry. The money made from surgery trickles down to other areas of the medical industry, such as the medical staff, hospitals, drug companies, medical equipment manufacturers, and medical-supply firms. Each surgery brings income to a string of people. So you see, it is not just the doctor who makes money when unnecessary surgeries are performed.

Because a physician in private practice has no boss or supervisor, the people who work in the office orbit around the doctor, who is in no danger of being fired for bad work.

In 1991, a doctor in California was investigated by state and federal authorities and consequently had his medical license revoked in that state for performing unnecessary eye surgeries. He claimed that a gift from the Lord gave him the ability to fix people's eyes and that this gave him the ability to earn millions. He earned the money by performing unneeded surgeries on dozens of patients and falsified medical records so he could be reimbursed by Medicare.

State medical licensing boards cannot take action against a doctor until the negligent actions have been reported. Even when someone who is guilty of the most atrocious mistreatment is reported to the proper authorities, it can take years for any disciplinary action to take place. Meanwhile, the doctor just keeps opening the door and letting the next patient in.

One gynecologist, a major shareholder at a hospital, who lost his license in California in 1992, was accused by the Medical Board of sexually abusing 69 patients over a ten-year period. More than 160 of the doctor's former patients eventually called the Medical Board with complaints about his sexual misconduct. The first known complaint against the doctor was received by the Medical Board in 1975. The Orange County Medical Association continued to refer patients to the doctor until March 1992, even though they were aware of possible inappropriate behavior. The county district attorney's office and the state attorney general decided *not* to press sexual abuse charges against the doctor because many of the alleged abuses occurred many years before and could not be prosecuted because of a one-year statute of limitations on such crimes. Many believe the doctor was able to continue his abuse for so long because he was a member of the board of directors of the hospital and no doctor would turn him in. The doctor, Ivan Namihas, eventually declared bankruptcy. He was convicted of mail fraud in June 1996 because he billed insurance companies for more than $10,000 in unnecessary surgery.

Some areas of medicine evolve so quickly that many medications, instruments, and surgeries quickly become outdated. Some of this is because certain treatments are found to be dangerous, damaging, or useless. Other changes occur after better treatments are found. Many surgical procedures now available have become popular within the last few years. This was after most of the doctors performing the procedures completed their training. Many of these procedures are taught at weekend getaways or are taught during day-long seminars. Some doctors learn new surgical procedures by watching a video and start doing the procedure as soon as they can obtain the necessary equipment.

Just because doctors say they are *qualified* to do an operation does not necessarily mean that they have had *experience* in doing the operation. Someone has to be the very first patient for the doctor to perform a newly learned technique.

Surgical procedures, unlike drugs, do not require approval from the federal Food and Drug Administration, so a doctor only needs a place to perform the surgery. If the hospital does not allow the doctor to perform the surgery within the hospital, the doctor can use a free-standing surgery center, or his own office surgical suite.

Specialists

> *I think that many Americans are going to be surprised and frankly quite alarmed to hear that any doctor with a medical degree and state license can go out and do everything from brain surgery to cosmetic surgery.*
> — Congressman Ron Wyden during Congressional subcommittee hearings on plastic surgery industry, 1989

Consumers should beware of doctors who are willing to do anything and everything to unsuspecting patients. When searching for a doctor to perform a particular type of surgery, it is best to hire a doctor who specializes in the surgery that might be performed. The doctor should be highly familiar with the anatomy of the area of the body that might be operated on.

Most every city phone book contains advertising placed by doctors who call themselves "specialists." Any doctor can legally call himself a specialist in any area of medicine, advertise himself as one, and start practicing in that area. Phone book companies do not have the time or resources to verify the credentials of the medical professionals who pay to advertise in their pages.

Among specialists there are some very good ones who have spent extra years studying and researching one area of medicine. There are specialists who limit their practice to the head and neck, and subspecialists or "superspecialists" who limit themselves to an even smaller area, such as the hands or eyes, or a certain disease. The superspecialists are usually associated with a university medical school.

As of July 1993, there were 39 specialty areas of certification and 71 subspecialty areas in which certification is authorized by the American Board of Medical Specialties. About 70% of American doctors are in specialty practice.

Some medical specialty boards require a recertification procedure to make sure that its doctors are up-to-date in the specialty. Not all specialties require their doctors to go through a recertification process.

The trend among today's medical students is to enter into a specialty area. One reason for this is that the vast majority of the professors in medical schools are specialists. These professors often persuade the students to specialize in one area of medicine rather than specialize in general medicine. Another reason is that new medical machinery and surgical techniques require special training to use and perform. Learning to do specific procedures takes time and skill, and once the skills are learned, doctors often stick to that one area of the medical field.

The discarded Clinton health plan sought to establish a National Council on Graduate Medical Education that would limit the number of students allowed to enter into specialty areas. The goal of these student regulations was to form a balance between specialists and primary care, thus widening the accessibility of primary care doctors while cutting the costs of healthcare by limiting access to high-cost specialty care.

While limiting the number of specialists and patients' access to them may be helpful in cutting healthcare costs, it does not necessarily provide for better healthcare, as some diseases and health problems are better treated by specialty doctors. The result might be that more patients who need specialty care will find that their health plans limit access to the needed care and that the patients' health can deteriorate while trying to cut through the red tape.

The Board Game

Doctors can have a lot of diplomas and certificates on their waiting room walls, and they can list all kinds of medical societies and organizations after their names, but the public just does not know which doctors are trained and competent in this field.
— Congressman Norman Sisisky, during Congressional subcommittee hearings on the plastic surgery industry, 1989

In 1993, approximately 60% of US doctors were board certified. Membership in a medical board is voluntary and is not a requirement to practice medicine. Although the primary goal of board certification seems to be to protect the public, just because a doctor is board certified does not guarantee that he is a good doctor. Nor does it guarantee that everything will go right with operations the doctor performs — or that he has even had adequate training to perform those surgeries. Because more and more consumers are seeking out board certified doctors, being board certified could mean money in the bank for the board certified doctors, and a do-anything-to-get-board-certified attitude may be the product of this.

WYDEN: Is it your view that, generally, in the cosmetic surgery field, not to take any one discipline or any one profession, that generally in the field the number of quacks and charlatans is growing and growing along the lines that the subcommittee has been told about?

CALEEL: I believe that there are individuals who abuse the privilege to practice medicine. I believe that in the current setting there are a significant number of them in the field of cosmetic or plastic surgery.

WYDEN: Doctor, do you believe that with the technological advances that have been made in surgical procedures over the last 30 years, a person who has a medical degree and a state license should be allowed to simply declare that they are a specific type of surgeon?

CALEEL: I do not believe that an individual with a medical license can declare themselves in any specialty area.

WYDEN: That is what goes on, though, is it not? We have heard widespread testimony that someone with a medical degree and a state license can claim to be a surgeon with a particular specialty. That can take place, can it not?

CALEEL: Yes; it can.

WYDEN: So you said that it does take place. Do you think that this is right, given the technological advances in the last 30 years?

CALEEL: No.

— Congressman Ron Wyden questioning Dr. Richard T. Caleel, president, American Academy of Cosmetic Surgery; president, American Society of Liposuction Surgery, Inc., during Congressional subcommittee hearings on the plastic surgery industry, 1989

Legally anyone with a medical license can do surgery. While some hospital staff privileges may limit what a doctor may do inside a hospital based on his experience, what a doctor does in his office surgical suite is not supervised.

The more common and more respected route for obtaining board certification through the American Board of Medical Specialties (ABMS) is to go through a program accredited by a Residency Review Committee sponsored by a specialty board. Other doctors can and have formed their own "boards" and sold certificates of membership to these "boards." Some doctors who are not board certified claim that they are. A 1987 study of Veterans Administration hospital doctors found 18% had improperly claimed to be board certified (*The Washington Post*, July 12, 1994, *What do the certificates on your doctor's wall really mean?*).

The ABMS was incorporated in 1933 and has become recognized as the official medical certifying group. Most medical professionals believe that only ABMS-approved boards are legitimate. The ABMS certifies only 23 specialties.

Doctors who are members of the ABMS have passed certain comprehensive oral and written exams for evaluating their skills. Before surgeons can take these tests they must have a medical degree, complete years of specialized surgical training, complete a residency, hold a valid registered full and unrestricted license to practice medicine in a possession, territory, or state of the United States or in a Canadian province, and must have practiced for two years. Before they can take the oral exam they have to submit a twelve-month portfolio case list of operations they were involved with and hold privileges in a hospital approved by the Joint Commission on Accreditation of Healthcare Organizations, or its Canadian equal.

If the doctor says he is board certified, do not assume that he is certified in the area of medicine in which he makes his living. Some doctors who perform surgery have no specialized training in the area of medicine they practice, are certified by boards unrelated to their specialized type of surgery, or are certified by boards that are not approved by the ABMS. They may have been certified in another area of medicine and then decided to enter into the surgery business. Some doctors are certified by more than one ABMS board. There are also many doctors who are not certified by any board.

> •
> *Some of these guys are pretty clever. They form boards, and they go to the printer and they have their little certificates made up and hang them on their wall, and these are all impressive.*
>> — Joyce Palso of California, testifying at Congressional subcommittee hearings on the plastic surgery industry, 1989. She had heart failure, a stroke, and had to have a valve in her heart replaced because of complications that arose after she was a victim of negligent medical care when she underwent a tummy tuck surgery.
> •

Consumers should not be impressed or intimidated by the fancy certificates, awards, licenses, and diplomas hanging on a doctor's office wall. Every doctor has one or more of them, including those who have injured, disfigured, raped or killed patients. Making a note of these papers can be helpful for checking on the background of the doctor. However, it can be easy to get the board certifications confused with other fancy-looking certificates that may simply be documents of membership or awards from societies, associations, academies or groups that have nothing to do with the doctor's education. Memberships in some of these societies have no bearing on professional skill.

Some allopathic medical societies give important continuing education classes, seminars, and workshops that improve a doctor's skills and increase knowledge, but just because a doctor is a member of the group does not necessarily prove attendance in any of the classes given by the group.

Some of the documents hanging on the doctor's wall may simply be certificates from a legitimate professional two-day seminar. They may also be from organizations any doctor can join simply by paying some money to the group. Some doctor associations do not check the credentials of the member doctors. The certificates may look fine as decorative items in the doctor's office, but as a representation of the medical care you might receive, they may be meaningless.

Some doctor associations may offer health, business, life, and other insurance plans to doctors. There are doctor associations that offer secured loans and other business-oriented services, such as opportunities to learn about public relations and marketing to help the doctor promote himself. Some of these associations offer pre-written press releases about specific health subjects to help a doctor gain valuable media exposure. The press releases are worded so that a doctor can add his name to them and send them out to the local media in order for him to become known as a source of information and an expert within the community.

There may be times when the proven talents of a particular doctor who lacks board certification can be what it takes to get the surgical result you are looking for, but usually choosing a surgeon who is board certified by the ABMS (not just board "eligible") is a much better gamble than choosing one who is not.

A person seeking a surgeon should not stop the background check of the doctor once it is found that the doctor is board certified. Being in good standing with the board could simply mean there has been payment of cash dues. It does not mean that all the operations he has performed have produced wonderful results.

To check whether a doctor is certified, contact the various medical boards listed in the *Research Resources* section of this book. Find out what the bylaws of the boards are and ask what the requirements are for a doctor to be in good standing.

To get a list of doctors in your state who have a history of medical malpractice, contact Public Citizen Health Research Group at (202)833-3000. Also, see the *Patients' and Consumers' Rights* heading in the *Research Resources* section of this book.

Licensing of Doctors

A state medical license can be obtained by taking examinations given by a state board, by mutual exchange of privileges if a doctor is licensed in another state, or by meeting the requirements of the National Board of Medical Examiners.

Each state has its own board with its own set of rules, and boards do not always implement established procedures (doctors who are in the military are federally licensed and in a league separate from doctors who are not in the military). The state licensing boards have also organized their own umbrella organization called the Federation of State Medical Boards.

State medical boards, many of which operate on very limited budgets, are composed largely of doctors and are meant to monitor and discipline or weed out bad doctors to protect the health and safety of the public. Before a state board can impose sanctions against a doctor, negligent actions or impaired performance must be reported to the board.

I think it is important to note here that getting involved in the medical delivery system is a risky business. It is as risky as driving on the freeway. Simply by the luck of the draw, you can get hurt and need additional care. That is costly, and not necessarily the kind of malpractice that one would associate with negligence, despite the number of patients who suffer from injury.

Here is another problem. Despite the number of patients who suffer an injury from negligence, few of the nation's 600,000 practicing physicians have had any disciplinary measures taken against them. For example, in 1991, state medical boards took only 2,800 disciplinary actions against physicians and they ranged from mere reprimands to a paltry few license revocations.

— Congressman Pete Stark, during subcommittee hearing on issues relating to malpractice, May 20, 1993

Some people think that if a doctor were dangerous he would not be allowed to be a doctor. This is not true. Many states fail to take disciplinary actions against doctors even after the Drug Enforcement Administration has revoked or put limits on their federal narcotics licenses and after the doctors have lost Medicare privileges. Because of laws, regulations, glitches in the system, and corruption in governing boards, bad doctors are not being cleaned out of the system the way they should be. In California, doctors do not even have to report malpractice settlements under $30,000 to the state medical board. To protect the doctors' careers, the awards over $30,000 that were reported to the California state medical board before January 1, 1993 (when a new law went into effect) are kept secret from consumers

— another result of lobbying by the doctor's group: the California Medical Association.

These boards that are meant to protect patients from dangerous doctors continue to inadequately investigate claims against doctors who are incompetent or impaired by debilitating conditions, such as alcoholism, drug abuse, or mental illness. Few of the bad medical professionals are ever disciplined, and therefore they continue with their careers. Many times the ones who are protected by the system of the state medical boards are the bad doctors, not the patients subjected to malpractice who are left to fight against the doctors in the battlefields of the courts.

Negligent and incompetent doctors are rarely disciplined or removed from practice. At most, about 0.5% of the nation's doctors face any action from their state medical boards each year. On average, only 3.44 serious disciplinary actions are taken for every 1,000 doctors.

State medical boards may take more than two years to even investigate complaints of doctor incompetence or misconduct, allowing the doctor to continue to treat other patients all during this time.

 — Excerpt from news release by Public Citizen Health Research Group, Washington, DC, 1993

After a doctor is convicted of a crime, the state medical board may take no action or may suspend the doctor's license pending an appeal on the conviction. After the conviction is upheld, the state may revoke the doctor's license after the sentencing. Even after all this the doctor may appeal his case, and the court can overturn any actions taken against him.

It is difficult for consumers to find out who the bad doctors are, because many of the records detailing bad doctors are for use only by state medical boards, licensing agencies, hospitals, insurance companies, and other professionals, and are not available to the public. If a doctor is recognized as being incompetent or negligent and is brought before a medical review board in one state and eventually loses his medical license there, he can move to another state and continue ruining lives in his "practice of medicine."

It is not unusual for a very bad doctor to have practiced in two or more states (or even other countries) where he has been disciplined by state boards for any number of violations, and where he may have left behind a trail of mistreated patients and malpractice lawsuits. Some doctors have gone so far as to change their names to avoid any problems their past may cause. The new state may or may not know of the doctor's history. The doctor's insurance carrier might, but these records are not generally available to consumers. Some hospitals fail to check up on the history of doctors they give privileges to. Even some hospital doctors have been found to be unlicensed.

2 • THE MARKETING OF MEDICINE

The News Media and Medicine

The business world is filled with people releasing self-serving calculated information to the media, especially in the medicine business.

One motive of those involved with new medical technology, drugs, or procedures is to attract the kind of attention that will help secure funding for more research, to promote professional careers, to increase stock value, or to otherwise increase profit margins. Attention can be had by getting the newspapers, news magazines, and news programs to mention a new device, therapy, procedure, or drug in a way that will look like something wonderful has happened — and this creates consumer demand.

Some of the people who appear in the news media to tell about a form of treatment for a health problem may be getting paid to say what they are saying in front of the camera. This includes doctors who just happen to work at a medical center where the treatment is provided; executives who work for a drug maker or medical device manufacturer; celebrities who work as spokespeople for a health organization or are being paid to "report" on how the drug or medical device helped them; and even a regular news personality who is telling the "news" about the form of treatment. We are not talking about those 30-minute infomercials here. We are talking about the people who appear on the regular national or local news, magazine news shows, and talk shows.

When reading about medical breakthroughs in the popular media, remember that the decision to report on an issue is based on audience interest, and the benefits of a so-called medical breakthrough may be exaggerated to gain the attention of a wider audience than would naturally be interested in it.

Journalists are always on the lookout for compelling stories. Just because the media make a new procedure, device, or drug appear to be magnificent does not necessarily mean that it is a landmark in the medical community. The media may have received their information about the procedure from a press release put out by a public relations firm hired by the researchers involved with the new technique, therapy, or drug. If the report is of a new medical device, the media may have received their information from the public relations firm hired by the manufacturer of the device. In other words, the medical information that the media present may be incomplete or flawed.

Changes in the Allopathic Trade

In recent years the medical industry has been forced to conform to cuts made by Medicare, intense pressure from insurers and employers to slash medical costs, and negotiations with HMOs to discount fees. All this has brought many independent doctors to join other doctors in group practices that belong to managed care programs that control millions of healthcare dollars and look at patients as commodities.

With the average American living longer and with increasing healthcare costs, the Medicare and Medicaid programs are the fastest growing part of the federal budget. Trustees of the programs foresee financial collapse of the programs in the not-too-distant future if changes are not made soon. Added to this is the ongoing talk about medical industry reform legislation that would change the way healthcare is financed.

The economic changes of the 1980s and 1990s combined with the growing popularity of cutting patient costs by letting patients recover at home (outpatient surgery), and with at-home care (where patients are treated at home by traveling therapists and nurses), has helped to bring national hospital vacancy rates up to 35% and more as the occupancy rates of hospitals continue the downward spiral that started in the 1950s.

Hospitals are expensive to build and operate. In Los Angeles in 1996, when the UCLA Medical Center looked at the cost of building a new hospital to replace the earthquake-damaged structure that currently exists, the engineers concluded that the cost of a new hospital would be about $1 billion. With costs like that, hospitals have to bring in the revenue.

Several hundred hospitals and medical centers have closed their doors since 1980. Rural hospitals have been among the hardest hit by recent economic changes because they cannot afford to update their equipment to keep up with the technological advances of today's medicine. In Los Angeles, where there are 79 private hospitals, more than half the hospital rooms are empty. Kaiser hospitals have reported that only 50% of their beds are filled on an average day. One hospital built in Baldwin Park, California, has never been opened.

To counteract the shortage of patients, the revenue-hungry medical industry has to develop new income sources to get people into their doors. This has led hospitals to become more profit-minded and manage their square footage like department stores, open the doors to their employee gyms to the public for a membership fee, and treat doctors like commissioned salespeople by offering incentives to them for bringing in new or more business. Hospitals are also competing with other hospitals and managed-care contracts by establishing strategic relationships with group practices and offering incentives to doctors in the surrounding communities to refer patients.

As more hospitals enter into managed-care contracts with insurance companies the hospital staff nurses feel the pressure of being responsible for more patients during a work shift. Hospitals are cutting costs by using fewer registered nurses. Instead, hospitals are hiring more nursing assistants that have limited training but cost less to employ. Many nurses believe these changes compromise the quality of patient care.

In efforts to recruit doctors who are likely to bring business into the hospital where the doctor works, some hospitals offer to pay a portion of the rent on doctors' offices, guarantee a minimum annual income for the doctors, and pay part or all of the doctors' malpractice insurance premiums. The costs of these are added onto the operating expenses of the medical centers and, in the end, figure into the bills that are sent to the patients.

Surgery Pushers

Two men chatting on a park bench got on the subject of their health and doctors. One was especially proud of his doctor.

"He never operated on me unless it was necessary. He wouldn't lay a hand on me unless he really needed the money."

There are more doctors than ever before competing for a share of the market. This has increased the consumer's odds of choosing the wrong doctor if he is not careful. Misleading and deceptive claims can be found in all forms of medical advertising and many forms of medical treatment are advertised as simple, low risk, and pain free when they often are not. A person reading a medical advertisement needs to keep in mind that advertising most often presents limited information stressing the benefits of a product or service.

The promises found in some of the ads for "surgery du jour" stoop to the level of those of turn-of-the-century traveling medicine salesmen who, in upbeat and animated presentations, claimed their all-in-one miracle cures would be effective in treating cancer, stomach aches, the common cold, female problems, bladder illnesses, sexual diseases, and dropsy. What the advertising often does is establish patient expectations that lead to post-surgical disappointments.

A doctor can take a weekend seminar on knee surgery or other area of surgery, purchase some new equipment and be in business the following week, advertising himself as a specialist in the field. A few operations will cover the cost of the new equipment and the surgeon can start making a profit within a week.

•

Some of these pseudosurgeons have realized huge profits in recent years, thanks to a laissez-faire FTC. The agency became an unwitting accomplice to the physical and emotional scarring of too many patients by failing to protect Americans from misleading advertising and cosmetic surgery hype.

• • •

Untold numbers of patients seeking the fountain of youth through a face-lift, a tummy tuck or an acid peel sometimes get more than they bargain for, suffering infection, stroke, and occasionally death following procedures that are advertised as safe, easy, and painless.

— Congressman Ron Wyden during Congressional subcommittee hearings on plastic surgery industry, 1989

•

Estimates of the amount of money Americans spend on surgery every year are in the hundreds of billions of dollars. It is not possible to get accurate figures of the amount of money spent on surgery because there are so many insurance companies, government agencies, hospitals, medical centers, and private surgery suites that have their own bookkeeping and record systems that are shut off from statistical analyzers, and because many smaller operations are paid for in cash. Many of the cash payments are untraceable because they are kept quiet for tax reasons.

Hospitals have started giving seminars about back pain, are holding weight loss programs, have opened sports medicine clinics, and are conducting health classes for the elderly. Some people in the surrounding communities may take advantage of these offerings as a sort of social gathering. It may be seen simply as good public relations for the hospital to get people familiar with the hospital as a friendly place. It is also a way for hospitals to introduce new patrons to the elective surgeries the hospitals have available. Many of the services are targeted toward elderly people who rely on Medicare because the 36 million Americans who are over age 65 and on Medicare bring a sizable amount of revenue into hospitals.

What all this boils down to is that the hospital is a business, and businesses need to make money. Medical facilities are bought and sold by corporations for their profit potential and, just as in any other business, the people who put their money into the facilities want to see a profit on their investment. If there is not a constant flow of patients going into the hospitals, the corporation is not making money.

American doctors have a history of performing unnecessary operations on unsuspecting patients. A perfect example of this is the number of tonsillectomies that were performed on children during the 1960s (15 per every 1,000 American children in 1965) that were of no benefit other than the financial gain seen by the doctors and hospitals who were involved with these operations. In the 1970s the overuse of cesarean sections to deliver babies was a bonanza for doctors, while most of the patients were again unsuspecting.

Some of the unnecessary surgeries are driven by consumer demand created by medical advertising and publicity. Just as people waste hard-earned dollars when they fall for any other sales pitch to buy a product they do not really need, it is an increasingly common practice for consumers to waste money on medical procedures that are not necessary and that can be dangerous. Whereas the greater portion of unnecessary surgeries are performed on women, both women and men should always question doctors who want to operate too quickly, and take precautions when entering hospitals that seem eager in marketing trendy operations that increase profit margins.

The Federal Trade Commission has made a decision that in effect permits unbridled advertising, and has failed to follow up on some of the really outlandish advertising claims. As a result, consumers find it very difficult in my view to make the best or the most appropriate choices for them.
— Congressman Ron Wyden during Congressional subcommittee hearings on plastic surgery industry, 1989

Whether it be done by a kindergarten dropout or someone with a doctorate in medicine, salesmanship is salesmanship and is done with the aim of getting money from someone else. Since the early 1980s when American doctors first started advertising, medical advertising has proliferated and saturated all forms of advertising media as doctors and hospitals clamor for a share of the market and plead with consumers for business. Hospitals have created marketing departments and doctors have hired publicists. Every possible angle is being used to get the attention of potential medical consumers as hospital administrators, and doctors use the tactics learned at seminars on how to advertise and market themselves. The results of this are sometimes extreme and weirdly humorous.

In Los Angeles there is a radio commercial with a woman's upbeat voice advertising the brain surgery unit at USC Hospital. The commercial mentions that shaving of the head for brain surgery is no longer necessary and the commercial includes a toll-free 800 number interested people can dial for more information.

I do not know what kind of profits are made from a hospital's brain surgery unit, but I have spoken with a few people in my life who have had brain surgery, and from what I can tell it is not something to look forward to. When I heard the commercial I thought it was some kind of joke, as if it were a skit from Saturday Night Live. *The pitch claiming that a person no longer has to shave his head to undergo brain surgery gave me the impression that a person can have brain surgery that morning and be out that evening with 500 of his closest friends at some posh restaurant and no one would even know. Who is it in the radio audience that the commercial was trying to reach? Are there actually people sitting around out there who would rush to the phone when they hear a toll-free number they can dial to schedule themselves for brain surgery?*

— The author

•

On any given day, medical advertising can be found in newspapers and magazines and on billboards, on radio and television, in junk mail, on door-to-door fliers, and through telemarketing. There are also "health" fairs held at malls and stands set up in supermarkets to give "free" tests to find people willing to spend their money on medical services (Medicare recipients are particularly sought out by hospitals because nearly all hospital bills are approved as they are submitted — hospitals know to inflate the charges on Medicare patient bills because Medicare payments are 50 cents or less on the dollar). In a business sense this is all done for good reason. According to the US Department of Health and Human Services, Americans spent about $900 billion on medicine in 1994 — give or take several billion. At 1995 levels of growth, that figure will exceed $1.7 trillion by the year 2000.

To earn money in their professions, mechanics need cars to fix, cooks need people to feed, painters need houses to paint, and surgeons need people to operate on. The surgeon, like everyone else, has bills to pay and has to make a certain amount of money every month. He has to feed his family and maintain his home, and is driven to maintain a certain lifestyle he has become accustomed to. He also has an office to run, taxes and rent to pay, office supplies and machinery to purchase, staff wages to meet, and medical supplies to purchase. On top of all this, he has to cover his malpractice insurance (if he has it). He may also be making payments on student loans or payments to a bank, professional organization, his family, or the local hospital to pay for loans he used to open his practice. Debt from medical school can easily reach $100,000. To make the money to cover these expenses, there needs to be a continuous flow of patients paying the doctor for his services.

It should always be remembered by the consumer that the doctor's office is a money-making enterprise. Because you are the patient — or a potential patient — you are their target revenue source. Just as in any other business, profit is the bottom line. Sadly, as is too often the case with other professions, a medical professional can often judge his success by his bank account. The doctor's career interests, his money-making capabilities, and the quest for luxury can become more important than the safety and health of the patients who seek his services. Developing marketing talents can then get in the way of acquiring curative skills.

Medical centers that are blatantly driven by profit have become a common sight throughout American cities. These surgery boutiques are usually located in highly trafficked commercial districts and have exteriors designed with the intention of inspiring confidence in the doctors who practice within the walls. With well-placed stylish signs letting every passerby know what surgical procedures are performed there, they do everything short of hiring mascots to stand out front to wave customers into the parking lots. Their newspaper ads are mixed in with ads for health clubs, dress shops, hair salons, and restaurants. They offer "bargain" prices and lure prospective patients with seductive promises. Some of the doctors who run these surgery boutiques had to settle for opening their own medical centers after no hospital would grant them privileges or after their privileges had been revoked. Their appointment books stack the patients one overlapping another, which creates a traffic jam in the waiting rooms, and the staff seem to have been hired on the basis of physical appearance and their sales ability to get the patients to sign the insurance and consent forms.

Of course this kind of blatant medical salesmanship couldn't exist without paying customers. But often these customers — the patients — are lured in by the advertising, and are then often misinformed, ill advised, and at risk of being taken advantage of.

Many people believe that medical advertising is screened by a government agency, and that therefore all claims about health products, procedures, and services must be truthful. This is not the case with most healthcare advertising. There is no federal, state, or local government agency that approves or verifies claims in advertisements before they are printed. There is no government regulator watching over the shoulders of every doctor and medical facility to direct the advertising and marketing materials these businesses put out. Law enforcement authorities can take action only after untruthful or misleading advertisements have appeared, but such actions are very rare.

How important is good publicity to a hospital? When a very famous person was seriously injured there were several medical centers hoping he would choose their facilities for his rehabilitation. A celebrity choosing a facility under such conditions can bring national attention to the facility. The credibility and reputation this establishes in the eyes of the public may increase business for decades. It may also attract financial donations from friends of the celebrity or from fund-raisers organized in cooperation with the celebrity.

Beyond doctors who network and hand out their business cards to potential patients at social events, the marketing of medical services has become a mini-industry all its own as various healthcare providers fiercely compete for a share of the market. American newspapers are filled with advertisements placed by surgeons, hospitals, and surgical centers enticing readers to undergo this or that surgical procedure. Many newspapers regularly contain advertorials (advertisements designed to look like a newspaper or magazine article) from doctors and medical centers. Toll-free telephone numbers are becoming a common offering by doctors, who are also now marketing themselves with videos and high-quality varnished full-color photo brochures. Free seminars are offered at hospitals and hotels where large groups are herded into conference rooms to watch some doctor give an upbeat marketing presentation. Some doctors have gone to the extent of hiring publicists to increase business by arranging interviews, sending out press releases, and placing articles in newspapers and magazines — as if getting the doctor's name mentioned in the right areas will prove he is a good doctor.

Because of my research with another book I wrote, Plastic Surgery Hopscotch, *I am now on several mailing lists of plastic surgeons and their groups. They have sent me videos, follow-up letters, questionnaires, postcards, newsletters, invitations to attend free seminars, and Christmas cards. One surgeon who has never met me has sent me numerous letters inviting me to come in for a free hair-transplant consultation. Another offered free limousine service to and from his office, and another (I am not making this stuff up) offered to serve a free three-course gourmet meal if I let him perform hair-transplant surgery on me. Glossy brochures from another hair-transplant doctor tried to lure me in by saying I can watch a video of my choice on his office television while he operates on my scalp. And my mail carrier must think I am an incredibly vain and insecure person.*

The manufacturer of collagen, Collagen Biomedical, sent me several coupons for $25 off collagen treatment injections at any participating surgeon's office, an offer for a free collagen skin test, and, to help me look my best, an offer to join the "Collagen Replacement Therapy Savings Plan Program" by purchasing a Collagen Replacement Therapy Savings Plan

Membership Card from a participating doctor. The Collagen Replacement Therapy Savings Plan Program Membership Card works just like the discount card that you can get at a Subway sandwich shop where you get a hole punched in your card every time you buy a sandwich and you get a free sandwich when there are no more spaces left. But with the Collagen Replacement Therapy Savings Plan Program Membership Card, the doctor validates your card every time you let him inject collagen into your face, and when the card is fully validated, he injects collagen into your face on the next visit . . . free! Of course, as the invitation mentioned, the savings will vary based on the retail price of the Collagen Replacement Therapy Savings Plan Program Membership Card. This offer differs from the sandwich shop, though, because the gloves the doctor wears when he is injecting the dead cow-derived collagen into your face are more expensive than the cheap vinyl gloves they wear at the sandwich shop when they are preparing your sandwich; the doctor also wears a face mask, and you are still hungry when the injections are over. Maybe if they offered a free three-course gourmet meal and some snacks and stuff after the collagen injections, such as the offer from the hair-transplant doctor, we could start talking business here. A complimentary limousine ride would be kind of neat too.

One particular cosmetic surgeon must spend a fortune on marketing and advertising every year. I attended one of his crowded seminars given at a fancy Beverly Hills hotel. The seminar reminded me of some kind of religious revival meeting. There were people there from all walks of life and the large conference room was filled to standing-room-only capacity. The audience paid attention to this doctor as if he were going to tell them some secret to life. The woman next to me wanted to have her eyes done. The mother in front of me brought her frightened son to see the doctor about making the teenager's nose smaller. The people in back of me asked me what I wanted done. When I told them I was just there to watch, they acted as if I were some kind of intruder or in denial.

The meeting included appearances by several people who claimed to be satisfied patients of the doctor. Along with these patients' testimonies there was an upbeat presentation by the happy doctor that included a slide show and a question-and-answer period. The seminar ended with strong encouragement to come visit the doctor. As we exited the conference room we had to walk past the doctor, who was smiling and shaking the hands of the attendees. Just outside the conference room we walked past tables where the doctor's office staff were selling a book the doctor wrote and scheduling consultation appointments.

The marketing letters I have received from this doctor are filled with encouraging words. The letters say that if I desire to "improve my appearance and experience the happiness that I will see" in his patients, then I should schedule a consultation with him. The letters mention his computer imaging system that will let me see the "new" me. The letters say that the doctor and his staff have helped many people just like me. Furthermore, I would receive a 20% courtesy discount on the price of the consultation if I bring the letter with me when I meet with the doctor. It did not mention anything about a three-course gourmet meal — or being able to watch videos during surgery.

Along with his letters, this doctor has sent questionnaires; fliers telling about the rather upbeat, vague and pro-surgery book the doctor has written on cosmetic surgery; a video; a lengthy list of his credentials; copies of articles that have mentioned him or that he has written; and postage-paid return postcards for me to fill out my name and address to request information from him.

I do not know what else he could possibly send me — maybe videos of him actually performing surgery (a few doctors did do this), or maybe he could send some of his former patients armed with copies of his book to come knock on my door and tell me how plastic surgery has changed their lives. Or, maybe he can offer discount cards that he validates every time I let him perform surgery on me and then offer some free procedure when the card is all validated. Just think, eleven plastic surgery procedures for the price of ten!

The latest postcard I received from this doctor was an announcement for another one of his free seminars. At the seminar, which the postcard noted would have a "capacity crowd," this doctor offered a free drawing for a $2,500 gift certificate for cosmetic facial surgery — to be performed by . . . guess who?!

After all this marketing material he has sent me, I took particular notice that one of his letters contains the following sentence:

"It is my intent to be of genuine, thorough help to each person — and NEVER to 'pressure' or 'sell.'"

I'm glad he included that sentence, because for a while there I was beginning to think he was trying to sell me something.
— The author

•

Some advertisements for surgery centers and surgeons feature photos of perky, smiling models who probably did not undergo the surgical procedure they are pitching. Some of the ads are so upbeat that you are sure surgery must be one of the most fun and entertaining experiences anyone could ever go through. Do not delay; call now; *operators* are standing by!

•

. . . All the people who are coming out of residency in the New York area will tell you flat out that what they are going to need besides the money to set up their practice is an extra $25,000 to $50,000 for their first year public relations and advertising or they are not going to survive.
— Dr. Mark Gorney, past president, American Society of Plastic and Reconstructive Surgeons during Congressional subcommittee hearings on plastic surgery industry, 1989

•

One of the marketing tools doctors are known to use are offers for free consultations. This consultation involves going into the doctor's office and filling out patient record forms. The patient then waits his turn and eventually is called in to visit with the doctor to be poked and prodded as if he were some lab specimen. Surely there is some "service," "technique," or "procedure" the patient can trust the doctor to perform on him. This is, of course, if the patient hands the doctor or the staff person who handles the "financial arrangement" some amount of hundreds or thousands of dollars, gets scheduled for a surgery sometime in the days or weeks to come, signs a consent form, and lets the doctor and his operating team cut away at his flesh. Such a deal.

The Real Drug Dealers

Pharmaceutical companies make drugs. To sell these drugs, they spend horrendous amounts of money on marketing and advertising — billions every year, and often more than they spend on developing the drugs. This includes buying full-page advertisements in medical journals, newspapers, and magazines of all types, creating TV and radio commercials and purchasing time on the airwaves to broadcast them, and by supplying stores with POP (point-of-purchase) store display cases.

Drug company salespeople are the most aggressive part of drug company promotion. The drug companies want all the doctors and pharmacists to know about their drugs. To do this, legions of salespeople are sent forth to hand out free samples of drugs to doctors, wine and dine them, give them tickets to sporting events, provide them free seminars, and cater lunches for nurses and doctors' office staff. Millions of dollars are spent on gifts, such as books, calculators, flashlights, and other useful items that bear drug company logos. These are handed out to doctors, nurses, hospitals, medical centers, and pharmacies. All this is done so that the drug companies can get their share of the estimated $70 billion Americans spend on prescription medications every year.

The drug company salesmen are trying to convince physicians that for every human problem the answer is the latest new drug.

— Dr. Steffie Woolhandler, associate professor of internal medicine at Harvard University

Besides the money spent on aggressive advertising and marketing activities, pharmaceutical companies also have to first spend money to research and develop the products they sell. The amount spent on these R&D projects alone comes to billions of dollars every year. Over half a billion dollars and a dozen years of research time may be spent on one drug before it is sold to consumers. Millions of dollars are spent just to get one drug through the FDA's approval process. Some of the money spent on developing drugs comes right from taxpayers.

Thanks to the strong political lobbyists working for the pharmaceutical industry, the US government spends millions to subsidize drug research through tax breaks and other measures.

A typical clinical research process that is done to test the safety and effectiveness of a drug is called a "double-blind, placebo-controlled trial." This is a situation in which neither the participants (the patients or individuals who are paid to participate in the study) nor the researchers know who is receiving the real drug. One group of participants may be receiving a simple fake pill while the other group of participants receives the actual drug. Depending on the drug and the condition or disease being studied, a trial like this may take days, weeks, or years. Bristol-Myers recently spent $30 million on this kind of study in Scotland to test a new cholesterol-lowering drug called Pravachol on 6,595 men.

Much money is invested on the development of drugs, because one drug that is successful in treating a common ailment could net billions of dollars in sales. For instance, Eli Lilly & Co. reaped $910 million in worldwide sales in 1993 from the antibiotic Ceclor. These types of profits can roll into pharmaceutical company bank accounts for years and years.

Patents on drugs used to last 17 years. Under the General Agreement on Tariffs and Trade, drug patents now last 20 years from the date drug makers file for a patent.

Drug companies are not interested in products that may help only a few people. Nor are they interested in substances that cannot be patented, such as vitamins or supplements commonly sold in healthfood stores. They are interested in drugs that will dominate market share. They want to develop drugs that will be bought in bulk quantities by health organizations. They are interested in drugs that can be sold to millions of people and that can bring millions and possibly billions of dollars in profit to shareholders. They want to have drugs in development that will give the company a strong financial forecast so that investor dollars will keep pouring in. They want money.

The massive advertising campaigns of pharmaceutical companies are designed to ensure that the drug companies can recoup the millions of dollars they have spent on developing the products, and make a profit. The FDA approval process for one drug can take several years and cost hundreds of millions of dollars. So when a drug is finally approved, the companies release huge publicity and marketing campaigns to introduce the new product to the medical community.

Many have accused the FDA drug approval process of being sluggish, expensive, and time-consuming. The FDA has always had the authority to allow compassionate uses for unlicensed drugs. Since 1991 the FDA has used an accelerated approval process to license experimental drugs faster for life-threatening conditions or serious disorders for which there were no existing drug therapies. In March 1996 President Clinton announced that the FDA drug approval process would be speeded up for medications that may benefit those suffering from AIDS or cancer.

Some praise a quicker approval process and say patients should be allowed to take informed risks. But others criticize faster approval for drugs saying that it benefits the drug companies by allowing them to put drugs on the market quicker while compromising consumer safety by allowing doctors to prescribe drugs that have not been thoroughly tested.

What the marketing departments of the drug companies often do is pump out so much biased promotional information that doctors begin to rely on the drugs more than they should and the patients end up with substances that are not beneficial to them.

More recently, companies are marketing prescription drugs directly to the public by placing advertisements in major newspapers, in magazines, on TV, and on radio shows in order to target the greatest number of consumers. They are even advertising drugs by using 800 phone numbers and on the World Wide Web. This has resulted in drug companies having a huge influence over how patients think about and treat their illnesses.

Pharmaceutical companies argue that advertising prescription drugs to consumers educates them and prepares them for the day the drugs are sold over-the-counter (*Internal Medicine News*, December 15, 1995). Some consumer groups say the advertising should be illegal because patients do not have the medical knowledge needed to make prescription choices; advertising to consumers makes patients pressure doctors into prescribing certain drugs; and that the drug companies' main goal is to make money.

A person needs only to browse through the business section of the daily paper to figure how much money can be made from a patented drug. The profit margins seen in the pharmaceutical trade are desirable to investors and are actually among the most profitable of any industry in the world. In fact, making money by investing in the medical industry is so much of a process in and of itself that a company in Berkeley, California, publishes a newsletter covering the subject: *The Medical Technology Stock Letter*. Evidence of the money that can be made in the drug business is also exhibited in every town and city throughout the US, where there is an abundance of pharmacies that supply the billions of overpriced and risky pills that Americans take every year.

Part of how the drug companies do their marketing research is by compiling information gathered from doctors, hospitals, HMOs, drug mail-order companies, and pharmacies (*Consumer's Report* October 1994). Records are purchased that include names and other data of people who were given the prescriptions. Some of this information can include Social Security numbers, as well as patients' age, sex, and names of physicians. All this can be used to do market research, figure out what products are selling and who is taking them, and guide the pharmaceutical companies on where to spend their advertising dollars. The cost of all these activities figures into the final costs charged to consumers for the products.

•

Generic drugs are less expensive to buy because they are produced using the same recipe as the original drug under guidelines of the FDA's Division of Generic Drugs. Generic drug manufacturers do not have to spend the money to develop the drug; they simply start producing it after the original patent has expired. Some pharmaceutical companies have purchased generic drug manufacturers to keep a hold on the profits made after their drug patents have expired.

•

University of Utah researchers conducted a study involving 13,000 patients in six HMOs and found that patients may experience prolonged illnesses and have more visits to doctors when taking generic drugs because they often differ in potency (*American Journal of Managed Care*).

•

In the past Americans could either get their prescriptions filled at the hospital or pay less by going to the neighborhood pharmacy — usually located at the back of a store so that the customers are exposed to a great assortment of "front-end" retail items as they walk through the aisles. Americans no longer have only two options of getting prescriptions filled. In recent years HMOs, managed care companies, and mail-order drug services have provided two more choices for consumers to get prescriptions filled. These additional choices have exposed a peculiar selection of prices.

•

According to the health consumer group Families USA, prices of the top 20 drugs rose 4.3% from 1993 to 1994, while overall inflation rose 2.7%. Profits of drug companies averaged 15% in 1993 while the profits of the average Fortune 500 business was 2.9%. Drug prices overall have risen six times the general inflation rate during the last decade.

•

Americans pay more for drugs than do people in England. Pharmacies found in drugstores and supermarkets often pay much more for drugs than hospitals, HMOs, mail-order prescription companies, and other institutions, but hospitals charge customers much more for drugs than do pharmacies. People who have insurance pay less for prescriptions than those who do not. HMOs tend to rely on generic drugs as a way to hold down costs. Home medical care services are probably the worst offenders in the area of price bloating — some charge patients hundreds of times above the wholesale cost for medications and supplies.

Price gouging is also done by middlemen who purchase drugs at low prices and then sell them to the retail market with a huge profit margin. In an article in the *Los Angeles Times*, Sara Fritz, a Times staff writer, revealed: "In some cases, the regular wholesale price can be many times the price paid by institutions. For example, Ciba-Geigy Corp. sells transderm-nitro patches for heart attack patients for $8.40 to institutional pharmacies, like those operating in nursing homes, and $39.89 to the retail druggist — a difference of 375%."

The Pharmaceutical Manufacturers' Association, which represents the nation's leading drug manufacturers, was opposed to the failed Clinton administration plan to level out the drug-pricing system. The PMA is one of the special interest groups that has hired high-priced lobbyists in Washington to court members of Congress and persuade them to act in the interest of the drug manufacturers.

Some of the drop in drug prices has been caused by discount drug distributors who map out competitive pricing strategies and negotiate steep volume discounts with drug companies, supplying employers' insurance groups and HMOs with prescription drugs. This is an industry trend that has caused a dramatic decline in pharmaceutical-industry stocks.

The arrangement with the discount drug distributors taking over some of the marketing of the pharmaceutical companies' products has provided an environment in which drug companies do not have to spend as much money on advertising. On the other hand, in 1993, two of the largest drug companies, Merck and SmithKline Beecham, purchased two of the largest discount drug distribution companies, MedcoContainment and Diversified Pharmaceutical Services. If drug companies then invest in HMOs and hospitals, everyone in the chain of delivering healthcare goods and services to the medical consumers will then be working for the drug companies.

It is because of these mergers that the Federal Trade Commission started keeping a close watch on these businesses. It is concerned about the competitive impact it can have within the medical industry. For these reasons, in 1994 the FTC placed restrictions on Eli Lilly's $4-billion purchase of PCS Health Systems Inc., a prescription management business.

•

In 1983, when Australian physicians Barry Marshall and J. Robin Warren first suggested that most ulcers are caused by the Helicobacter pylori (H-pylori) bacteria, they were laughed at and called heretics by other doctors. Their conclusions challenged what the medical community had believed to be the cause of ulcers: stress, spicy foods, and alcohol, in combination with stomach acids. Their suggested treatment of what amounted to an average two-week antibiotic program that cost about $300 per patient also challenged the $4 billion spent annually to treat ulcer patients. Traditional medicine used two of the world's biggest-selling prescription drugs, Zantac and Tagamet, to treat ulcers (with prescriptions lasting about eight weeks). In the past it was not uncommon to perform surgery on ulcer patients, sometimes to the extent of removing their stomachs.

•

The prescription drug industry is tainted with a checkered past that includes the marketing of too many drugs that not only failed to accomplish what they were meant to relieve or cure, but were also believed to cause additional health problems. Birth defects caused by DES, and cancer believed to have been caused by the breathing disorder drug Organidine, are two examples. Organidine, made by the pharmaceutical company Carter-Wallace, was withdrawn from the market in June 1994. In August 1994, Carter-Wallace also had to place warnings on its epilepsy drug, Felbatol, after it was found to cause liver failure and a rare, and frequently fatal, form of anemia in ten patients. On the day Carter-Wallace made the announcement of the possible side effects of Felbatol the price of the company's stock dropped by nearly one-third on the New York Stock Exchange.

•

Bristol-Myers Squibb Co. said it halted a clinical trial of a heart drug, d-sotalol, after more patients taking the drug died than those taking a placebo. They were testing d-sotalol on heart attack victims at risk for cardiac arrhythmia, an irregular heartbeat. Bristol-Myers found 54 patients died our of 1,373 given the drug, compared to 28 deaths of 1,389 placebo patients.

•

In a survey of foreign exchange students conducted at Santa Monica City College in California, students were asked what their first impressions of living in America were. One German student said that if she were to judge America by what she saw on television she would think that everyone here is in pain because there are so many commercials for aspirin and other painkillers. (Americans spend over $2.9 billion a year on over-the-counter painkillers.)

3 • INDUSTRIAL WASTE

Health Insurance

Healthcare is the number one profit industry in the US and employs more workers than any other industry. No country spends as much on healthcare. In 1995, American healthcare represented 13.9% of the country's gross domestic product. The average of $3,299 spent on healthcare per person per year is the highest of any developed nation, and the 7.8% growth rate in 1993 for health spending in America was higher than the national inflation rate of 2.7%, and greater than the growth of the gross domestic product.

According to the Department of Health and Human Services, the federal government paid 31.7% of the nation's healthcare bill in 1993, and spending in the federal Medicare program grew more rapidly than private insurance in 1992 and 1993. In 1994, Medicare, which is available to 35 million Americans who are 65 or older, and some disabled persons, spent roughly $164 billion and spent about $180 billion in 1995. (Medicaid, which serves approximately 38 million poor, blind, and disabled Americans, cost $89 billion in 1995.)

America is also where the most up-to-date and advanced forms of medical science and technology are found. It is the home of the Cleveland Clinic, the Mayo Clinic, and all of what are considered to be the world's top allopathic medical schools and hospitals. These facilities are used by many world leaders and wealthy citizens of the planet who jet to the US whenever they are experiencing serious health problems.

Today, with all the modern developments in medicine and with what is believed by many to be the best medical care present, many Americans do not have easy access to medical care even when an emergency takes place. Some people argue that the US has the best healthcare delivery system in the world and that it should be left alone. Others argue that the system needs to be changed because it only works for those who fit into the puzzle when they are able to afford private health insurance or receive their health insurance through an employer.

The system can work for those people who are able to maintain insurance. On the other hand, there are the others who work at jobs that do not offer health insurance or are unable to work (reportedly 37 to 39 million Americans were without any type of health insurance in 1994, and about half of those were children. That figure grew to 41 million by 1995). Many people without insurance, when experiencing a health problem, delay seeking treatment if they receive any treatment at all. Teenagers appear to be at the greatest disadvantage in this area. A Congressional Office of Technology Assessment report found one in five teenagers has at least one serious medical problem. Teens who are not covered by health insurance often do not seek medical attention until their ailment has progressed to its latest stages.

Although some people have ways of receiving treatment, such as through Medicare, or at county hospitals, for many people these options do not work and they are left without healthcare, or receive it only when it becomes an emergency.

The city of Los Angeles has more uninsured people than any metropolitan area in the US and tuberculosis is 2.5 times more common there than in the rest of the US. Many of the uninsured people of Los Angeles often rely on the services of County-USC Hospital. There are approximately 650 emergency visits each day to that hospital, the busiest in the country, and a person can end up waiting more than ten hours for emergency care. Many patients arrive at the emergency room with ailments that are not generally considered urgent, or that could have been treated earlier and at a lower cost if the patients had been able to afford medical care. There has been talk that the hospital may have to be shut down because Los Angeles County is experiencing a financial crisis, and also because of the condition of the aging, earthquake-damaged facility.

You want health care for sure? Get on welfare, go to jail, get elected to Congress, or get rich. Be a federal employee. Be the President.
— President Bill Clinton, speaking before a group of Latinos in Miami, July, 1994

My friends, the threat is here today to our national security. It won't do us any good to build all these heavy instruments of war in the name of defending our people if we can't protect our people's health, if we can't protect our people from disability. And that is where the real enemy is. It is within our borders.
— Senator Mark Hatfield, speaking at a conference of the National Health Council, July 20, 1995

Managed healthcare programs were started in the 1920s to take care of farmers. Henry J. Kaiser started providing prepaid healthcare to his shipyard workers in the 1930s. In the 1940s, unions started negotiating health benefits for workers in their labor contracts. In 1948 the Taft-Hartley Act made health benefits a legitimate item for union negotiations with company management. From the 1950s through the 1970s employer-provided health insurance became increasingly popular. The elderly began receiving health coverage in the 1960s through a new government program called Medicare. President Nixon signed the *HMO Act* in 1973 and this gave HMO companies more power in negotiating contracts with companies. Third-party administration of employee health coverage began in the 1970s when 3M started paying an insurance company to administer company health insurance. The boom in HMOs and preferred provider organizations was not seen until the 1980s. In the 1990s companies that provide insurance for employees are signing contracts with HMOs because it is believed that they provide less expensive medical insurance than health insurance plans of the past. Over 50 million Americans were members of HMOs nationally in 1995. With a membership of nearly seven million in 16 states in 1995, Kaiser was the nation's largest HMO.

In a land that many consider to be the best place to live on the planet, people who do have health insurance, do not even have the guarantee that they will have health insurance tomorrow. The time when Americans worked for the same company for decades has passed. Today Americans switch jobs the way they change cars, and job security no longer exists. Along with job security went health insurance. Employee cuts, corporate mergers, bankruptcies, and divorces leave millions of previously insured people without health insurance. Many people who do have health insurance carry an inadequate amount of it, and, according to the Commerce Department, in 1990 20% of American people lost their health insurance for at least a few weeks during the year. With an increase in the use of temporary laborers, many more people in the workforce are living without health insurance, as most of these temps are not covered by company health plans (about 2.5 to 3 million workers were temporary in 1994 and the Bureau of Labor Statistics predicts a million more people will be working as temps by the year 2000).

Even among the people who thought they had good insurance, there are those who have found that health insurance companies have lifetime reimbursement limits. If a person comes down with a sickness that uses up all his health insurance coverage, he can end up being uninsured and unable to obtain health insurance unless he pays a huge increase in his premiums.

Anyone who has ever had to struggle with the benefit restrictions of a health insurance company knows the problems with the current system. Pre-existing conditions place additional burdens on millions of Americans. The discovery of defective genes that can show a person is predisposed to a certain type of health problem will place more people under the label of having a pre-existing condition. (In California, health insurance companies are prohibited from using genetic testing to turn down people who carry the gene for a disease but who show no symptoms of the disease. This is a good law, but it does not cover the many people who do have symptoms, and it continues to leave them in the cold.)

The most common types of health insurance:
- **Fee-for-service plan.** This is the old type of insurance that allows the patient to choose any doctor.
- **Health maintenance organization** (HMO). This is when health insurance is paid for if the patient goes to doctors under contract with the HMO. Some HMOs employ doctors who work only for the HMO. Other HMO plans have doctors under contract who may also be seeing patients with other types of insurance, or no insurance at all.
- **Independent practice association** (IPA). This is an HMO that has contracted with networks of doctors. Members of the plan are covered only when they see HMO doctors.
- **Preferred provider organization** (PPO). An insurance plan whereby members choose from doctors under contract with the plan. Members can also go to doctors who are not in the plan but the member must pay a higher copayment (this is called a "point-of-service option").

A conflict that exists in the profit-making adventures of the HMO industry that insures over 50 million Americans is that of deciding who gets what treatment, on what basis the decisions are made, and of who should have the final decision on treatment options.

Most people believe a doctor or other healthcare worker is and should be the one who decides on what treatment a patient should receive, with the patients' approval. What we are seeing is that insurance company employees, who are acting to protect the profits of the insurance companies, are overriding the decisions of doctors. They do this by refusing to pay for certain types of treatments, encouraging doctors to prescribe less expensive therapies, directing what types of medications may be prescribed, dictating what doctors may and may not do, and otherwise dominating medical decision-making processes and treatment procedures.

Insurance companies are not charities concerned with doing good for mankind, they are businesses concerned with money, and their key executives typically receive million-dollar salaries. Their focus on money makes some people joke that HMO stands for "honor money only."

Insurance claims representatives often deny payment because the insurance company literature in front of them says the company does not cover, or discourages coverage of, the particular therapy, and often this insurance company policy is based on cost. By doing this, the insurance company employees, who do not examine patients and often have little or no medical training, are intruding with patient health needs by changing what a doctor has prescribed based on cost rather than on patient need based on patient symptoms, disease stages, and other conditions. If the insurance company representative has a college degree it is likely to be a business degree, not a healthcare degree. This is why it is said that managed care companies do not manage care, they manage cost. Managed care may be sufficient for the majority of the people because the majority of the people are relatively healthy, but for many others there is a hook in the managed care web.

Patients are caught in this web because their insurance plans detail the range of treatment options and access to doctors. If the patient does not follow insurance guidelines, the insurance company does not pay for treatment. Also, if a patient is prescribed a drug that is not on the HMO's list of approved drugs (called "formularies"), the patient may have to pay for the drugs out of his own pocket. Even the list of formularies is created with financial interests in mind. Similarly, if a patient is found to have a rare disorder, and needs to see a certain type of specialist practitioner, the patient may also be left to pay for this out of his own pocket if he does not succeed in achieving reimbursement from his managed care company. In this way the patient is not receiving the treatment that is best for him, but is receiving the treatment that is best for the financial health of the insurance company.

The doctors are caught in this web of insurance industry control because they rely on insurance companies to provide them with patients, and thus their income. Insurance companies offer doctors a contract without negotiation. The doctor can either sign it and be in the loop, or not sign it. HMOs place value on a doctor's economic performance, and even if he signs the contract it doesn't mean he is a permanent provider. Some doctors say that their ability to keep costs low seems to be more important to insurance companies than medical skills. HMOs often offer doctors year-end financial bonuses for keeping expenses to a minimum. Some doctors are going back to school to earn master's degrees in business administration with the goal of improving their profit margins and strengthening their negotiating skills with insurance companies.

A controversial element in many contracts doctors sign to become associated with an HMO is that of "disparagement" or "gag order" clauses. These gag orders may prevent a doctor from telling a patient information that is pertinent to the type and quality of care that the patient may receive. A situation that may be difficult for the doctor and not in the best interest of the patient is when an HMO tells a doctor he will have to treat his patient using a less costly but riskier type of drug or surgery because the HMO will not cover a more expensive treatment that may be better for the patient. If the doctor tells the patient this confidential information, the doctor may have his referral privileges suspended, or may even lose his contract with the HMO. When Harvard University medical professor David Himmelstein criticized gag clauses on the *Donahue* television show, he was eliminated from an HMO provider network he had a contract with.

Gag clauses are truly an obstruction of care. Even the American Medical Association and state medical societies have condemned gag clauses. The AMA position is that gag clauses are "an unethical interference in the physician-patient relationship."

If the doctor does not follow insurance company guidelines and costs the insurance company money, he may have his contract with the company canceled. An article that appeared in the *Wall Street Journal* (December 30, 1993) told of insurance companies terminating dozens of contracts with doctors who did not keep patient care expenses to a minimum. Having an insurance company cancel the contract it has with a doctor will damage the doctor's income because all patients he has through that insurance company will have to abandon him for another doctor, unless the patients want to pay the doctor out of their own pockets.

The same vulnerabilities that affect doctors also affect group practices and medical centers that have contracts with insurance companies. There are occasions when doctors, group practices, and hospitals absorb the costs of patient treatments with the goal of avoiding conflicts with insurance companies.

•

When the parents of a nine-year-old girl with a rare form of kidney cancer went outside their health maintenance organization's network of authorized doctors to find a surgical specialist experienced in the type of cancer with which their daughter was afflicted, the HMO refused to cover the $57,000 medical bill. The HMO reasoned that the parents violated their HMO agreement by going outside the network without approval. The parents argued that they did not have sufficient time to seek the HMO's approval and that they also did not want to hire a doctor with insufficient experience to treat their daughter. The parents then fought with the HMO to seek compensation for the medical bill. On November 18, 1994, in the largest financial penalty ever levied against a health plan by the California Department of Corporations, which regulates HMOs, state regulators fined the HMO $500,000 for failing to provide adequate medical care to the child. The HMO is appealing the fine.

•

In June 1994, a Monticello, New York, man who had been approved for a heart transplant by his medical insurance carrier was told three weeks after the transplant, and $300,000 in medical bills later, that the insurance company erred and would not pay for the transplant. The *Washington Post* quoted the man as saying, "I guess they thought I'd just die and they wouldn't have to deal with me any more."

•

A California teacher filed a lawsuit against her HMO when the company rejected her claim to cover the cost of delivering her baby, including the ambulance ride and hospital stay, because she delivered her baby at a hospital that was in the HMO contract but was not her home facility. The HMO reasoned that the policy forbade pregnant women who were in their ninth month from traveling more than 30 miles from their home medical facility. An HMO spokesperson said, "The medical consensus says women should not travel in the last month of pregnancy."

•

Many insurance plans had placed 24-hour limitations on the amount of time a new mother could spend in the hospital after giving birth. After stories circulated about a three-day-old New Jersey baby dying two days after being released from the hospital, public outcry prompted states to start passing bills guaranteeing mandatory minimum hospital stays of at least 48 hours following a vaginal delivery, and 96 hours for a cesarean delivery. In May 1996, when President Clinton endorsed legislation that would require health insurance companies to guarantee at least a 48-hour stay for new mothers and their babies, Richard Coorsh, a spokesman for the Health Insurance Association of America, argued that such legislation was unnecessary. Coorsh noted survey findings that newborns discharged from hospitals after 24 hours are no more likely to return for health problems within their first month than babies who are allowed to stay longer. Some insurance companies have advocated releasing mothers as early as eight hours after childbirth.

•

A Washington, DC-area man was denied coverage by his HMO when he sought emergency hospitalization for treatment of his lymphoma while he was staying with his brother in New York. The HMO plan included a provision that excluded care for foreseeable medical problems outside of the HMO's service area. The HMO argued that the man's AIDS diagnosis made his need for medical care foreseeable. The case was taken to court and the court ruled in favor of the HMO. A federal appeals court rejected the earlier court ruling and sided with the patient.

•

In October 1995 an arbitration panel ruled that Health Net, the second-largest HMO in California, pressured doctors at UCLA Medical Center to deny a bone marrow transplant to a woman with breast cancer. The woman, a mother of two young children, eventually died. Her family was awarded $1.3 million, and Health Net changed its procedures for deciding on coverage for bone marrow transplants. The estate of a woman who died under similar circumstances was awarded $12 million when the court ruled against the HMO (*Wall Street Journal*, December 28, 1993).

•

Healthcare is the biggest expense for people who are disabled, and this can interfere with employment. People without health insurance are far more likely to die of serious illnesses because health insurance is often put ahead of people's health. The staffing cutbacks driven by the profit motives of managed care companies bring another set of horror stories to the picture. Health insurance fails in these ways because the current US healthcare system is a profit industry and the people who make the profits have been very successful at protecting them. One way that helps people do this is by purchasing lawmakers in Washington.

Medical Lobbies

Lawmakers' workdays are filled with meetings with lobbyists, many of whom represent giant corporations. . . . When lawmakers travel to give speeches, they rarely address groups of poor people. The big-money lobbies often pick up the tab, and their representatives fill the audiences, ask the questions, and occupy the luncheon tables. . . . Lobbyists provide the prism through which government officials make their decisions.

— Jeffrey H. Birnbaum, in his book, *The Lobbyists: How Influence Peddlers Get Their Way in Washington*, Random House, 1992

Hundreds of billions of dollars are spent every year on healthcare in the United States — more than in any other country. The medical industry spends millions of those dollars on an army of influence-peddling hired guns called lobbyists. Lobbying groups spend millions of dollars to pump out their propaganda in the form of persuasive, and often confusing, TV, radio, and newspaper advertising to incite the American public to support their special interests. When dealing with politicians, lobbyists talk about wanting favors from politicians, and politicians talk about wanting campaign contributions from lobbyists. Lobbyists successfully encourage, entice, manipulate, and enrich lawmakers to pass laws in favor of the act of making money in medicine — laws that protect doctors, medical insurance companies and other healthcare interests.

Political action committee money is given to individual politicians. Soft money is used to build the strength of a political party.

According to a study released in December 1995, by Washington, DC-based Common Cause, the American Medical Association gave $13.7 million in PAC and soft-money contributions in the past decade.

Collectively, the report showed that PAC and soft money from doctors' and health insurance groups totaled $48.6 million over the past decade.

Many bills introduced to protect medical consumers and improve medical standards have been stifled by medical lobbies. The laws that do get passed may protect and improve some standards, but usually protect only doctors' standard of living. Just as candidates for office win because they have the most amount of money backing their campaigns (in 1992 the candidate who spent the most money won in 388 of 435 House races), the bills with the most money backing them often pass into law.

Two of the most active lobbying groups involved in national healthcare issues currently are the American Medical Association (AMA) and the Health Insurance Association of America (HIAA). Then, in each state there are state associations of doctors, such as the California Medical Association; these state groups lobby heavily and are very successful.

In September 1994, the Annenberg Public Policy Center at the University of Pennsylvania estimated that $60 million had been spent on healthcare advertising, largely opposing reform. Millions were also spent on campaign contributions to the appropriate opinion-molding politicians and also on catered closed-door negotiations, lobbyist-financed social events, and weekend getaways to resorts for the politicians and their families. Before recent lobbying reforms, these campaign contributions, gifts, and cushy trips were the legal way to buy votes in Washington and in every state capital.

The medical lobbies are so universally strong, and have been so successful in getting laws passed protecting the medical industry, that it would seem that doctors are in a nation all their own with their own set of rules. Unfortunately, when you look at some of the laws that do protect doctors, one can understand such a statement. In this situation there are doctors doing things to people that would result in a prison sentence for anyone who is not a doctor.

The groups that fund the medical lobbies consist of well-paid individuals who fill the top positions of companies and associations that provide medical supplies, medical services, and medical insurance. These individuals, the lobbyists they hire, and the politicians who make the laws enjoy health insurance at reasonable cost. As they make pronouncements about creating or not creating a national health plan, they do not know what it is like to be refused emergency treatment, nor do they know what it is like to be faced with a decision of whether to buy food or medication, or what it is like to struggle with medical bills that can take years to pay off, and that cause many people to go into bankruptcy. They, their children, and others in their socioeconomic class will always get medical care when they need it.

Healthcare Reform

In the beginning of 1993, as the Clinton Administration went about devising its plan to overhaul the American medical system, it was estimated that politically powerful lobbying groups financed by the doctors, nurses, hospitals, medical equipment manufacturers, pharmaceutical companies, and other medical interest groups would spend over $100 million in their efforts to influence lawmakers and the American public through lobbying and advertising and publicity.

When healthcare reform became an issue of the 1992 presidential election, it was certain that there would be a collision of concerned self-important politicians, lobbyists, medical executives, and lawyers elbowing each other for a say in what changes any landmark health reform plan would bring about. Everyone seemed to want to get in on the act. There were dozens of different healthcare reform plans presented, including the Catholic Health Association Plan, the Jackson Hole Group Plan, the Heritage Foundation Plan, the Garamendi Plan, and the Senator Kerry Plan. What happened was that so many people reached for the pie at one time that none of them got what they wanted.

Some of the groups that expressed some level of support for the Clinton health plan included the American Academy of Family Physicians, the American Academy of Pediatrics, the American College of Physicians (which later withdrew its support in favor of another plan), the American College of Preventative Medicine, the American Medical Women's Association, the American Society of Internal Medicine, the American Thoracic Society, the National Medical Association, and the National Hispanic Medical Association. Among the other major players in the medical lobbying game that gave varying degrees of support to the goal of creating a national health plan, but not necessarily the Clinton plan, were the American Dental Association, the American Hospital Association, the American Nurses Association, the American Pharmaceutical Association, the Health Insurance Association of America, and the Physicians for a National Health Program.

Then there was the American Medical Association, which has occupied itself with successfully swaying American politicians and laws that govern healthcare since the AMA was founded in 1846. According to the consumer research and advocacy group Citizen Action, in efforts to defeat the Clinton administration's plan for comprehensive healthcare reform, the AMA contributed $1,363,474 to members of Congress.

In September 1993, when the Clinton administration revealed its national healthcare reform plan, the AMA, which, with about 296,000 members (nearly half of America's doctors), is the nation's largest and most influential organization of physicians, announced that it would neither endorse nor oppose the Clinton plan. Later in the year the AMA showed some opposition to the Clinton plan when it denounced the requirement that employers pay 80% of employees' health insurance premiums.

Along their way, the AMA also said it would actively lobby Congress for a number of changes in the proposed national health plan, including tougher limits on the amount of money that could be awarded to patients who win lawsuits against doctors. (The survivors of people whose lives have been ruined by, or who are related to people whose lives have been ended by, sloppy medical care should be asked what they think about this issue.)

The AMA agreed that there is a need for some type of health system reform and that some portions of the plan were good, such as the part that guaranteed healthcare for all Americans. The AMA had begun a campaign for universal coverage years before the Clinton proposal. With the Clinton proposal the association believed it could play a broker role in constructing the details of the final health plan — and the way the government works — to secure the future of AMA members.

Those actions appeared to be quite different from what the AMA had done in the decades prior to the Clinton healthcare reform proposal. For decades the AMA had successfully played a major role in defeating attempts to reform American healthcare, including those plans proposed by Franklin Roosevelt, and in 1945, 1947, and 1949 by Harry Truman. Still, it is generally the case that when the AMA takes any action, it is in favor of the doctor's profits and not necessarily for the benefit of medical consumers.

The AMA did, however, like one part of the Clinton plan that was good for consumers, and that is the part that would let people choose their own doctors. This would reverse the trend set by HMOs that limit where a person can go for medical care, a situation that is a financial threat to hospitals and doctors who are left out of HMO contracts. (According to the Group Health Association of America, more than 50 million Americans, about one in five, belonged to an HMO in 1993. That figure grew to about 57 million by the beginning of 1996. In 1982, fewer than 10 million Americans belonged to an HMO.) This is the threatening trend that has brought many in the healthcare industry to favor adopting a healthcare delivery system similar to that in Canada, which also allows patients to choose their own doctors.

To get its viewpoints across to the American people, in 1993 the AMA sent letters to thousands of doctors and medical students to tell them what it is the AMA did not like about the Clinton health plan. Doctors were encouraged to persuade their political representatives to push for substantial changes in the Clinton proposal. The association also sent literature to the media and to county and state medical societies and encouraged doctors to explain to their patients what they thought was not right with the proposed national health plan.

The threat implied in the literature sent out by the AMA and various other self-serving medical industry-related groups was that overhauling the American medical industry would create an uncontrollable healthcare delivery environment where some people would be dying and others would be unable to find the medical care they needed — as if that situation did not already exist.

The AMA stumbles over itself in its pursuit to discredit anyone or any group engaged in anything that might interfere with the amount of money allopathic doctors can make. The AMA actions appear to consider any legislation insulting that would lower doctors' helium-filled rates or would require doctors to work on salary (as many other people do). As long as the American public continues to believe the clever tactics these medical industry-funded groups shovel out in efforts to keep a grip on the huge profits the medical industry enjoys, many people will remain without easy access to healthcare, and most will pay too much for it.

.

When it was seen that Congress obviously was not going to approve a healthcare reform package in 1994, Senator Harris Wofford of Pennsylvania proposed cutting off the tax-financed health insurance coverage enjoyed by members of Congress until they passed comprehensive reform. Wofford argued that "Members of Congress shouldn't take from the American people what they won't guarantee for the American people." He said that it was "a good, clear, fair proposition that people will understand."

It did not happen.

.

The Clinton healthcare reform plan now stands as another example of how lobbyists manipulate Congress and the guy in the White House. These political folks' compromising positions left them bending over backwards to please the medical and insurance lobbies while virtually ignoring citizen groups.

Many believe that the Clinton plan would have not been good because it relied too heavily on insurance companies and that as long as insurance companies, their discriminatory practices, and their profits are a major force in the healthcare delivery system, the system will continue to fail the people.

Many people who were not for the Clinton healthcare reform plan believed that it basically missed the boat on correcting defects in the present system. Some speculated that the Clinton plan was allowed to fail so that another form of health reform could go into effect. The idea behind this was to extend Medicare to cover those who do not have medical insurance by creating a new "Medicare Part C" program.

The Medicare system was established in 1965 as part of Lyndon Johnson's Great Society plan. It uses a few dozen insurance companies that are hired to sort, evaluate, and pay doctor bills by using a schedule called the Resource Based Relative Scale that was introduced in 1991.

Payments under the Medicare system are not determined under set guidelines by a government-run office. Depending on what insurance company is covering your region, you could be denied or approved for a treatment based on the whims of the insurance company covering your area.

Medicare currently serves 32.4 million Americans who are 65 or older and 4.4 million disabled persons. Ranking behind interest on the national debt, Social Security, and defense spending, the Medicare program is the fourth costliest activity of the federal government. The program cost $164 billion in 1994 and the cost of it is growing 10% or more annually — about twice the rate of overall healthcare spending. The growth of the nation's elderly population is causing the price tag of the Medicare program to escalate.

An increasing number of people seem to be for a single-payer health insurance system. One of the major deciding factors is that a single-payer system would eliminate health insurance companies, their commissioned salespeople, insurance company profits, and the time consuming paperwork that insurance companies generate, and cut medical advertising — which all figure into the final costs of medical care that companies and consumers end up paying.

Many people who are against a single-payer health plan are not aware of, or do not take into consideration, all the taxpayer money that is already spent on healthcare. Hundreds of billions of dollars are spent on Medicare and Medicaid. The government also spends billions to run the Veterans Hospital system and on medical care for US servicepeople. In addition to those expenditures, the government spends about $10 billion every year to subsidize American medical schools and teaching hospitals. On top of that money, the government spends money to provide health insurance to government employees. A single-payer system could consolidate much of these expenses and eliminate extremely wasteful duplication of services and administrations that handle the separate systems.

Some people thought that switching to managed care insurance programs would save money. Despite the continued trend of companies to join managed care systems, employers' health care costs rose again in 1995. The 1994 Insurance Directory published by the American Medical Association contains over 5,000 third-party payers and self-administered corporations. According to a report by the California Medical Association, paperwork, advertising, multimillion dollar executive salaries, and other non-medical expenses account for approximately 30% of every insurance premium dollar. With so many new companies entering the field and so much money at stake, the fast-growing HMO industry is beginning to look a lot like the savings-and-loan industry of the 1980s.

A single-payer plan would lower auto insurance rates by eliminating health coverage from auto insurance. It would alter workers' compensation costs, saving taxpayer and state budget money in that area. It would cover dental care, eyeglasses, and long-term nursing-home care. It would allow you to go to the hospital and doctor of your choice (just as the Canadian, Swiss, French, and German systems do) and would allow you these benefits if you lose your job or are between jobs, are a seasonal worker, become divorced from the person who carries your insurance, become too sick to work, or decide to go back to college for more education. It would not contain pre-existing condition limitations. It would give people more choices than they are currently allowed under current healthcare plans. It would lower the cost of healthcare in America and prevent rationing.

Under a single-payer system a single agency would collect the health tax and pay everyone's healthcare bills. This would do away with consumers' out-of-pocket payments. It would also release companies of their responsibilities for insuring employees and let businesses concentrate on doing business.

The single-payer systems of Canada and Australia have much lower operating costs than the insurance company controlled system of America, where nearly everyone is one serious illness away from financial ruin. Many people believe that with the health and other forms of security a single-payer system would provide for Americans, the money for the single-payer plan would be well spent because it would improve overall public health, help prevent contagious diseases from spreading by providing a way for people with these diseases to obtain care early in the disease process, and result in a more productive work force.

It seems the only way a dramatic change will occur in the US health system is if the citizens place unwavering no-nonsense pressure on the Washington establishment. Anything less than a single-payer plan may be similar to putting a Band-Aid on cancer.

Malpractice Laws

Besides being opposed to the cost-controlling measures in the Clinton health plan, the medical interest groups, and specifically the insurance industry groups, were and are concerned about the way any national health plan would deal with lawsuits patients file against doctors. When Donna Shalala, the Secretary of Health and Human Services, met with a group of doctors and told them the Clinton proposal to limit medical malpractice was not in keeping with what the doctors had hoped for, the doctors reportedly booed and hissed.

•

There is not any relationship between the cost of healthcare and medical malpractice costs, so we do not understand why this is even being discussed.
— Attorney Barry Nace, president of the Association of Trial Lawyers of America

•

Consumers who have been harmed by medical malpractice face an arduous and by no means certain battle for justice. . . Seeking to discourage lawsuits by victims of malpractice and to deny full compensation for malpractice deaths and injuries, the medical/insurance lobby portrays victims as cheats, judges and juries as dupes, and the judicial system as a bonanza for greedy consumers.
— From the book *Silent Violence, Silent Death,* by Harvey Rosenfield; Essential Books, 1994

•

As the money-making activities of the medical industry have been debated throughout the offices of lawmakers and the media, the medical industry has turned and placed blame for the high cost of medical care on the court system and on consumers for what the medical interests say are an overabundance of malpractice suits with large court awards. These claims are weak. Placing blame on consumers for the inflated prices charged by the medical community is ridiculous. And anyone who believes in this type of propaganda pumped out by the medical interests is being misled by these interests. It is not the fault of the patients that malpractice cases are filed. When patients do win malpractice cases, the jury awards for the damages are often reduced because of state laws that have been created to protect the doctors.

While I was working on this book I spoke with many people involved with malpractice cases, including lawyers, doctors, nurses, and patients. One comment that struck me came from a doctor who claimed that some patients enter a doctor's office and look for areas to sue the doctor. Now, I think I am pretty knowledgeable about the subject, and I have never met anyone who enjoyed being involved with a malpractice lawsuit. What that doctor was doing was blaming the victim.

Some of the people from the medical establishment that have been involved with this healthcare reform issue have claimed that patients who sue doctors are aiming for something comparable to lottery winnings. I find that comparison to be absurd. Though some patients may blame doctors for things that are not the doctor's fault, I don't know anyone who wakes up in the morning with plans to go find a doctor to sue, and the big awards do not come easy. Their chances of winning big money are much greater if they play the lottery.

In January 1996, a publication out of Boston called Lawyers Weekly USA *reported that medical malpractice verdicts accounted for five of the ten largest court awards of 1995. The amounts ranged from $40 million to $98.5 million. Three of the biggest awards involved injuries to babies during childbirth. These statistics do sound impressive, and they will be used by medical groups to lobby for their interests, but they are also misleading. Awards like that are rare, given when there was gross negligence that ruined a person's life, and after obsessive legal battles. Then the battles continue through the appeals process. The awards are not what they appear to be at first glance at the figure, and cannot make up for a situation in which a patient is left in a wheelchair or is so brain-damaged that he cannot care for himself and his life has been destroyed.*

— The author

What some of these large, influential medical interest and insurance industry groups want are more laws that will protect doctors, medical workers, hospitals, drug companies, medical equipment manufacturers, and insurance companies by limiting the rights of malpractice victims by making it harder for the victims to sue and by limiting the amount they can be awarded by a court. Specifically, they want a national law similar to the controversial Medical Injury Compensation Reform Act (MICRA) that was passed by the California state legislature in 1975, when those legislators gave in to the pressure of the medical/insurance lobbies working in that state's capital.

MICRA limits damages for "pain and suffering" to $250,000. MICRA also permits those doctors found liable of malpractice to pay awards over $50,000 on an installment basis. It includes a sliding scale of attorney's fees that starts at 40% for awards up to $50,000 and goes down to 15% for awards over $600,000. MICRA does not take into account the victim's age or lifetime medical costs caused by the negligence. This law has not reduced healthcare costs in California. In fact, no law limiting malpractice awards will reduce healthcare costs, but will benefit doctors, hospitals and especially insurance companies — and should be declared unconstitutional, as it is an injustice to the rights of the general public.

When the lobbyists for the insurance industry were pushing legislatures to pass MICRA into law, it was being sold as a way to reduce doctors' insurance costs and thus protect doctors who are, by definition, small businessmen. As Harvey Rosenfield says in his book *Silent Violence, Silent Death*, ". . . the price of medical malpractice liability insurance in California had increased dramatically since the passage of MICRA. In fact (according to a General Accounting Office study) premiums for physicians increased from 16% to 337 % in Southern California . . . between 1980 and 1986." So you see, the malpractice caps were put into place and the insurance companies still raised their malpractice insurance rates.

The group that really benefits from MICRA, and which spent a lot of money to get it passed into law, was the insurance industry. The financial benefits the insurance industry enjoys because of MICRA, and laws similar to it, are precisely why the insurance industry spends so much money on lobbyists and campaign donations — lobbyists who get laws passed that help the insurance companies make more money, and campaign donations that can make a politician.

> *The regulation of malpractice has traditionally been left to the states. In the past 15 years, every state has enacted some type of reform in an effort to limit the increasing costs of malpractice or malpractice insurance. Yet there is still no evidence that these tort reforms have had any effect on the methods in controlling healthcare costs.*
>
> *In your testimony, I think you indicated that California's malpractice reform had helped to control the state reform costs. The evidence was quite to the contrary. It may have held down the premium, but we (Californians) still have the second highest per capita cost and as stiff a growth rate as any state.*
>
> *So there is precious little evidence that the malpractice reforms in California have done anything. While they may have lowered the premiums (doctor's cost of having malpractice insurance), the effects certainly didn't pass through to the benefit of the beneficiaries or to your patients.*
>
> — Congressman Pete Stark, chairman of Subcommittee on Health, during Congressional subcommittee meeting on issues related to malpractice, May 20, 1993

> *I think federal solutions would do two things: Number one, it would protect our California law because attempts will be made to dismantle it, we are sure; and secondly, there have been numerous attempts throughout the*

rest of the country to adopt the California model which have met with only extremely limited success.

And what we would advocate would be the combination of California MICRA law, and if the Maine experience bears out to prove to be as beneficial as it is hoped to be, adding that to it on a nationwide basis.

— Dr. Richard F. Corlin, American Medical Association, during Congressional subcommittee hearing on issues relating to medical malpractice, May 20, 1993

•

The $250,000 cap has been heavily eroded by inflation since 1975 when MICRA was enacted. In order to provide the same level of compensation in today's dollars, the cap would have to be approximately $630,000.

• • •

The $250,000 cap is a hidden time bomb that will drastically restrict the legal rights of healthcare consumers.

— Ralph Nader, 1994

•

Regardless of whether a health insurance reform plan that does or does not go into effect — one similar to the Clinton administration's unproved controlled competition plan, one similar to the Canadian, Australian, or German single-payer plans, or one similar to Israel's multiple health-fund plan — the limits on the legal action that patients can take against doctors will likely be left to be determined by political bargaining.

•

JOHNSON: Let me go on to another problem. America is the only country that allows people to sue on the basis of contingency payment. And that has been one of the things that has driven medical malpractice suits. Would you be willing for us to not allow contingency suing in this area?

BECKHAM: Well, this is the process. You know, if you close the door to the courthouse you are going to save all these things. If you don't allow people to litigate, you are going to eliminate malpractice, and you save it all. If you take additional steps to cut people off from their rights, you are going to reduce exposure and premiums and are also taking away from our people the basic rights that they have from the founding of our democracy.

To say that you are going to abolish contingency fees, when this is the only way that many people can get a chance for redress, will make it so that you deny those people the opportunity to have a chance to be heard.

JOHNSON: I certainly have been one who has supported subsidies to make legal aid available to everyone, but contingency fees ————

BECKHAM: Have you ever had a legal aid lawyer represent you, as opposed to a good personal plaintiff lawyer, ma'am?

JOHNSON: Many of them are very, very conscientious.

BECKHAM: I am not talking about that. I am talking about their ability to handle medical malpractice cases in which they have limited experience and which require large amounts of time and expense to successfully litigate.

• • •

BECKHAM: . . . *people have a right to go to court if they desire to do so. And I think the more penalties you put on people if they go to court, the more you deny justice to people.*

— Dialogue between Congresswoman Nancy L. Johnson and Walter H. Beckham, Jr., of the American Bar Association during Congressional subcommittee hearings on issues relating to medical malpractice, May 20, 1993

•

I read a letter (that was written) to New York *magazine recently, unfortunately unsigned, by a physician who had been malpracticed upon when she was giving birth and her baby was very severely brain-damaged. And she herself is a physician. She ended the letter by saying, "If you take away my right to sue, you had better give me the right to shoot." And there is a lot of truth there.*

A lot of what gets lost in this debate is justice and fairness and that people who have been wronged want a forum in which to go and prove that they have been wronged and then to receive their just compensation. And that is what our court system is there for, and if you take away all the rhetoric, it is really not used all that often. It is used by a very small percentage of injured victims, but when they choose to use the court system, it really shouldn't be curbed except for a very, very good strong reason.

— Pamela Gilbert of Public Citizen's Congress Watch, during Congressional subcommittee hearing on issues relating to medical malpractice, May 20, 1993

•

. . . *The more you cut down people's rights to go to court, the more you cap their damages, the more you cut them off by statute of limitations, the more money you save, and if you don't allow any of it, you save it all.*

• • •

. . . *I might say this on contingent fees, it is interesting to me that the clients don't protest contingent fees. They see how hard the lawyers work. They know how hard medical malpractice cases are. They know the conspiracy of silence (between medical professionals not wanting to testify against each other). And they know that only about 25% of medical malpractice cases result in any recovery, and there are not any clients protesting. The only people who protest contingent fees are their adversaries. And that has always been a very interesting thing to me. And when they want to cut down on lawyer's fees, I think it would be very helpful to remember that 34% of each dollar goes to the defense costs, including defense attorneys' fees.*

I have never heard anybody say they should cut defense lawyers' fees in order to save money in the system. The medical profession wants the best lawyers to defend them, but they want to cut down on the caliber of the lawyers who represent the other side by reducing fees.

— Walter H. Beckham, Jr., American Bar Association, during Congressional subcommittee hearing on issues relating to medical malpractice, May 20, 1993

•

Most attempts to address the problem of medical malpractice have been embodied in attacks on victims and their right to recover damages from negligent (healthcare) providers, not on solving the problem at the source: ensuring quality care and eliminating medical negligence.

Limiting the ability of people to bring lawsuits is even more inappropriate when you look at the small number of malpractice victims who ever bring a claim or get compensated through the courts. The fact is that Americans rarely use the courts for accident compensation.

If you look at the Harvard study, only one in eight negligently injured patients filed a claim to recover damages. And 16 times as many patients suffered an injury from medical negligence as there were patients who received compensation from the malpractice system.

• • •

Even so, there is currently an effort under way to use the upcoming proposal to address the national crisis in healthcare as a vehicle for the same shopworn proposals that the American Medical Association has been pushing for two decades.

They claim that limiting the victims' rights is a solution to the skyrocketing cost of the healthcare system. In fact, nothing could be further from the truth.

> — Pamela Gilbert, director of Public Citizen's Congress Watch, testifying before Congressional subcommittee hearing, May 20, 1993. She was referring to the *Harvard Medical Practice Study*, conducted by the University's School of Public Health, which reviewed more than 31,000 records of patients discharged in New York State in 1984.

Defensive Medicine

Actions taken by the doctor to order tests and perform procedures and prescribe medications that do not provide any benefit to the patient but are done by the doctor to avoid malpractice claims are known as "defensive medicine."

Public Citizen's Health Research Group reported that in 1991, doctors' medical malpractice insurance premiums were about $4.8 billion, or 0.6% of total healthcare costs. In 1992, doctors and hospitals spent about $12 billion on insurance premiums to protect themselves from malpractice claims. During that same year, doctors ordered about $20 billion worth of unnecessary procedures to protect themselves from being sued (some estimates are much higher).

•

Although the medical industry argues that "defensive medicine" — what it defines as medical malpractices that are not in the best interest of the patient but are performed to avoid liability — is driving up healthcare costs, there is no evidence that so-called defensive medicine would be reduced by restricting medical liability.

It would be legislative malpractice for the President and Congress to restrict malpractice victims' rights in the face of the overwhelming evidence that the malpractice liability system should be strengthened, not weakened.

> — Ralph Nader

•

My view is that to the degree that defensive medicine is practiced, it is done as a way — at least physicians believe — to keep from ever being sued.

• • •

While we can't assess the exact amount of excess utilization that may be attributed to fear of medical malpractice suits, we estimate that defensive medicine costs resulting from these procedures alone is close to $4 billion.

Claims of total available savings on defensive medicine, made by various members of Congress, range from zero to $52 billion annually. Our middle range estimate of potential savings, and the one that we believe is reasonable, would be roughly $4.3 billion in 1994, or a total of $35.8 billion between 1994 and 1998.

> — From statement of Robert J. Rubin, MD, president, Lewin-VHI, Inc., a healthcare consulting company, presented to Congressional subcommittee on issues relating to medical malpractice, May 20, 1993

•

Other than the fear of malpractice actions, a doctor could have a variety of reasons to over-prescribe, including financial gain from the tests and procedures, patients' demands, misdiagnosis, requirements of the organization for which the doctor works, insurance company guidelines, and the doctor's habits or training.

•

A 1991 study by the state of Florida found that physicians in that state own the vast majority of certain healthcare facilities, and that these ownership agreements have led doctors to order unnecessary tests and questionable treatments in order to increase their profits. The report, commissioned by the Florida Healthcare Containment Board, found that at least 40% of the practicing doctors in the state have invested in facilities to which they can refer patients. In the case of diagnostic-imaging centers, the study found that doctors own 93% of such facilities. In addition, the study reported that the number of tests per patient is almost twice as great in doctor owned labs than in those not owned by doctors. Likewise, the average per patient charge in a joint venture facility was more than twice the charge in a non-joint venture lab.

> — Taken from testimony of Pamela Gilbert, Public Citizen's Congress Watch, presented to Congressional subcommittee hearings on issues relating to medical malpractice, May 20, 1993

•

Next to people requiring medical care to treat illnesses created by lifestyle, what drive up the nation's healthcare costs are unnecessary testing, excessive drug prescriptions, and unnecessary surgeries, along with dishonest claim forms.

On a physician level, costs may be lowered when doctors communicate well with their patients and become aware of their needs. Doctors often do not spend enough time working with patients to make proper diagnoses and spend little time instructing patients on what they can do to become healthier.

4 • BAD MEDICINE

Health Criminals

When a doctor commits white collar crime, the local police do not show up at the doctor's office, drag him away, and toss him in jail. The medical lobbies have helped to create so many laws that protect the doctors that when a law is broken, there needs to be an investigation of some sort and evidence needs to be gathered by one or more of the authorities who govern the medical industry.

In 1993, a manufacturer of medical devices, C.R. Bard Inc., pleaded guilty to criminal charges filed by the federal government that the company illegally sold heart catheters that had not received FDA approval. The company admitted conducting illegal testing of equipment on patients.

In 1994, the US government announced that it settled federal securities and fraud charges against the Santa Monica-based hospital chain National Medical Enterprises (NME) for a record $379-million fine after the company pleaded guilty to eight federal criminal counts. The network of medical crime was believed to be the most massive health fraud scheme ever. The lawsuit exposed millions of dollars in kickbacks and bribes given to doctors, referral services, and others so they would refer patients to 61 NME-owned psychiatric and substance-abuse hospitals in 30 states. NME then fraudulently billed Medicare, Medicaid, and other programs for those services.

NME was accused of making false statements in required federal filings and annual reports, and of misleading investors by improperly recording its sales and profits. The company was also accused of admitting and treating patients unnecessarily, keeping patients hospitalized longer than necessary to take advantage of their medical insurance, and billing insurers several times for the same service or when no treatment was given.

Evidence was uncovered during the investigation that showed NME bribed school counselors to send children to psychiatric hospitals, where the youths were held against their will, and doctors were paid to keep the patients longer than necessary. Evidence was also exposed by investigators that showed NME hospital employees used computers to track illegal payments to doctors and to measure how successful each doctor was at providing bogus referrals. Investigators explained that doctors who fell below a certain productivity level were cut off from the bribes. One former NME "administrator of the year" pleaded guilty in a Dallas federal court to paying at least $20 million in bribes to gain patient referrals to facilities run by NME.

In agreeing to the record financial settlement with the federal government, NME neither admitted nor denied wrongdoing.

Separately, the company paid more than $200 million to settle civil suits filed by former patients and insurers. Nearly 150 lawsuits were filed alleging cases of patient mistreatment and abuse. In one out-of-court settlement the company admitted responsibility in the death of a 13-year-old girl who committed suicide at the NME-owned psychiatric facility in Chula Vista, California.

In 1995, National Medical Enterprises merged with American Medical International of Dallas, and changed its name to Tenet Healthcare Corporation. It is now the second largest investor-owned healthcare company in the US. (The largest is Columbia-HCA Healthcare Corporation of Nashville, Tennessee. That firm operates 335 hospitals and 125 surgical centers in the US and Europe.)

•

In October 1994, T2 Medical Inc. agreed to pay $500,000 to end a federal investigation of fraudulent business practices. The investigation focused on whether the company, which does business in 38 states, was paying doctors for referring patients to company-run medical centers the doctors had a financial interest in by way of preferred deals on company stock.

•

Whether a Fortune 500 defense contractor delivers substandard equipment, or a large healthcare supplier lies about its costs to obtain inflated federal reimbursement, or a doctor falsifies a diagnosis to get paid by Medicare, or a businessman lies on an application for federal funds, we will seek to recover every dime and more on behalf of the taxpayers.

— Frank Hunger, assistant attorney general for the Justice Department's civil division

•

Let the message be very, very clear: We've made healthcare fraud a major law enforcement priority, and we're going to pursue it as vigorously as we possibly can.

— Attorney General Janet Reno, June 1994

•

The General Accounting Office estimated in 1995 that Medicare billing fraud may amount to as much as 10% of the entire budget of Medicare.

•

In February 1996, a person wearing a black hood was escorted through the halls of the Dirkson Senate Office Building in Washington, DC. The person was there to testify as a star witness in the case exposing the fraudulent Medicare billing practices for lifesaving medical equipment. The witness testified behind a screen and through a voice modulator that Medicare rules were routinely violated and the lives of patients were often jeopardized by the use of experimental medical devices. The witness also said that doctors were rewarded by the device manufacturers with cash, stock options, and royalty contracts.

The case was the result of a probe of the records from 131 major hospitals that were subpoenaed by federal agents working for the Health and Human Services Department. Officials testified that evidence suggested that most, if not all, of the hospitals submitted bills for experimental devices. The illegal billings for experimental medical devices may have been as much as $1 billion over the past decade. The charges came from hospitals that were billing Medicaid for high-tech medical devices, such as cardiac catheters, that were still undergoing clinical trials. The case against the hospitals was that the hospitals knew they were billing illegally, and allegedly with the encouragement of the medical device manufacturers.

The hooded witness, an employee of a major medical institution, was the one who blew the whistle on the illegal billing practices. The witness had filed a sealed whistle-blower suit under the federal False Claims Act of 1994.

The hospitals allegedly used the unapproved devices and then billed Medicaid for approved devices, then hid the illegal billings from federal regulators. The witness testified that during angioplasty procedures doctors often covered themselves by inserting the correct device, taking an x-ray photo for the patient file for billing and records purposes, and then proceeding with the procedure using the experimental device. He testified that doctors who use the experimental devices are motivated to do so by the financial rewards that are given to them by the medical device manufacturers.

Hospitals claimed that they were unaware of the policies restricting the devices that were used, that the rules were vague, confusing, and flawed, and that the patients were provided with the devices because the devices were the best that were available. One hospital that settled with Medicare by paying $1.3 million claimed that the unapproved devices were used in the best interest of the patients and that the approved devices would have cost about the same price. Others defended the actions of the hospitals by pointing out that lives may have been saved by using the newer technologies and that anything less would have been unfair to the patients.

A group of 22 hospitals filed suit against the Health and Human Services Department claiming that the terms of the rules governing the use of the unapproved medical devices were not defined or effectively revealed. They are also seeking to overturn the regulations.

Some lawmakers who have been lobbied by the medical industry want the rules revised and the new rules made retroactive so that the investigations and lawsuits would all be dropped.

Some new laws were enacted that allow Medicare to be billed for experimental devices.

The medical device industry has annual sales of $57 billion.

•

The Department of Health and Human Services defines medical fraud as the obtaining of something of value through intentional misrepresentation or concealment of material. The Justice Department has investigated fraudulent activities among hospitals, laboratories, nursing homes, ambulance companies, medical equipment dealers and manufacturers, doctors in private practice, and healthcare workers in group practice.

One of the more common criminal acts by doctors is drug abuse and misuse of Drug Enforcement Administration-granted licenses to prescribe controlled substances. Medical professionals can get drugs very cheaply and use them to feed their own addictions, or turn around and sell them to addicts and drug dealers.

•

It would be greatly remiss of me to omit the problem of substance abuse among doctors. Doctors have among the highest rates of drug abuse, alcoholism, divorce, depression, suicide, and sundry other forms of social pathology of any professional group. Within the profession those who are drunks or junkies are cryptically referred to as "impaired physicians."
— From the book *Morphine, Ice Cream, Tears*, by Joseph Sacco, MD; William Morrow & Co., 1989

•

We have been involved in fraud convictions in most sections of the healthcare industry. I would like to take a moment and share an example of one of the most diabolical schemes.

A defendant in another case tipped us off that controlled substances were being dispensed by a podiatrist. A quick drive by his office substantiated this claim. There were literally lines of people waiting outside his office to go inside.

This Detroit podiatrist generated three-quarters of a million dollars through a conspiracy that included Blues' subscribers and pharmacies. The podiatrist would use runners, that is a sort of street salesman, to encourage subscribers to visit a podiatrist. The podiatrist would then subject the subscribers to hundreds of unnecessary diagnostic and surgical services for which he would bill. I use the term "surgery" loosely, since the podiatrist's only intent was to create a scar. He believed that as long as he performed surgery of a sort, he would be untouchable by fraud charges. His definition of surgery was to pierce the skin and sever the tendon that controls the toes.

In return, the subscriber would receive a prescription for a controlled substance. Dilaudid, a synthetic form of heroin, and Percodan were the most popular. They sell on the streets for $25 to $50 per pill.

The prescription would then be filled at a local pharmacy that was friendly to the operation. The drug store would charge the subscriber cash, as well as bill the insurance company, including billing for an expensive antibiotic that was never actually dispensed.

The original runner investigative technique in this case involved surveillance to identify the runners. We then made undercover drug purchases from the runners, who in return introduced us to the podiatrist. Eventually the podiatrist issued illegal prescriptions to one of our undercover operatives.

Ultimately, the podiatrist pleaded guilty and was sentenced to 10 years in prison. He paid restitution, was departicipated from the plan and had his license revoked.

— Gregory Anderson, director, Corporate and Financial Investigations, Blue Cross and Blue Shield of Michigan, during Congressional subcommittee hearing on issues relating to all-payer fraud and abuse, March 8, 1993

•

STARK: What are your three largest areas, or two largest areas, of fraudulent activity?

MOREY: Well, I certainly think the number one is billing for services not rendered. We are continually amazed at the claims that we get where the services were never rendered, and it is just false on its statement.

The next area that seems to inflict the most pain on us is patient referrals. We are in a society where the competition is such that there is a degree of activity out there to solicit patients, so we are experiencing a lot of problems with patient referrals.

STARK: What would be third?

MOREY: Well, we certainly have a lot of hospital and clinical tests that are run that just probably were not necessary to begin with.

STARK: So on the one hand, it is just absolute stealing, fraudulent billing, might as well be akin to counterfeiting or issuing phony stock certificates. I mean sending you a bill for something that never happened.

MOREY: That is true.

STARK: What percentage would you guess, Larry?

MOREY: Oh, I would say it is high. In our fraud area I would say that is at least 50% of it.

STARK: And then referrals are just necessarily raising the price of something by giving a commission or a kickback or sharing the fees?

MOREY: Yes. What it generally does is it leads to over utilization.

— Pete Stark questioning Larry Morey, Deputy Director Inspector General for Investigations, Office of the Inspector General, US Department of Health and Human Services, during Congressional subcommittee hearing on issues relating to all-payer fraud and abuse, March 8, 1993

•

Healthcare fraud and abuse encompass a wide range of improper billing practices that include overcharging for services provided, charging for services that were not provided, accepting bribes or kickbacks for referring patients, and providing inappropriate or unnecessary services. Of particular concern is that healthcare fraud has moved beyond a single activity to organized healthcare programs affecting both the government and private insurance sectors.

For example, one fraudulent scheme that has troubled public and private payers in California for the past decade is alleged to have involved over $1 billion in fraudulent billings from about 90% of all the insurers in California and involved about 200 physicians and other providers. The scheme centered around soliciting people with health insurance who go to mobile labs, called rolling labs, for noninvasive tests, such as heart and blood pressure measurements. Frequently, the laboratories and the referring physicians then used phony diagnosis in submitting the insurance claims.

• • •

Because these fraudulent providers are very clever and they can figure out if you split your bills across different insurers, you can do a lot of things, and it is very difficult for insurers to pick up that this same doctor is double billing them, billing Aetna, billing CIGNA, billing Medicare.

— Taken from statements of Janet L. Shikles, director, Health Financing and Policy Issues, Human Resources Division, US General Accounting Office, during Congressional subcommittee hearing on issues relating to all-payer fraud and abuse, March 8, 1993

•

For example, we went to the outpatient hospital expenses with the hopes that it would reduce the inpatient hospital costs, and what we have found is that the fraud has followed the patient home. Now we are experiencing fraud in our home infusion programs. We are experiencing fraud in home therapy programs. So this is a great challenge for us, and as we look at the industry, we see that fraud is occurring in home infusion companies as they pay kickbacks for patient referrals, and we are noticing an excessive cost in the treatment that is received in our homes.

• • •

We have encountered a number of schemes in the laboratory industry: (1) billing for services never rendered, (2) unauthorized or excessive tests, and (3) disguising billing procedures in which the carrier (insurance company) is actually billed twice (by the doctors or medical facility). In the last five years, almost 50 convictions and civil actions have been obtained as a result of our laboratory investigations.

— Larry Morey, Deputy Director Inspector General for Investigations, Office of the Inspector General, US Department of Health and Human Services, during Congressional subcommittee hearing on issues relating to all-payer fraud and abuse, March 8, 1993

•

Healthcare fraud is acknowledged increasingly to be a crime problem — and I emphasize that — of rather alarming national proportions. By the most conservative estimates among our members, who comprise the private sector health insurers and the public sector law enforcement organizations with jurisdiction over healthcare, we are losing between a minimum of 3% to perhaps as much as 10% of our national healthcare expenditure every year.

This year the Commerce Department tells us we will spend just under $940 billion on healthcare. So by our math, we are looking at a minimum loss to fraud of $28 billion to perhaps as much as $94 or $95 billion. And again, that is to outright fraud.

I mention that it is a crime problem, because there has been discussion about the healthcare arena in which this activity takes place. In our feeling, we are looking at what is essentially a crime problem that takes place in the healthcare system.

• • •

As you have noted, it is anything but a victimless crime. When we look at the kind of financial loss we are sustaining, the insurers and the government may be the immediate victims of the loss, but there is no mistake that in the end it is all of us around the table here and in this room, and our families and associates, and employers who pay the cost of healthcare fraud, one way or the other.

> *As I mentioned, in some cases people's health is put at risk. That is something that can't be overlooked in the process; nor can the interest of employers who pay the cost of healthcare for their employees be overlooked. They represent a critical constituency in any effort to make us all better consumers of healthcare services and better watchdogs against healthcare fraud. Those businesses are sustaining enormous annual increases in the cost of providing healthcare insurance to their employees, and they need to be alert, as we all do.*
>
> *. . . we all need to pay as close attention to the insurer's statements of what is paid on our behalf as we would to a monthly credit card bill or a Sears bill to make sure that what was paid for was, in fact, what was provided. No question, we need to be better consumers.*
>
> — William J. Mahon, executive director, National Healthcare Anti-Fraud Association, during Congressional subcommittee hearing on issues relating to all-payer fraud and abuse, March 8, 1993

Lax regulation and peer review with unclear standards are not enough to catch every case of misconduct. Many of the doctors who regularly commit fraud do it in a way that is difficult to identify because they have developed credible lies and skills that evade the system. Even when they are caught, some doctors continue to commit the same crimes with a "laws be damned, catch me if you can" attitude — as can be expected from anyone who lacks good judgment or who has a drug addiction and has to work with drugs as part of his job.

A Beverly Hills, California, doctor, Mark Kaplan, 55, was sentenced to eight years in state prison after pleading no contest to one count of conspiracy and three counts of insurance fraud. His wife, Polina Ioffe, pleaded guilty to a single count of conspiracy and was sentenced to a two-year prison term. The couple also were fined $7.5 million — the largest amount ever recovered from a state fraud case.

From 1988 to 1992, the couple had recruited thousands of laid-off workers and persuaded or fooled them into making false on-the-job injury claims. Some workers who were legitimately injured and who sought treatment at the doctor's clinic did not receive the care they needed. Some people went to the clinics after seeing advertisements placed in foreign-language media and were led to believe they were going to an employment agency that required medical tests for job placement. It is believed the couple had scammed at least $30 million from the state workers' compensation system. Seven of the doctor's employees pleaded guilty to charges filed against them and subsequently received short jail terms.

If you suspect your doctor or another health professional of insurance fraud (giving untrue information — listing a fake "more bankable" diagnosis on insurance papers given to an insurance company in order to get money from the insurance company or government agency), then you might want to, under the guidance of an attorney, contact your state attorney general's office, the fraud bureau of the state department of insurance, and an in-house fraud investigator at the headquarters of your insurance carrier. (For further advice, contact one of the consumer awareness groups listed in the *Research Resources* section of this book under the heading *Patients' and Consumers' Rights*.)

Under the federal Medicaid and Medicare guidelines, payment for patient referrals is illegal for companies and individuals receiving reimbursements from the government-run healthcare programs. For more information on Medicaid and Medicare guidelines, a person should contact his local Social Security office.

To report a doctor who is abusing drugs or illegally selling them for profit, contact the local office of the US Drug Enforcement Administration. The DEA can revoke the doctor's certificate of registration that allows him to prescribe narcotics. Without a DEA permit the doctor will have a difficult time practicing medicine, and any hospital where he works may subsequently dismiss him.

Surgery Nightmares

Medical procedures are subject to mistakes, and not all mistakes are the result of doctor error. A patient's dissatisfaction with the outcome of an operation is always a possibility. A patient may be dissatisfied with the results of the surgery even when the doctor considers it to be a good result.

Some surgeries do not turn out right because the surgeon did sloppy work. For various other unforeseen reasons some surgeries do not result in what the patient was expecting. In his book *The Making of a Surgeon* (Random House, 1968), William Nolen explains that all doctors make errors, that medicine is not an exact science, and that symptoms cannot be added into a computer to get a calculated treatment. Under the unpredictable and uncontrollable conditions present during all medical treatments it should be expected that surgery will not always be successful.

An unsatisfactory surgery result can have a very negative effect on every area of the patient's life, cause public embarrassment, be a drain on the patient's emotions and relationships, and lead to financial difficulties as the patient spends time and money trying to correct, or at least attempting to improve, the results of a bad surgery. A patient who goes in for surgery to improve his health can become angry, irrational, depressed, and even suicidal if the operation does not turn out the way he expected. These emotions can be amplified if the change causes a physical condition that alters the normal appearance, movement or function of the body.

When all is said and done, it is the patient who needs to be satisfied with any surgery, since it is he who will have to live with the results.

As when a person goes to the grocery store, when he goes to the surgeon he should want to know what he is getting for his money and should make sure he gets what is best for him. Giving the surgeon too much power can be compared to going to the grocery store, handing the cashier money and telling him to get the amount of food that can be purchased for that amount of money. The cashier may have very different tastes in food and buy all sorts of things the customer does not like. When going to the surgeon, the patient has to make sure he gets what is best for him; if he does not do this, it will be too late to realize he made a mistake and, unlike the grocery store scenario, he cannot return the item for a new one.

> *Sometimes what happens in the hospital is not any different than what happens on the street. In both cases, the man with the knife wants your money — and he might be willing to risk killing you for it. Let me warn you, if you think the hospital will police the doctor, you better hire a bodyguard for yourself.*
>
> — From the book *Doctors Are Gods*, by David Jacobsen and Eric D. Jacobsen; Thunder's Mouth Press, 1994

Dr. James Burt, a gynecologist who practiced in a prominent hospital in Dayton, Ohio, was surgically redesigning the vaginas of some patients without their permission or previous knowledge. These women awoke after giving birth and other surgeries to find they had been maimed. Dr. Burt believed the female genitalia were naturally positioned at the wrong angle and that his surgical procedure would bring greater pleasure, or enhance a woman's sex life. This "love surgery" included altering the clitoris and rearranging the vagina. Many of these women experienced pain during intercourse, incontinence, bleeding, infections, bowel movements through the vagina, and other complications. These surgeries were done for more than twenty years before Dr. Burt finally gave up his medical license in January 1989. He then retired to Florida.

A doctor in New York who advertised himself in subways as "Dr. Tush" used laser surgery to correct hemorrhoids. His ads mentioned benefits, such as fast healing and a quick return to work. He performed many botched surgeries, and a number of his patients underwent additional surgery to try to repair what this doctor did to them. Many of them sued. The doctor was driven out of business, no longer practices medicine, claimed bankruptcy, and now lives in Washington State.

One California woman who had a tummy tuck complained of ongoing sharp pains in her abdomen. Her doctor told her it was typical to have discomfort after such a surgery and that she needed to be patient while her body healed. Months went by and the woman was still having more pain than she thought should be expected. A relative took her to see another doctor, who ordered x-rays. They found that the doctor had left surgical scissors inside the woman's abdomen. This required another surgery to remove the scissors. (In another messy operation that took place at a military hospital, a towel was left in a man's torso during surgery.)

•

Many thousands of people who have bad surgical results go in for additional surgery to try to correct it. Some of the originating doctors offer to do operations over free or at a discount price. Sometimes the second surgery does not correct the problem and leads to further disappointment. Other dissatisfied patients cannot afford to get a second surgery, may not be able to handle the trauma of going through another surgery, may find there is no way to correct their problem or feel they cannot trust another doctor. People caught in this situation who were interviewed for this book repeatedly said the same thing: They would give anything to have their original body back.

The doctor who performed the surgery may become rude, and his compassion for the patient may quickly disappear when he hears the patient criticizing his work. There have been patients in this situation who have been physically pushed out of the doctor's office and told never to return. Those who have had unsuccessful surgery can, in addition to living their own nightmare, find the doctor and his staff very unsympathetic. The doctor and his staff may simply ignore the disappointed patient and the patient's phone calls, hoping the patient will "get over it." The doctor who has a dissatisfied patient knows to become silent and to say as little as possible. This silence comes into play because any admission of negligence or malpractice can become a part of a lawsuit and interfere with the physician's malpractice insurance and career.

Those patients who have been victims of negligent surgical disasters often experience coping problems similar to, or more intense than, those of people who have been raped or likewise violated. These symptoms, which can emotionally cripple a person, include feelings of helplessness and of being deceived, revolving thoughts, insomnia, sleepwalking, nightmares, night terrors, loss of appetite, loss of concentration, loss of integrity, an overabundance of anger, and a feeling of being attacked during simple confrontations. They may feel vulnerable and trespassed against. Thinking that they should have known better may result in overwhelming guilt and shame.

Relationships may be damaged because the person emotionally clings too tightly to the people around him or withdraws into depression. The toxic thoughts may play out in the person's body language, the tension of his muscles, his breathing patterns, and the pitch of his voice. The long-term effects may be posttraumatic stress disorder, when the person's reactions to everyday occurrences have more to do with the triggering of intrusive traumatic memories than with present situations.

Probably for as long as there has been surgery, there have been dissatisfied patients who entertain thoughts of violent revenge. There have also been dissatisfied patients who have gone to the extreme of murdering their surgeons, and some dissatisfied patients have committed suicide. People in this predicament who are thinking these types of thoughts should promptly seek some type of psychological therapy.

If you are in the position of seeking to have a botched surgery repaired, it is probably a bad idea to trust a doctor and let him operate on you again if he has already botched one operation. You also may find it hard to find a doctor who will give you a second operation. A patient who was dissatisfied once is likely to be dissatisfied again. Why should a doctor spend time on you when he can take on other, less complicated jobs?

A person planning a surgery to correct a bad result from a previous surgery should avoid becoming an eager victim. Each succeeding surgery on the same area can become technically more difficult to perform, and the outcome is less predictable. He should abstain from having the operation too soon. Usually a healing period needs to take place. All options should be looked at and research should be done. Medical books may be helpful in studying the actual structure of the body part. The various types of surgery that are available and the various ways the surgeries are performed should be studied. Prudence should be taken when looking for the right doctor, and caution taken when consulting with doctors who seem too enthusiastic about doing the operation.

Anyone considering surgery should aim to receive the best care possible with the original surgery so time and money will not be wasted and physical, mental, and financial health will not be risked in trying to repair a bad job. He should do whatever can be done to attain the best results on the first try, because this is the most important one of all.

The California Medical Board

> *. . . last year, California took less than two disciplinary actions per thousand physicians. In Florida, it was almost 10 disciplinary actions per thousand physicians, and about 8.3 in Maryland. It would take a leap of faith, I think, to imply that California doctors are seven per thousand better than those practicing in Florida or Maryland.*
>
> — Congressman Pete Stark during subcommittee hearing on issues relating to malpractice, May 20, 1993
>
> *. . . there is an obstetrician-gynecologist in Los Angeles, an extremely litigious person who wound up already suing seven or eight different doctors who testified against her, so I will confine my comments to what is in the public record. She was accused of charging as much as $40,000 for hysterectomies, that is not an error in my reporting. It is an error in what she did, obviously.*
>
> *The medical board held a hearing for a variety of reasons including which she had been kicked off the staff of more than one hospital and they concluded there were at least six reasons, any one of which would result in her losing her license and for all six of those reasons, they ordered her license revoked.*
>
> *By playing various games with the courts, which are beyond my ability to understand the detail of, 3 1/2 years later, she still is practicing in a little dinky hospital that I wouldn't let my dog go to, but she is still practicing, including going on television and TV talk shows and so on.*
>
> — Dr. Richard F. Corlin, American Medical Association, during Congressional subcommittee hearing on issues relating to medical malpractice, May 20, 1993

An internal report that was released in August 1993 by the California Medical Board questioned the quality of the medical expertise used by the state in its disciplinary cases concerning doctors. The report, the result of a six-month investigation, stated that in too many instances, the doctors used by the state as experts against other doctors were themselves not qualified for their roles. It stated that investigating physicians were sloppy in the way they reviewed cases, or lacked up-to-date medical knowledge or expertise in the specialty of the physician they were examining. The report was a serious blow to the medical board, which had repeatedly been criticized by consumer groups, prosecutors and legislators for failure to take timely or adequate action against bad doctors.

In the spring of 1989, a lengthy report criticizing the California Medical Board was released by the University of San Diego's Center for Public Interest Law (CPIL), which monitors state licensing boards. The report rebuked every step of the system that was supposed to process consumer complaints against bad doctors and claimed the people paid to run the system were not properly trained and lacked medical or legal expertise. The report, which recommended substantial structural and administrative changes, concluded that the board was ineffective, had not been protecting consumers for a number of years, and was letting bad doctors, including ones who had killed patients, continue practicing medicine. As an example the CPIL cited the case of one Los Angeles-area obstetrician who killed nine babies and was charged with 45 felony counts, including nine counts of second-degree murder, before the board took action against him.

In 1990, the assistant director of the board told state legislatures that there was a backlog of 600 uninvestigated cases of public complaints against doctors even though he knew the actual figure was about 800. Investigators with the board witnessed top officials destroying hundreds of files containing these consumer complaints. Outraged investigators complained to their union and the CPIL, which in turn filed complaints with the state governor. An investigation by the state was called for. Since the attorney general's office declared a conflict of interest because it represented the Medical Board in actions against doctors, the California Highway Patrol (CHP) was brought in to do an investigation.

The investigative report, which was released by the CHP in January 1993, accused the board of lax administration, misconduct, corruption, and appalling mismanagement. The report detailed the destruction by the board of the files containing inadequately investigated consumer complaints against doctors. Several of the cases involved a string of patient deaths in a Los Angeles hospital. Among the deaths was one patient whose colon was ruptured during surgery to remove an ovarian cyst. In a subsequent operation performed to repair damage from the first, the patient's heart was punctured and she died. In another case, an accident victim was given an over-the-counter painkiller and discharged, only to die later from fractured ribs and a lacerated liver.

The CHP report also alleged that a diversion program created to rehabilitate doctors who had drug, alcohol, or psychological problems had been improperly used as an alternative to disciplining unfit physicians. One administrator accepted gifts from a doctor he was overseeing in the rehabilitation program. The program was accused of lax monitoring of doctors and was described by some critics as a money-making scheme that benefited clinics connected with the program's staff.

Top staff members of the board were accused of misusing government cars, gasoline credit cards, cellular phones, and frequent flyer credits, and of being generally dishonest in performing their responsibilities.

All these allegations brought lawmakers to introduce legislation that would strip the board of the power to investigate, prosecute and discipline its own profession. They believe that, as a way of making the state physician disciplinary system more responsive to consumer complaints, the power should be given to an independent unit of the attorney general's office.

Public Citizen's Health Research Group ranked California 34th out of the 50 states' disciplining of doctors in 1994. That amounts to 3.28 actions for each 1,000 doctors in the state, compared to the national average of 4.3 actions per 1,000 doctors. The disciplinary actions that were taken affected only 0.3% of California doctors.

The study was based on records from the California State Medical Board, federal healthcare agencies, and the US Drug Enforcement Administration. It took into consideration the actions taken against doctors for such offenses as sexual misconduct with patients, drug and alcohol abuse, incompetence, and criminal convictions. Actions that were taken against the doctors included revocation or suspension of medical license, probation, and other forms of professional discipline. (For a copy of a book containing the report and a list of disciplined doctors, contact Public Citizen's Health Research Group in Washington, DC. Their address is listed under the *Patients' and Consumers' Rights* heading in the *Research Resources* section of this book.)

When a Doctor Was Negligent

The following is a very small portion of the information one may need to consider when malpractice occurs. If you are a victim of medical malpractice, read books on the subject, and consult with at least one attorney who specializes in malpractice and who is familiar with the laws in your area.

Some people approach a doctor's office as if it were a haunted house where life-threatening occurrences take place. To make a visit to a doctor's office seem more inviting, the medical community presents advertising with images of happy and caring medical professionals.

In 1976, the Department of Health, Education and Welfare's Malpractice Commission estimated that one-half of one percent of all patients entering hospitals are injured there due to negligence. That estimate would indicate 156,000 such injuries and deaths resulted from doctor negligence in 1988.
— DHEW Malpractice Commission information from *Journal of Legal Medicine*, February 1976. Calculations by Pamela Gilbert, director of Public

Citizen's Congress Watch, in a prepared statement for a Congressional
subcommittee hearing, May 20, 1993

•

As children we are taught, at least through action, that there are
certain authority figures we can trust; one is the teacher, one is the
police officer, and one is the doctor. Probably the majority of the
people who work in these positions are trustworthy and represent
their professions to the best their circumstances will allow.

Doctors are different from the other authority figures. This is
because children are told it is okay for a doctor to touch them where
no one else is allowed to touch. People depend on that
trustworthiness when they turn to doctors in times of need. In the
process of being a patient a person lets a doctor see more of his
physical and emotional sides than what people are used to exposing
in everyday life. That is when a person is vulnerable to violation as
he places his health in the hands of a medical professional who
may sell himself as a caregiver although he may be negligent. As
with other persons who use their authority to violate another
person, doctors who commit gross negligence are often very bright and
seek to hide their dark side from those who would expose them.

•

A Los Angeles doctor was sentenced to thirteen years in prison for
sexually assaulting four female patients. Prosecutors wanted the judge to
impose a 37-year sentence. The decertified orthopedic surgeon was
convicted of ten felony and criminal counts of sexual battery and rape, and
penetration with a foreign object while the victims were unconscious.

•

mal•prac•tice (1671) **1**: a dereliction from professional duty or a
failure to exercise an accepted degree of professional skill or learning
by one (as a physician) rendering professional services which results
in injury, loss, or damage **2**: an injurious, negligent, or improper
practice : MALFEASANCE
mal•prac•ti•tio•ner (1800): one who engages in or commits malpractice
— By permission. From *Merriam-Webster's Collegiate® Dictionary* ©1993 by
Merriam-Webster Inc., publisher of the Merriam-Webster® dictionaries.

•

There is a virtual epidemic of medical malpractice in this country.
Public Citizen has looked at the results of three different studies and we
estimated that between 150,000 and 300,000 Americans are injured or killed
each year by doctor negligence. If you extrapolate from the 1991 study by
Harvard (School of Public Health) *that has been discussed already today,*
approximately 80,000 deaths occur annually due to doctor negligence. That
is more than twice the number of motor vehicle occupants killed every year.
— Pamela Gilbert, director of Public Citizen's Congress Watch, testifying
before Congressional subcommittee hearing, May 20, 1993

•

Iatrogenic disease is defined as disease caused by a doctor or by a
hospital. The number of people who die in the US as the result of medical

treatment is equivalent to three Boeing 747 crashes, with fatalities, every two days.
— Deepak Chopra, MD

The tragedy of popular elective surgery procedures is that many people who went in for operations they thought would make their lives better ended up having their quality of life, and sometimes the entire fabric of their existence, disheveled when the surgeries were not successful. Sometimes this is the result of maloccurrence (situations out of the doctor's control) and does not necessarily mean the doctor was negligent. But other times it is caused by the faulty actions (malpractice) of the medical caregivers.

Should one of us go into an emergency room and be asked all the questions that a doctor would ask after an accident, including "Are you allergic to anything?" And you answered, "To the best of my knowledge I am not allergic to anything." The doctor proceeded to give you a shot of penicillin. The reaction caused you to go into shock and spend an extra day in the hospital. That, in fact, is malpractice, but it is not negligent. It is just one of those accidents.

On the other hand, had we gone into that same emergency room wearing one of those little medallions that say, "I am allergic to penicillin," and told the person receiving us that we were allergic, they then proceeded not to tell anybody and they still jabbed you with the penicillin. After you had the same reaction, that would be negligent malpractice.
— Congressman Pete Stark, testifying before subcommittee on issues relating to malpractice, May 20, 1993

If you become a victim of medical malpractice, do not expect to be told about it by anyone involved with your medical care. That would be like handing you an invitation to sue them. Unless it is blatantly obvious that medical malpractice has occurred, you may not know it has occurred until you or someone in your family notices something is not right. Filing a lawsuit will likely be the only way you can get any of the medical professionals involved in your care to talk about any bad medical care you received.

In November 1994, Lissette Nukida, a nurse who worked in a Carson, California, rehabilitation center, pleaded guilty to injecting insulin into the intravenous solutions of two women patients. She explained that she did not intend to kill anyone but wanted to be sent to prison because she believed doctors there could cure her recurring headaches. The two patients fell into comas and were treated for dangerously low levels of blood sugar. Nukida also admitted to injecting insulin into unused medications being kept in a storage room.

A male nurse who worked in the surgical recovery room of a hospital in Tampa, Florida, was charged with raping four unconscious women who were recovering from surgery. After his photo appeared in a newspaper, twenty more women came forward with accusations that the nurse had also raped them. He had worked at three other area hospitals. The 45-year-old man tested negative for HIV.

Actions of a doctor that can be considered negligent:
- Doing things to a patient against the patient's will.
- Failing to inform a patient of common risks in a manner meant to deliberately alter the patient's ability to make an educated decision on whether to undergo surgery or other treatment.
- Performing an operation without the necessary equipment, medicines, or staff.
- Performing an unnecessary operation after misdiagnosing a condition.
- Performing a surgery with the knowledge that it is unnecessary.
- Causing injury to a patient through faulty practices.

    An illness, disease, or injury resulting from a doctor's actions is called an iatrogenic illness or injury.

    An infection that is acquired during a hospital stay is called a nosocomial illness. Nosocomial illnesses are often the result of unclean operating tools, contaminated hospital items, or unsanitary medical workers. Even sweat or body hairs from the arms and faces of the members of the surgery team can cause a post-surgical infection.

    Birth defects caused by medications are called teratogenesis or teratogenicity deformities.
- A doctor who is treating patients while he is under the influence of drugs or alcohol.
- Approaching a patient sexually.
- Fondling or raping a patient while the patient is drugged or unconscious.
- Prescribing or administering the wrong medication.
- Creating a situation that leads to the death of a patient who did not have a life-or-death condition. This includes complications that result in a suicide.
- Lying to a patient.

    Many doctors believe it is acceptable to misinform a patient if it is done to avoid upsetting or frightening him in a way that would interfere with his health and deprive him of any hope for a cure.

    Some types of doctors regularly have to deal with how to inform a patient of a terminal illness or injury. It can be a delicate balance of when, what, and how to inform the patient in a way that provides for realistic hope. The doctor has to take into consideration what type of person the patient is, how he will accept the prognosis, and the patient's capabilities of calculating the information in a way that is in his best interest. And the doctor has to be prepared for the types of questions the patient might ask while recognizing that statistics do not always dictate how a patient will react to forms of treatment or how long a patient will live.

    In September 1993, the California Supreme Court ruled that doctors must give seriously ill patients enough information to make intelligent decisions about treatment but that doctors are not obligated to disclose the statistical chances of dying — even if the patient asks to be told the truth about a health condition. The court ruling also held that doctors do not have to inform patients on pertinent details related to patients' non-medical interests, such as survival rates and how much time the patient has to put his affairs in order. The ruling stated that doctors need to provide statistical mortality rates only if it is a common standard of practice in the medical community.

While misleading a patient or withholding information from a patient might be helpful in certain instances where the patient's health would be endangered if he reacted adversely to the truth, it might also alter the patient's ability to focus on the threat to his health. When a potentially life-threatening condition exists, valuable time can be wasted that the patient otherwise could have spent exercising his right to make decisions, doing research, getting second and third opinions, and considering various available options.

•

What are the specific damages?
- Pain.
- Suffering.
- Altered abilities.
- Emotional trauma.
- Psychological trauma.
- Endangerment.
- Economic burden.
- Altered lifestyle.
- Decreased life expectancy.
- Damaged or strained personal and professional relationships.
- Wrongful death of a companion or relative who did not have a life-or-death condition.

•

Even after a doctor has been found guilty of gross negligence that resulted in the death of one or more of his patients, he may still be able to continue being a doctor. If a state medical board investigates a doctor for unprofessional conduct and finds him guilty, the board might only send him a letter of reprimand to formally acknowledge his guilt. This reprimand probably will not affect the doctor's practice, nor will it be filed in the national database that collects information on disciplinary actions against doctors. It basically does little if anything as far as altering the way the doctor treats patients. It probably will not affect the doctor's standing with insurance companies, or his hospital privileges.

•

Remember, in America you are innocent until proven guilty. Then you appeal for nine years.
— Andy Rooney

•

If you think a doctor who treated you was negligent, one of your options is to consult with a lawyer (before the statute of limitations has run out) who specializes in and is well experienced in malpractice law, and who has substantial jury trial experience. You may want to consider taking the doctor to court, not only for personal reasons, but also to protect other people from having done to them what was done to you. (People's Medical Society, Public Citizen's Health Research Group, the American Trial Lawyers Association, the Center for Medical Consumers, the National Center for Patients' Rights, and Safe Medicine for Consumers are groups listed in the *Research Resources* section of this book that can provide you with information about taking legal action against a medical professional, medical center, or hospital.)

If you are a member of a union you may be eligible for free, or reduced-rate, legal representation through a union staff attorney or through a law firm that is under contract with the union. Some credit card companies also sell legal insurance benefits. Some companies offer legal insurance plans to their employees. These plans may try to steer a person into more costlier legal services once he contacts them for legal advice that should be covered under the plan. A person may simply want to take advantage of the free consultation that many of these plans offer, and decide from there if he wants to use the law firm to handle the case.

Be careful when choosing a lawyer. In the same fashion wherein some doctors sell themselves in a particular specialty when they have not had any special training in that specialty, there are lawyers who market themselves as malpractice lawyers when they have not done any significant amount of research on malpractice law. (Ask for the lawyer's resume. Ask if he has malpractice insurance and ask to see the certificate of insurance provided by the insurance company.)

Upon hiring an attorney, set a requirement that any bill you receive from him must be itemized with dates, reasons for charges, and receipts of any outside charges. Do not let the lawyer charge you for things such as meals, valet parking at restaurants, and recreational activities. If the lawyer is hungry he will eat whether or not you let him add food charges to your bill. If he wants to play golf he should play golf, but you should not be charged for his golf game on the basis that he was thinking about your case while he played golf. Keep on top of the bills so you do not end up challenging substantial overbilling charges before the fee dispute service of the county bar association or in a jury trial. (Your chances of winning are greater if you go to a jury trial to dispute overcharges by a lawyer. The fee dispute service of the county bar association is made up of lawyers, and some say the setup there is simply a good old boys' club where the club members always win.)

In choosing a lawyer, experience and fee should be related. One lawyer may charge an hourly rate that, at first, looks cheaper than another lawyer's.

> However, because of a lack of experience in some area, the less expensive lawyer may charge a larger fee in the long run. Ask for a resume and check references. If you feel overwhelmed, take a trusted friend to the initial meeting to help you keep track as you interview the lawyer about services and fees.
>
> If you retain a law firm, be sure you understand who will work on your case and who will supervise the work. If junior lawyers will handle your work, the fees should be lower. That is fine as long as you know an experienced attorney will be reviewing the case periodically.
>
> Let your lawyer know that you expect to be informed of all developments and consulted before any decisions are made. You may also want to receive copies of all documents, letters, and memos written and received in your case, or have a chance to read them in the lawyer's office.
>
> — From US Small Business Administration booklet *Starting and Managing a Business from Your Home*, by Lynne Waymon, in cooperation with the American Association of Community and Junior Colleges

Be cautious about whom you discuss your feelings with concerning a negligent doctor. The doctor may countersue for trade disparagement (lowering of professional rank), libel and defamation of character. It would be wise to seek legal counsel with an experienced malpractice lawyer before writing any letters or taking any action relating to a negligent doctor or what a negligent doctor did to you.

With the lawyer's guidance, write and send a letter of complaint to the state medical board, and any other governing body, briefly detailing the situation. This may include administrators of every hospital the doctor is associated with, any school where he teaches, and also to your state legislator who may be working on, or familiar with, medical regulations. (It is not required to have legal advice when filing complaints against a doctor, medical professional, hospital or medical center, but remember that any letter you write may be dug up, taken out of context, and presented as evidence against you in a courtroom.)

Do not bother writing letters to associations the doctor belongs to, such as the AMA. The AMA is a political lobbying and allopathic doctor education group and has no licensing or disciplining authority over doctors. Doctor associations, such as the AMA, exist to advance the standing of doctors. Some doctor associations have raised money to help pay defense funds for doctors who are being sued by patients. The association will likely hand your letter over to the doctor for use in his defense.

Many doctors now work in an employee-type arrangement with HMOs and other medical groups. This provides a doctor with a steady income and a more secure work arrangement as the doctor becomes part of a system. HMOs are very cost-conscious, and part of the way they judge a doctor is on a scale of what his way of practicing medicine is going to cost the HMO. If the doctor you are taking legal action against is a member of an HMO, you may also want to write to an administrator of the HMO. If you are accusing the doctor of performing a surgery that was unnecessary, the HMO may take notice. Any suggestion that the doctor could lose his HMO contract is a serious threat to the doctor's future income. (If the HMO is or may become involved in the lawsuit, writing a letter to it may not be a good idea. Consult your lawyer.)

If the doctor's actions amount to what could be considered criminal activity (drug abuse, rape, and other such offenses), you may want to contact the county district attorney's office or the state attorney general.

The state medical board may tell you what steps you should take in filing a complaint against a doctor, and it may ask you to fill out specific forms. A letter to the state medical board might trigger disciplinary actions against the doctor and can help pave the way for the doctor's medical license to be taken away — but the state medical board may also hand your letter over to the doctor. Disciplinary actions taken against a doctor by a state medical board may only entail talking to him, and nothing more. (The process of revoking a doctor's license to practice medicine is rare and usually takes years. State medical boards are composed mostly of doctors. Do not be surprised if your concerns are dismissed by them. In 1994, twelve of the California State Medical Board's nineteen members were doctors.)

•

Concerning medical errors and its prevention, the profession has, with rare exceptions, adopted an ostrich-like attitude.

— Dr. David Blumenthal, *Journal of the American Medical Association,*
December 21, 1994

•

Reasons another doctor or a hospital might not report or take actions against a bad doctor:

- Fear of being sued.
- Financial interest — the bad doctor may be referring a large number of patients to the knowing doctor, or may be bringing the hospital a significant amount of business.
- The doctors may get their insurance through the same insurance carrier.
- The doctors may be members of the same medical group, HMO, or have other professional/financial links.
- Fear of attracting negative attention to the profession.
   This can result in media reports, or stronger regulation by insurance companies or the government.
- Fear of attracting negative attention to the hospital or medical center.

Hospitals spend large amounts of money to build community trust. Like any business, hospitals do not want bad publicity. If a doctor has committed gross malpractice, the hospital may take steps to eliminate him from the hospital staff while keeping the negligent act from hitting the news media. These steps may include an agreement between the hospital and the doctor whereby if the doctor moves out of state, the hospital will not report him to the state medical board and will not take any action to restrict his practicing elsewhere. This is known as "sundowning." The negotiation may also include an out-of-court settlement with a patient who has been violated. The settlement may restrict the patient from talking about the negligent act. These actions prevent the hospital from becoming a media spectacle and allow the doctor to continue working in his profession with a clean record — no matter how incompetent he may be.

- Fear of retaliation from a state medical board that may dislike tattle-tale doctors or doctors who work as expert witnesses for a patient who is suing a doctor.

When a hospital just lets a physician with a competence or professional conduct problem leave his or her employment with the facility and fails to send (a hospital disciplinary report) to the medical board, the physician can simply ask for staff privileges elsewhere. Then we have no means of accountability or tracking a problem physician.

— Dixon Arnett of the California Medical Board, *Professional Licensing Report*, May 1995

Be prepared to supply the lawyer with your medical history and any information you have to solidify your case. You and your lawyer have to prepare for appearing in the courtroom when you exercise your right to present evidence. During this time of preparation, remember that everyone deserves a defense and a fair trial, and to protect the innocent from being wrongfully denounced, you must prove that the doctor is at fault.

In a trial in Simi Valley, California, a nurse's aide, who was accused of molesting two female patients, acted as his own lawyer in court. The two women, one a developmentally disabled 32-year-old and the other a frail but otherwise mentally capable 72-year-old, were cross-examined by the defendant in the courtroom. Because the defendant was working as his own lawyer, although he had been accused of threatening one woman at the time of the crime to track her down and assault her again, he was given access to the women's phone numbers and addresses.

If a doctor is seriously negligent in the treatment of one patient, chances are that he has a record of indiscretions and there may be other patients he has mistreated. In California when stories of one bad doctor made their way into the local news, several dozen of his former patients came forward and filed complaints against the doctor. If you know of other people who have had bad experiences with the same doctor, you may want to have a meeting with them and your lawyer.

An important question a patient involved in a malpractice case should ask himself is:
Did any of my actions play a part in the malpractice?

A jury may rule that you were partly responsible because you misinformed the doctor about medications you were taking, did not follow the instructions of the doctor, or that your own actions were paramount for part or all of the undesirable outcome of your medical care.

If the doctor finds you are taking any type of action that questions his professionalism, he may foresee a possible lawsuit and prepare himself accordingly. He may contact a lawyer with whom he is already associated through his past negligence, one who is associated with the group practice of which he is a member, or one who works with the hospital or other facility with which he is associated. He may also contact the American Association of Hospital Attorneys, which is associated with the American Hospital Association. Or he may choose to contact another association for an attorney referral, such as the National Health Lawyers Association, or the American Association of Medico-Legal Consultants.

Be aware that any letters you send to state medical boards or other governing bodies might be shown to the doctor by the people who receive the letter(s). That can be enough to start a campaign to discredit you as the doctor proceeds to defend his credibility and career. Remember this: If for no other reason, it is important that you do not write any letters, hold any conversations, make any phone calls, send any faxes, or otherwise take any actions that can alter your case, without first consulting your lawyer.

If you decide to take the doctor to court, be forewarned that a lawsuit can get very involved. The doctor you are suing does not pay legal counsel to make you look like an angel. The other party can dig into your past to find things about your character that may be unflatteringly presented in court to prove your claim is frivolous, your findings are inaccurate, your reasoning is questionable, and possibly that you are mentally incompetent. It is like putting your life under a microscope. Your judgment, morals, memory, honesty, stability, personal history, and reputation can be presented in the most unflattering manner, dissected, and questioned — all with the goal of portraying your claim as weak, faulty, or unfounded.

Attorneys are trained to be speculative. The defense will use any means possible to gather information needed to persuade the jury to rule against you. Private investigators can be hired to spy on and photograph you, and seek out and question people who know you (or think they know you) to find information that may be damaging to your case. Any information that makes its way into court records is then public record, and other people, including the media, can gain access to it.

Lawsuits against doctors can be very expensive. Before the case goes to court it has to be prepared for the court. This preparation includes filing fees, using the services of other professionals, such as court reporters, obtaining and copying records (good luck getting the doctor to turn over all his records on you), travel, postage, word processing, and library and computer research. You will also be required to respond to written questions (interrogatories) from the doctor and his lawyers. Then you will have to go through a deposition where you and your lawyer sit in a meeting room with the doctor's lawyers, a court reporter, and possibly the doctor, and answer many questions from the doctor's lawyer under oath. The expenses for all this are usually your responsibility and can add up to thousands of dollars. It will be expensive for you and it will be expensive for the doctor's malpractice insurance company as it takes actions to defend the doctor. For this reason it would be better for the insurance company if you had died undergoing the surgery, because it is likely that it would have been cheaper for the company.

Although there is something seriously wrong with a justice system that can be influenced by money, anyone involved with a lawsuit will quickly learn how much influence money can buy in the court system. Chances are that the doctor has more money than you, and one of the privileges of having money is the ability to pay for expensive legal counsel, private investigators, and jury consultants. The doctor or his malpractice insurance carrier can probably get a better lawyer than you can — and one who knows how to play all the manipulative legal games. Malpractice insurance is expensive, insurance companies are big money, and big money plays tough.

> . . . there has always been a concern about the relatively low rate of official actions against physicians by state boards and a concern that physicians' colleagues were not coming forward, or the state boards were not being as aggressive as they ought to be in dealing with negligent providers [doctors]. Perhaps, even that they weren't outreaching to get the information necessary to find out there was a problem [with a doctor].

One interesting development recently is that, as a result of malpractice crises of the mid-1970s, physician-owned insurance companies were developed to provide malpractice insurance.

My understanding is they now provide more than half of the insurance. These companies, owned by doctors, have underwriting committees comprised of doctors and have begun to be somewhat more aggressive in denying coverage, or in putting restrictions on the practice of people they insure, or in putting surcharges on the physicians they insure. I saw an estimate about that in 1985, of the physicians who sought insurance under these physician insurance companies, 3% in that year were under some sort of a restriction. This implies that when you get a group of doctors who have a financial incentive as they own the company, to take a hard look at their peers, they look a little harder than maybe the state boards do.

— Lawrence H. Thompson, assistant comptroller, General Human Resources Division, US General Accounting Office, during Congressional subcommittee hearing on issues relating to medical malpractice, May 20, 1993

•

In most states, drivers have to prove they have liability coverage. But in medicine, doctors can practice cosmetic surgery without insurance coverage at all, and many do.

— Congressman Ron Wyden, during Congressional subcommittee hearings on plastic surgery industry, 1989

•

Do not expect to win your case on the basis that it resembles a malpractice case where another victim of medical negligence won his case. Each case is judged on its own merits.

If the doctor does not have malpractice insurance (is "going bare"), you may have a difficult time getting a lawyer and you may end up negotiating a settlement with an uninsured doctor. Even if the doctor has malpractice insurance, if he is performing an operation that is outside his expertise and not covered under his insurance contract, the insurance company may then disclaim responsibility for him and not represent him in the lawsuit. In this scenario he is essentially uninsured, liable for his own actions, and will have to pay for his own legal counsel.

If you do get a lawyer to fight your malpractice case, your lawyer (if he is not one of the few lawyers who also has a degree in some area of medicine) will have to consult with a doctor who will explain what it was that was done to you, and what was done wrong. You will also need this consulting doctor or another doctor to testify for you, and this could cost money (expert witness fees).

•

In its efforts to educate doctors in the legal aspects of medicine, the American Medical Association sells a book titled *Medical Malpractice: A Physician's Guide,* and a videotape titled *How to Be an Effective Medical Witness.* The cover of the tape says the tape will teach a doctor to qualify as an expert witness, prepare for testifying, use the available evidence on which to base his opinion, answer questions about his fee, properly state his opinion using "magic" legal words, prepare for and testify at his deposition, deal with trick questions and trial tactics of attorneys, effectively describe complex medical issues, humanize his testimony, deal with conflicting medical reports and opinions, and deal with an abusive attorney.

A doctor does not spend years in medical school to have some random patient ruin his career and financial stability with a lawsuit. The doctor, his lawyer, or his insurance company will probably have no difficulty in finding (paying for) another doctor who will testify (as an expert witness) that the surgery was within acceptable standards, and testify to whatever else the negligent doctor wants the jury to hear. He may find such a doctor to testify in his favor through the American Association of Testifying Physicians. Legal magazines are also filled with ads placed by experts in every conceivable specialty willing to hire out for court cases. There are "jukebox doctors" who make good money by saying whatever they are coached to say when someone deposits the right amount of money in their pockets. It is your word against theirs, and they may be fraudulent, but they have the medical degree, and you do not.

On your side of the fence, you may have difficulty finding another doctor to act as an expert witness. You may learn why some people use the phrase "fraternity of physicians." Many doctors are unwilling to testify against another doctor, because they then may be accused of libel or slander, or because of some financial interest. If you do find a doctor who recognizes the damage that another doctor has done to you, this doctor might back down from testifying against the negligent doctor based on the fact that both doctors get their malpractice insurance from the same insurance company. The insurance company, through its representatives, may suggest that the doctor's insurance can be canceled if he agrees to be your expert witness, or the company may hint about higher insurance premiums. Finding a doctor to work as your expert witness may also be difficult because you may be thought of as just another crybaby who did not get what you wanted and who does not understand the risks of medicine. A doctor who sticks up for you may feel he is defaming his profession. On the other hand, you may be seen as the unknowing little guy fighting against the sneaky medical establishment, and this can play on the jury's sympathies.

Binding arbitration agreements:
Your insurance plan may have limitations on the legal avenues you can take in suing a doctor, including an arbitration clause that limits your

right to a jury trial. If you are a member of an HMO, your membership contract probably stipulates that any disputes be resolved through third-party arbitration and not in court. The paperwork you signed when you initially went to the doctor might also contain a binding arbitration agreement. If a patient dies because of negligence, the family may also be bound to the arbitration agreement. A pregnant woman who signs this form may bind the rights of her unborn child. A person who changes his mind after signing an arbitration contract has 30 days to cancel the agreement in writing.

If you signed a pre-surgery arbitration agreement at the doctor's office, or when you entered the hospital, this may prevent your case from being presented before a trial jury. Instead, you may be limited to an arbitration panel of three people who are usually lawyers or retired judges who will listen to your case and decide whether any negligence took place and what, if any, award should be given. Each side picks an arbitrator and together they select a third. It is often the third, "neutral," arbitrator who casts the deciding vote. Large awards are rare in the arbitration process and, because arbitration is done in private, there is no public record of the proceedings. Therefore, the malpractice award may not show up on the doctor's state records.

To win your case, you have to prove to a supposedly fair and impartial jury that the medical care caused harm or some type of damage to you or otherwise deviated from the accepted standards of practice that exist within the medical community. You may be dealing with a jury who thought you got what you paid for. The jury members do not need to be intelligent or educated; they need only be eighteen years old. Even though people in court are supposed to tell the truth, and nothing but the truth, anyone who has been involved with any kind of serious lawsuit knows that lies exist in courtrooms like wet exists in water. Often a person can get the feeling that the crooks in the courtroom are not the ones on trial, and these feelings may be legitimate.

The court case can become a display of the expert knowledge held by all the characters present in the form of legal and medical professionals involved with the case, and the interests of the victim can become lost in this cast of characters who may be using the case to help define their careers. Do not be surprised if the doctor blames you for the malpractice because of your demands on the doctor. There have been many malpractice cases where the doctor claims he performed the surgery only after the patient demanded it against the doctor's better judgment. (Did these doctors also not want the money they made by performing the surgeries?)

The American Hospital Association, along with other organizations, believes that the medical liability compensation system currently fails to meet its own goals of adequately and fairly compensating injured patients, and at the same time effectively deterring bad healthcare practices.

Many of our healthcare providers are afraid to practice their trade because of anticipated liability claims and, as a result, resort to defensive medicine, over prescription of tests by providers, etcetera.

Many providers are unwilling to practice in their specialty area, such as obstetrics and emergency room care, because of increased malpractice premiums and the threats of unfounded lawsuits. As a result, many communities are left underserved with little or no access to appropriate healthcare services.

People injured by poor quality of care are entitled to fair and prompt compensation for their injuries, but our present system costs far too much and works much too slowly, and fails to provide fair compensation to most patients injured by medical malpractice, while providing exorbitant lottery-type awards to others.

> — From statement of John D. Leech, member, board of trustees, American Hospital Association, at a Congressional subcommittee hearing on issues relating to medical malpractice, May 20, 1993

Duke University Law School's Medical Malpractice Project recently completed a study that attempted to review every malpractice suit filed in North Carolina between July 1, 1984, and June 30, 1987 — 895 cases. The project also collected information on more than 300 other cases filed in a sample of North Carolina counties between July, 1987, and December, 1990. The study found that medical malpractice juries are not consistently pro-plaintiff, nor do they award excessive damages.

According to the study, about 40% of the cases reviewed were terminated without any payment to the plaintiff, and about 50% were settled. Only about 10% of the cases, or 117 cases, were decided by jury.

Out of the 117 cases that went to trial, there were only four large jury awards, ranging in size from $750,000 to $3.5 million (subsequently reduced to $2.9 million). These judgments were awarded in cases involving severe brain damage, permanent paralysis and brain damage, death from suffocation by an intubation tube improperly placed, and a child who suffered brain damage at birth. The study found that the average damage award in cases that plaintiffs won was $367,737. But this number was much inflated by the four large awards discussed above. The median or mid-point award, on the other hand, was only $36,500.

The Duke study also found that juries are not biased in favor of injured patients. In the cases that went before a jury, the plaintiff prevailed in just one out of five. Furthermore, the juries found in favor of defendants in 18 out of 19 cases that insurers expected to win, and 13 out of 17 cases that insurers rated as questionable. And juries even ruled against plaintiffs in a majority of cases — six out of eleven — that insurers thought they would lose.

> — From prepared statement of Pamela Gilbert, director of Public Citizen's Congress Watch, citing Duke University Law School project,

and with information from *The Unfair Criticism of Medical Malpractice Juries*, Neil Vidmar, *Judicature*, October/November 1992, and *Still Warring Over Medical Malpractice*, Kenneth Jost, *ABA Journal*, May 1993.
Presented at a Congressional subcommittee hearing on issues relating to malpractice, May 20, 1993

A US General Accounting Office study of claims closed in 1984 found that the average time to resolve the claim was 25 months. Some took as long as 11 years. In over half the cases, plaintiff legal fees exceeded 30% of the payments to the injured party. In addition, the insurers also paid $800 million to investigate and defend the claims closed in 1984, as compared to $2.6 billion that they actually paid in the claims. If you add it all together, it turns out that the lawyers and the overhead account for about almost half of the payments made.

— Lawrence H. Thompson, assistant comptroller general, Human Resources Division, US General Accounting Office. Testifying before Congressional subcommittee hearing on issues related to malpractice, May 20, 1993

Although malpractice victims usually need money immediately, lawsuits can take years to make it through the court system. The medical boards might not take any action against a doctor until there is a ruling against the doctor. During the years it takes to get a ruling, the doctor can harm many other people. The person who was victimized can be awarded a settlement, but this does not mean collection of the judgment is certain. If the doctor has no insurance company representing him and the patient is suing a doctor directly, and if the doctor's assets are hidden in financial closets, such as living trusts, the patient may not be able to collect a dime.

The patient who sues a doctor can end up owing a lot of money because of lost income and, among other things, legal fees, medical bills and other debts. These costs may amount to more than what was won in the lawsuit. If your medical bills were paid by an insurance company and you win a malpractice lawsuit, the company can recover the amount it paid to cover your medical bills — but not more than what the court awarded you. During your trip through the legalities of malpractice hell, you can burn out, which could be what the defense wants so that you drop the lawsuit or take an out-of-court settlement. This could be a good thing, or you may simply be getting taken advantage of again.

The architects of the Clinton health plan considered a proposal that would bar patients from directly suing doctors and instead would allow patients to sue the health insurance providers. The limit, known as "enterprise liability," was designed to mirror other industries where consumers sue the company and not the person or persons who work for the company.

Even if a malpractice victim wins his lawsuit, there is no way to reverse what was done to his body or mind and return it to its original state. It is similar to rape. The victim is the victim because of the negligence, is treated like he is victimizing someone else during the lawsuit, and remains a victim. If there is an out-of-court settlement it can end up protecting the doctor, because it will include a secrecy clause that keeps the patient from talking about the settlement. In all, the road to justice (if any is actually built) can make you compromise your goals, can be so time-consuming that it interferes with every area of your life and, in the end, can be unsatisfying.

5 • ALTERNATIVE AND HOLISTIC HEALTHCARE

A Natural Approach to Caring for the Body

People often neglect their bodies and, after years of not taking care of themselves, expect doctors to break out some magical pills or find some surgical procedure to make right what was a preventable ailment. The result of unhealthy living is that more than 300,000 heart bypass surgeries are performed every year and this brings millions of dollars into hospitals.

Pharmaceutical companies are making billions of dollars from the approximately 25 million Americans who are taking blood pressure medication. Millions of other people are taking prescription drugs for health problems that could have been avoided if the very same people had taken better care of themselves. If those taking prescription drugs changed their eating habits and started to exercise regularly, many of the drugs could be eliminated.

> According to a panel of experts assembled by the National Institutes of Health, physical activity and regular exercise reduces the risk of heart attack, stroke, obesity, diabetes, osteoporosis, and some cancers. The panel recommended that healthcare providers encourage their patients to exercise.
>
> — National Institutes of Health Federal Advisory Panel Report, December 20, 1995

People who do not take responsibility for their health often unfairly place doctors in the position of rescuers. Many of these people look to doctors as some kind of magical healers and depend on them to find the only sure cure for sicknesses. Some people enjoy the attention they receive from doctors so much that going to a doctor becomes more of an emotional/social boost than a physical need. Although there may be doctors who believe the rescuer position is their proper place, at least in the case of chronic diseases this kind of positioning has become a financial burden on the US medical system because too many people have turned to big-dollar medicine to try to cure lifestyle-induced illnesses.

When it is taken into consideration that allopathic healthcare workers focus much of their attention on treating sick people, what they do may be described more accurately as "sick care."

Much of the US system spends its time fighting already established diseases and intervening near the end of the disease process when it is most expensive to heal. Medical schools focus too much of their attention on fighting already established diseases and using risky chemical drugs and technologic-intensive medical equipment in the process. Patients with unrealistic expectations of modern medicine fill doctors' waiting rooms. Instead of preventing disease formation early in life, the US healthcare system wastes billions of dollars and contributes to a lower quality of life for millions of people every year.

Patients often blame doctors for not curing their illnesses. Doctors can play some part in bringing people to good health, but people would be better off if they took more precautions to avoid chronic health problems. Rather than expect doctors to cure what is the result of unhealthy living, there are things a person can do throughout his life that can eliminate the causes of the symptoms, rather than wait for symptoms to arise and then, often at great cost, try to treat the diet- and lifestyle-induced illnesses.

While conventional medicine may be vital when a person is experiencing a medical emergency, the surgery, drugs, and technology used in conventional medicine are not the only options when an emergency is not at hand.

Much of what Americans refer to as non-conventional medicine are forms of medicine that have been in use for hundreds and even thousands of years and are now becoming accepted as an alternative to, or in addition to, the traditional Western medicine that is most popular in the United States.

These "natural healing arts" include such methods as those that are commonly practiced in China, Japan, and India (ayurveda), other types of medicine, such as homeopathic and chiropractic care, and mind-body approaches, such as meditation and yoga. Together these are often referred to as holistic forms of medicine. Although some of these holistic specialists are occasionally allowed into a hospital to treat certain cases and often have patients who are allopathic doctors, in large measure they practice outside the hospital setting.

Allopathic therapies are usually based on science, and this has its limits. Science-based therapies tend to treat the body like a machine, working on one part and expecting that part to respond in a certain manner. Although science-based therapies may have a place in treating certain physical conditions, they are not where all the answers to health maintenance are found. What science-based therapies do is give the patients scientific care, and this is not how the human being functions.

Alternative therapies recognize that the human body has a healing pattern and that the mind is a part of this system. Alternative therapies are referred to as holistic because, rather than treat the body in segmented scientific experiments, they often focus on the whole inter-reactive system that makes up the human — physical, emotional, and spiritual. Many people do not like to refer to them as "alternative" therapies because this title seems to indicate that a patient would have to choose between traditional Western therapies and alternative holistic therapies, although an either/or choice is not the case.

Holistic therapies assist the body in healing by supplying it with the resources it needs to become healthy and by improving the quality of the patient's health.

The therapies used by holistic practitioners are normally non-toxic and noninvasive and provide assistance to the life forces of the body and mind by way of nutrition, manipulative therapies, exercise, and botanical remedies. This assisting in the natural defenses and healing capabilities of the body is why holistic therapies are also known as "complementary therapies." Many of these therapies work to eliminate toxic substances from the body, negative thinking and unhealthful emotions from the mind, addictive and damaging substances from the diet, and immune-system suppressing and disease-inducing factors from life.

Your health: It is what you eat, and what you think, and how you move . . .

The five leading causes of death and disability in America, high blood pressure, cancer, heart disease, diabetes, and obesity, are often related to unhealthful eating, stress, and lack of exercise.

A person's health is affected by his attitude, self-image, social activities, genetic predisposition, environment, fitness level, diet, support network, family structure, and affection.

As many people repeat the scenario of getting sick and going to an allopathic doctor who too often relies on big-profit toxic chemical drugs and surgical scalpels, and who offers little if any patient education, holistic therapies treat ailments using less invasive programs and often show the person how to avoid becoming sick by recognizing and changing the things in his life that may be causing illness. Holistic therapies call for patient participation and patient responsibility in maintaining health through dietary, exercise, and lifestyle modification. Because the therapies involve educating the patients, the holistic practitioners often spend much more time with their patients than conventional doctors do.

Many people are now recognizing that the risks of chemical pills and the drama and danger of surgery are not always the answer to health problems. Rather than rely on medical science, technocratic computerized medical machinery, chemical medications, and surgery to try to repair what has gone wrong with the body, many of the holistic forms of medicine are a back-to-basics approach to healing.

Much of the holistic focus is on staying well in the long run through maintaining a healthy lifestyle. This is a switch from the rather common pattern of events where a person leading an unhealthy lifestyle is forced to change because health problems brought on by long-term unhealthy living have threatened the person's life.

In efforts to reap benefits where benefits can be found, many people are choosing both allopathic and holistic approaches to prevent and treat ailments. Some allopathic doctors now prescribe holistic therapies in combination with traditional allopathic therapies to treat, or assist in the treatment of, chronic conditions. Some holistic therapies are being accepted by the mainstream gatekeepers because many holistic therapies make patients "feel better," and when patients feel better they heal better. As holistics have become a multibillion-dollar industry, and continue to gain prominence, many insurance companies are starting to provide reimbursement for holistic therapies.

A nationwide telephone survey directed by doctors at Boston's Beth Israel Hospital, Harvard University's teaching hospital, suggested that as many as one-third of all Americans seek out alternative treatments to manage their health (*New England Journal of Medicine, Unconventional Medicine in the United States,* January 28, 1993). Dr. David Eisenberg, the primary investigator of the study, is setting up the Center for Alternative Medicine Research at Beth Israel Hospital. According to a media release from the center, its principal objectives are to "design and implement clinical and basic science investigations of commonly used alternative therapies, and to evaluate the financial implications of their use."

In 1992, the National Institutes of Health in Bethesda, Maryland, allotted a rather slim but recognizable $2 million to the new Federal Office of Alternative Medicine (FOAM). The office then began to fund studies of unconventional forms of medicine. In June 1993, the Office of Alternative Medicine was established as a permanent office of the National Institutes of Health. In 1994, the budget of the office was increased to $3.5 million, and thirty researchers and institutions were given grants to study treatments, such as acupuncture, hypnosis, massage therapy for surgical patients, dance movement for cystic fibrosis, macrobiotic eating habits for cancer, biofeedback for diabetes, and yoga for heroin addiction. In 1995, the budget for the FOAM was increased to $5.4 million. As of 1996, the office has funded about ninety alternative medicine studies and is helping to support ten specialty research centers to study the way various ailments respond to alternative therapies.

In the private sector, one of the nation's oldest medical schools, Columbia University, announced in 1994 that it was starting a school of alternative and complementary medicine to teach doctors about diverse strategies for maintaining health. Additionally, prestigious medical schools at UCLA and Tufts, Georgetown, and Harvard universities have introduced alternative medicine training to their curricula, and other schools are in line to do the same.

Divided They Stand

Many allopathic doctors still continue to assert that the holistic therapies are not based on scientific fact when their own bags of tricks also contain many dubious practices. Some of those in the allopathic field have an arrogant disregard for any approach to healthcare that differs from their own. Some allopathic doctors accuse holistic practitioners of quackery, as if the allopaths know all and are the only ones who have the right to treat health problems. The truth is, there are many ways of treating ailments, and when something does go wrong with the body, all the responsible treatment options should be considered.

Whereas the forms of treatments on both sides of the fence have been refined over the years, many holistic or "non-conventional" types of treatment are still considered by many people to be bogus and not worthy of investigation. Although some of these assertions may be true, and there are some bogus treatments practiced by overly enthusiastic individuals who hold limited knowledge, this should not result in a blanket attitude toward every area of holistic medicine. Many conventional treatments are also bogus, while others offer little benefit, are of questionable effectiveness, create stress, and a rather large number of them are potentially dangerous. One thing holistic and allopathic medicine have in common is that they are populated by people trying to market various kinds of treatments and gizmos that carry questionable promises of improving health.

Many of the negative views toward holistic medicine have been influenced by conventional allopathic doctors, their groups, pharmaceutical companies, and others who may be driven by financial interests or who refuse to consider the benefits of treatments that were not taught in the schools these individuals attended. Also, because some of the holistic forms of medicine come from non-white nations of the world, prejudice has played a part in suppressing the acceptance of these types of therapies in the US. In turn, this has limited the knowledge of allopathic doctors as to what the various alternative treatments are and what they are capable of doing.

One reason one form of curative theology is more popular than the other is that American hospitals and the major university medical schools have been occupied and dominated by allopathic doctors and have been assisted with money from the pharmaceutical drug manufacturers.

Allopathic doctors are the "traditional" doctors who specialize in such things as cardiology, radiology, urology, emergency medicine, proctology, pulmonology, plastic surgery, anesthesiology, dermatology, rheumatology, endocrinology, gynecology, ophthalmology, hematology, nephrology, otorhinolaryngology, pathology, and neurology.

Although not all allopathic schools are alike, they do require their graduates to have a science background, and they all teach the same type of therapeutic approaches based on drugs and surgery with few lifestyle-based therapies thrown in. This group of individuals largely think of themselves as the "real" doctors — and many do not like the term "allopathic medicine" because it categorizes them as just one of many types of doctors. Allopathic doctors often consider their training to be comprehensive, but when they have received their training from medical schools influenced by drug company money, and have not studied the variety of other forms of health care, how comprehensive can their training be?

What is taught in the medical schools influences what therapies patients are exposed to within hospitals. Locked out of mainstream hospitals are those individuals who practice holistic or functional forms of medicine, such as homeopathy, chiropractic care, acupuncture, ayurveda, herbology, vegetarian nutrition, and hypnotherapy. Another is naturopathy, which uses various alternative modalities along with some Western practices. These forms of medicine are largely not taught in US medical schools.

Holistic practitioners do not hold any position with the major medical journals — which are often filled with studies that have been financed by the drug companies or some big business associated with the allopathic medical community. The medical journals carry advertising placed by the drug companies to influence the doctors to prescribe the drugs to their patients. The journals rely on the advertising dollars from the drug companies to stay in business. The seed money that funds the studies appearing in the medical journals may also come from the government offices that are strongly influenced by the allopathic medical trilogy, consisting of the big-money and politically powerful allopathic doctor associations, chemical drug companies, and medical device manufacturers.

When one considers that many holistic therapies challenge the safety and effectiveness of allopathic treatments and high-priced drugs, it may be easy to see why holistic groups are kept out of this trillion-dollar loop. It has all been a tightly woven cloth, but the edges are beginning to fray. What has been occurring lately is that more and more consumers are becoming enlightened about what alternative medicine has to offer and are choosing alternative therapies. By doing this, the consumer money is going toward the holistic side of the fence, much to the dismay of the allopathic establishment. The economic and therapeutic successes of holistic treatments have motivated the allopathic organizations and the drug industry to engage in some very questionable activities.

The holistic practitioners have had to practice their medicine in an environment where the allopathic industry is constantly attacking them with propaganda and using money from the allopathic establishment to influence government activities. Allopathic groups, such as the American Cancer Society, the American Medical Association, the National Health Council, and the Arthritis Foundation have ganged up with the Food and Drug Administration, the Federal Trade Commission, the US Postal Service, and the Office of Consumer Affairs to remove alternative therapies and products from the market. These are products and therapies that the allopathic and drug groups have determined to be dangerous to the public. These groups have engaged in financing, planning, and helping federal agents to carry out such activities as raiding the offices of physicians who prescribe alternative treatments, healthfood stores that sell alternative health products, and the companies that manufacture and distribute the products.

The FDA is able to engage in these kinds of medical policing activities because the agency, which is a branch of the Department of Health and Human Services, has authority to regulate foods, drugs, cosmetics, and medical devices that are imported or sold between states. FDA authority covers the shipment of both raw materials and finished products across state lines. The FDA is also responsible for regulating the content of products and certain processes by which products are manufactured. The agency also may require pre-marketing testing of these products. When a product does not go through the FDA approval process, the FDA can take action to confiscate products and take action against any company engaged in the manufacture, distribution, or sale of the product.

The activities the FDA has taken against alternative practitioners and companies that manufacture, distribute, and sell alternative health products have been carried out even though there is often a lack of evidence that any harm had been done. While the allopaths and the federal agents may claim that they are doing these things in the interest of consumer safety, a more accurate conclusion may be that they are out to suppress the alternative therapies that take money away from allopathic practitioners and drug companies by removing the competition from the marketplace, or limiting alternative therapies, and damaging the credibility of alternative practitioners.

By harming the businesses of alternative practitioners by removing their office records, confiscating products such as herbal remedies and dietary supplements from the shelves of alternative health stores and warehouses of distributors and manufacturers of the products, and labeling alternative therapies as "quack" medicine, these federal agents, who are influenced by and working for the financial interests of the allopathic trilogy, are limiting treatment options and altering and endangering the lives of people who can benefit from alternative therapies.

The actions of the FDA have led to much controversy because the FDA and the other government agencies have been participating in campaigns financed by the pharmaceutical industry and allopathic organizations to attack their economic competitors. For instance, the money flow from consumers is more likely to go toward the allopathic establishment when the FDA limits the use of a natural therapy, such as evening primrose oil for the treatment of eczema, and provides the news media with propaganda warning the public against the use of natural products that are actually harmless and effective. The public, after having the allopathic propaganda successfully construct a negative view of alternative therapies in their minds, is then more likely to rely on therapies prescribed by the allopaths and manufactured by the pharmaceutical industry. This is true even though the allopathic treatments may be more expensive and not as effective as natural remedies. Additionally, the people who work for the FDA stand to make a profit because many of the top officials with the FDA have been employees of pharmaceutical companies and many of them take jobs with pharmaceutical companies when they leave the FDA.

Regardless of all the actions of allopathic groups and the drug companies to do economic damage to the alternative practitioners, product manufacturers, distributors, and stores, the alternative therapies continue to become more and more popular. This is because people are finding that not only do many of the alternative therapies work, but they are also often less expensive, less invasive, more reliable, and carry less risk than many of the allopathic therapies. The cost issue has also played a major part in alternative therapies being accepted by some health insurance plans.

In addition to having to contend with the allopathic and pharmaceutical propaganda and the biased policing of the FDA, the main gripe the alternative practitioners have against the toxic and invasive drug, surgery, and technology emphasis of allopathic therapies is that the allopaths simply treat or suppress symptoms and do not give attention to the underlying cause of ailments that lead to the symptoms. There is also much evidence that many allopathic treatments are of questionable effectiveness and often unnecessarily harm patients.

While it is true that alternative medicine has a history of bizarre and sometimes dangerous remedies, the mainstream doctors are not without their own questionable "cures." They once advocated vomiting as a cure-all; bleeding to purge diseases out of ailing patients; using toxic substances to treat common ailments; and they preached against exercise and sports that caused physical exertion. More recently the allopaths treated acne with x-rays, performed hysterectomies to "cure" anemia, and gave a drug called Thalidomide to pregnant women who then had severely deformed babies.

Currently there are many surgeries and other allopathic medical interventions that are done for reasons other than for benefiting the patients. Examples of this are the doctors who perform surgery so they can meet their board certification quotas or otherwise perform surgery for the doctors' convenience, such as for financial gain; doctors who take the risks of using a drug (the synthetic hormone pitocin) to induce pregnant women into labor so the doctors will not have to be inconvenienced by having to stay up all night waiting for the baby to be born; doctors who perform unnecessary episiotomies (an incision to widen the birth canal) to benefit from the fee-for-service arrangement; and doctors who give in to patient demands for drugs or surgery when it is clearly not in the best interest of the patient. There are also the bottom-feeders of the allopathic groups, those who sell themselves as magical cosmetic surgeons and make fortunes by preying on passive people who have low self-esteem.

While there will be those who will continue to ignore the successes of holistic therapies, the holistic approaches will continue to become more and more popular. As a result, we are seeing some allopathic doctors accepting, studying, and practicing holistic therapies so their practice conforms to what is called "naturopathy," or "naturopathic medicine."

Herbology

In some parts of the world the knowledge of herbal medicine was considered to be sacred. Using roots, stems, leaves, seeds, juices, and resins — or extractions from them — as medicine had a relationship with nature and spiritual matters, and was administered by "medicine" men and women who, with their ability to prescribe various plant-based treatments, were believed to have magical powers. This is one reason herbal medicine has been disregarded by much of modern medicine, because some people believe spirituality has no place in the healing of the body and treating of the sick.

Besides being uncomfortable with the history of herbal medicine, the big money people have not been behind it because it is low-tech, inexpensive, easily available, and cannot be patented, and therefore it shows no promise of large returns for financial investors who instead keep their money in high-tech, big-payback allopathic medicine facilities, machinery, and chemical drugs.

Although there are times when allopathic drugs are necessary, what many people are beginning to realize is that the new and expensive chemical drugs often carry serious side effects, such as stress, addiction, depression, birth defects, tissue deformities, and other ailments and illnesses. People now know that dismissing all the herbal medicine therapies because some have a relationship with a few things they disagree with or are uncomfortable with has been the equivalent of tossing the baby out with the bath water. Even with allopathic drugs that are made from plants, there may be an important component of the plant that was lost in isolating and synthesizing the most active ingredient.

Herbs and extractions of them have been used for thousands of years in all parts of the world to make botanical medicines that treat everything from skin abrasions to sleep disorders. In fact, herbal medications were the only kind available until man started making synthetic drugs in the last century. Even some of the most common drugs used today are made from plants. These include cocaine from the coca plant; morphine from opium, which comes from poppies; and even aspirin from willow bark. Newer drugs, such as digitalis from the foxglove plant, taxol from the Pacific yew tree, and vincristine from the rosy periwinkle of Madagascar are more examples of drugs derived from plants. Some people estimate that 50% of allopathic drugs prescribed today contain plant ingredients or are synthesized forms of them.

Herbal gardens with both culinary (food) and medicinal (medicine) herbs have been a common sight in Europe for hundreds of years. These herb gardens were duplicated by Europeans who settled on the American continent. Some of these gardens, many incorporating plants that were used for medicinal purposes by Native Americans and that were brought over from other parts of the world, can be seen in preserved and duplicated historic sites in the eastern American states.

For centuries the Chinese have made use of medicines that have been made from herbs to assist and stimulate the body to heal. Today there are many Chinese herbalists practicing in the Chinatown sections of major cities, and they often use formulas that have been employed for thousands of years. These herbalists are helping to revive the use of plant-based medicine. There are also many non-Chinese herbalists, homeopathic doctors, and naturopathic doctors who have incorporated herbal remedies from other areas of the world, such as Germany, where the Federal Health Agency has studied hundreds of herbs since the 1970s, and from the American Indians. These modern herbalists have helped turn the botanical medicine field into a billion-dollar industry.

Among the botanical medicines used more and more by Americans are the saw palmetto berry to reduce enlarged prostates; echinacea to stimulate the immune response and fight infection; feverfew for treating headaches; a tea treatment to relieve the inflammation of eczema; and a mixture of herbs to use in place of prescription sleeping pills.

One of the many reasons the destruction of the rain forests is so despicable is that many species of plants are being destroyed before they can be tested for medicinal content that may be needed for the diseases of today and will be invaluable to future generations. According to the National Cancer Institute, only about 0.5% of the world's known plants have been investigated for their medical value. As Norman Myers explains in his book *The Primary Source*, one-fourth of the medicines available today owe their existence to plants.

One way of extracting the constituents of the plants is with a solvent that is a mixture of alcohol and water, and sometimes glycerin or vinegar. Non-alcoholic extracts are available for those persons who are sensitive to alcohol. These herb extracts are prepared by mixing them in water, tea or juice — although some herbal preparations are taken as drops under the tongue, and others in powder or pill form. Other derivatives of plants are used in teas, lotions, ointments, baths, and as soothing aromas.

For more on herbs, books about them, and companies selling them, see the *Herbs and Plant-Based Medicines/Therapies* section in the *Research Resources* section of this book.

Homeopathy

Homeopathic medicine is a natural medical science that uses ingredients of animal, plant, or mineral origin. The modern popularity of homeopathy is attributed to the German physician Samuel Christian Hahnemann (1755 – 1843). Hahnemann, who graduated from medical school in 1779, worked to standardize the German *Pharmacopoeia* and wrote a standard textbook titled *Apothecary's Lexicon*. After leaving the practice of medicine, he worked as a translator of medical journals. It was during this time that he started experimenting with and developing medicines made out of highly diluted substances that, when given in large doses, produced symptoms identical to the symptoms of the ailments that small doses of the substances cured.

While many allopathic drugs are derived from the same sources as homeopathic drugs, and homeopathic doctors may use laboratory tests and x-rays to help diagnose and monitor problems, the difference is in the way homeopathic therapies are used with the goal of stimulating the natural defenses and healing powers of the body. Treatment may be preceded by taking a complete health history of the patient — including eating habits, emotional background, and questioning the patient's reactions to seasons and other factors. The complete environment of the individual is taken into consideration, and therefore it is truly a holistic form of medicine. The patient's physical, emotional, and mental responses to each applied substance are noted.

Homeopaths believe there is a vital force in all living things and that sickness is a disturbance of this force. The symptoms that a person is experiencing are signs or expressions of how the body is dealing with or fighting against the disease. Homeopathic remedies use a very small dose of a naturally occurring substance to stimulate the natural defenses of the body to rid itself of the disturbance. The basic law behind homeopathy is that if a substance, when given in a large dose, produces symptoms of a particular ailment in a healthy person, that substance will also cure the ailment in an unhealthy person who is given a small dose to enhance the symptoms. This is known as the "Law of Similars." The word homeopathy is from the Greek words "homoios," for similar, and "pathos," for suffering. Enhancing the symptoms is central to the person's becoming well because the symptoms are the response the body is using to fight the disease.

In addition to the development of the medicines based on the Law of Similars, Hahnemann developed a theory about the cause of chronic illnesses. This reasoning is based on what he called the theory of "miasms." This theory addresses the question of why a person suffers a certain ailment based on a weakness, or as what can best be described now as an inherited tendency to experience a certain disease. Treating these miasms involves strengthening a weakness.

Homeopathic medicine was brought to the US in the early 19th century. The American Institute of Homeopathy was founded in 1844, two years before the allopathic medicine group called the American Medical Association was organized with the help of drug manufacturers. Homeopathy is currently popular in Europe and other parts of the world. The British National Health Service covers homeopathic treatments. Homeopathy is once again becoming popular in the US. In 1994, the National Institutes of Health's Office of Alternative Medicine gave two funding grants to researchers studying homeopathy.

A key reason why homeopathic remedies have not received financial backing is that the remedies use inexpensive, readily available substances. This has kept big pharmaceutical companies from becoming interested in conducting research on the remedies, because the companies cannot place a patent on the remedies to make money from them. This shows one reason why a person should not place value on a remedy based on how much money is behind it. It also may explain why the hospitals and medical centers that need to provide investors with impressive profits typically practice the more profitable allopathic approaches to healthcare.

Although there are laws regulating the practice of homeopathy, homeopathic medicines may be purchased without prescriptions at many healthfood stores and an increasing number of homeopathic pharmacies.

Acupuncture

Acupuncture, an ancient Chinese form of treating ailments, has been practiced for thousands of years and is rooted in Taoist philosophy. It is done by inserting thin disposable needles into the skin at one or more of the over 1,000 points that control the flow of qi (pronounced "chee"), an energy in the body. The belief is that any imbalance or interruption in the flow of qi creates illness. The acupuncture needles are used to stimulate the pathways of the flow.

An acupuncturist will treat a patient only after an exam to learn the ailments of the person and determining which points along his energy flow are out of harmony and need to be worked on. An exam will include questioning the patient about his medical history as well as inspecting his tongue, listening to his body, and smelling the body odor. Needles are inserted at the specific acupuncture points and, depending on the strength of the qi, remain in place for anywhere from a few minutes to more than an hour. During the treatments the acupuncturist may also burn an herb called moxa. The burning moxa may be in stick form and waved around the body or in cone form and placed on top of salt or a slice of ginger on the skin.

It is now known that the body responds to acupuncture because stimulating the points alters neurotransmitters in the body. As acupuncture is being adopted into the modern world, some acupuncturists now apply a weak electrical current to the needles. They believe this is more effective than just plain needles. Others apply laser light and different colors of light to the acupuncture points for what they believe is a more potent effect.

Acupuncture-based drug detoxification programs are being assigned to treat substance abusers more and more by prosecutors, judges and public defenders in the United States and in other countries. These programs give drug offenders the option of addiction treatment along with counseling instead of jail. Acupuncture is used before or after counseling to reduce the agitation and physical withdrawal symptoms experienced by drug abusers (*Alternative Medicine Journal*, September/October 1995). Many people have also received acupuncture for chronic pain, weight loss, and to assist in relieving cigarette addiction.

Acupuncture schools provide education in physiology and anatomy. Acupuncture organizations established in the United States include the American Association of Acupuncture and Oriental Medicine, the National Council of Acupuncture Schools and Colleges, the National Commission for the Certification of Acupuncturists, and the National Accreditation Commission for Schools and Colleges of Acupuncture and Oriental Medicine.

Massage

Massage is being used in physical therapy to help treat victims of accidents, sports injuries, and strokes, and to treat people who are experiencing chronic pain. Massage can help correct body alignment and, because it reduces stress, has a beneficial effect on the function of the internal organs.

Massage utilizes the important aspect of touch in the healing process, something that seems to have been lost in many healthcare facilities between the high-priced medical equipment and lab tests.

Manipulative therapies have not been favored by certain individuals because of the issue of touch. When some people hear the word "massage," they think of massage parlors, prostitution, and illegal and impure activities. This is to their loss. The professional and licensed massage therapists of today are legitimate, well educated in their approach to the healing arts, and can play a major role in helping deal with stress and those in recuperation from injury. Massage therapists work in physical therapy centers, chiropractic offices, and health spas.

Massage works to help eliminate stress and alleviates pain because it stimulates the release of endorphins that can provide a feeling of well-being, and increases the level of serotonin, which suppresses pain. Massage stimulates the blood to flow more freely, and this increases the oxygen level in the skin and throughout the body. Massage also assists in the flow of the lymph so that it removes impurities from the tissues. Ingesting a large amount of water before undergoing a rhythmic massage to the back can help the inner organs eliminate impurities. Massage may also prompt a person to release emotions he has not dealt with, and that may also be central to the experience of stress.

Clinical research studies conducted at the Touch Research Institute at the University of Miami School of Medicine have concluded that massage can induce weight gain in premature infants, and that it alleviates depressive symptoms, reduces stress hormones (norepinephrine and cortisol), alleviates pain, improves circulation, and positively alters the immune system in children and adults who have various medical conditions. Massage has a positive effect on patients with such ailments as AIDS, arthritis, asthma, diabetes, and sports injuries. The studies have also found that massage therapy enhances alertness, improves nighttime sleep patterns, and releases a serotonin-like substance (the primary ingredient in most pain killers). The institute has concluded that it may be as beneficial for a person to touch as it is to be touched.

The skill of the massage therapist and the comfort level of the patient play a major role in what may be accomplished in a massage session.

Massage may irritate some skin conditions. A person who has an unhealed burn injury or sunburn should refrain from getting a massage. Persons with certain injuries, diseases, infections, and other conditions may not be good candidates for massage.

Chiropractic

Although bone adjusting has been used for centuries, the modern chiropractic treatments originate from the teachings of a 19th century American named Daniel David Palmer and his son, Bartlett. Chiropractic has been considered to be quackery and a target of severe criticism by the American Medical Association. It is now accepted by many insurance plans because it may sometimes be beneficial for such ailments as back and neck pain, and in treating injuries.

Chiropractic therapy focuses on the alignment of the spinal column and bones of the body in order to keep energy sources of the nerves open and to keep the body in balance. Chiropractic adjustments may be combined with massage, stretching, yoga, and other exercises to help relax and realign structures.

Chiropractors limit themselves to manipulating the structure of the body and do not prescribe, and are often opposed to, drugs and surgery. Chiropractors often refer patients to other types of doctors and vice versa as patient needs may indicate.

Currently 41 states require private health insurance to cover chiropractic care and seven require coverage for acupuncture. According to the Group Health Association of America, the number of HMOs offering chiropractic care jumped from 28.4% in 1992 to 46.6% in 1993.

— From *Advance*, a publication of the Foundation for Chiropractic Education and Research, May/June 1995

Minding Your Health

The body and mind are interrelated, and the body responds to the way the mind thinks. That is why paying attention to the spiritual side of health can assist in curing people of physical ailments. Whereas popular medicine has nearly disregarded the strength of the mind in bringing a person to good physical health, holistic therapies incorporate the powers of the human spirit and recognize the importance one's emotions, thoughts, social interactions, and frame of mind play in the healing process.

The body is sensitive to the way the mind feels. Negative thoughts and feelings have a negative effect on the way a person feels, and a potent, distressing, and toxic effect on a person's immune system and overall health. The reactions within each cell of the body have strong influences on how a person feels physically and each cell has a relationship to what is going on in the mind. Thought processes release messenger chemicals (neurotransmitters or neuropeptides) through the body, and these communicate emotions to the physical body by hooking up to receptors on cell membranes. The study of these physiological processes and how changes in mind can suppress or strengthen the immune system is called "psychoneuroimmunology."

The emotional state plays a part in all forms of recovery. If a person feels better as a whole, he is likely to be healthier. Getting a person to release his anxiety and experience positive emotions can be particularly helpful in somatic illnesses (ailments thought to be caused by emotion) and also in treating any type of sickness. A person's emotional state may be helped by practicing some form of mind relaxation, such as meditation.

Although when some people hear the word "meditate" they may envision wild chanting and contortionist posing, or monks secluded in cavernous sanctuaries, there are less intense ways of finding a calm sense of being and increased awareness. While there are different opinions about what meditation should be, and some people may be into the humming or chanting mantra of Transcendental Meditation (introduced by Maharishi Mahesh Yogi in 1958), others may simply sit quietly in a silent room with their eyes closed and visualize themselves sitting by a clear running stream.

Meditation is something that comes from within. One of the goals of meditation is to find a tranquil harmony with the spiritual side of life that will assist in self-discipline and build self-dignity. Preferably it would bring a person to experience something quiet within him, to enable him to free his mind from the babble, cares, prejudices, confines, hostilities, cynicism, insignificant details, role-playing, and opinions of daily life. The goal should be to experience feelings, such as compassion, peace, love, and courage.

Meditation does not have to be a ritualistic adventure. Providing comfortable surroundings for escape once each day and have a quiet time to ponder deep and positive thoughts are all that is needed. It may be in a bedroom, in the bathtub, on a patio or porch, in a sauna, or outside in a safe place. During this time a person may play music that relaxes or inspires him, surround himself with scents that he enjoys, and dim the lights or light candles to plan for calmness. Some people spend this time reading something that enlightens or listening to tapes that uplift them.

While not everyone can sit alone in a room or find motivation to do so on a daily basis, there are people who find comfort and inspiration in a hobby, such as painting, playing an instrument, or creative writing. Others take this time to perform exercises, such as dancing, yoga, or tai chi, or by swimming when there is access to water. Others may find motivation in other more involved exercises, such as jogging, karate, or weightlifting.

Other ways to create harmony between the physical and spiritual are through hypnosis, biofeedback, massage, discussing feelings in group therapy or with friends and family, and interacting with nature, such as by gardening or caring for animals.

People interested in mind-body medicine may want to read books written by Norman Cousins, or doctors Bernie Siegel, Andrew Weil, Larry Dossey, and Deepak Chopra. A positive attitude may be coached by reading books by inspirational authors and by attending motivational speaking seminars (as in any area of health, a person should be careful about where he spends money in this area).

Finding Holistic Practitioners

There are many ways to treat the ailments of the human body. When seeking any form of therapy, consumers should investigate their options, scan treatments for safety and benefits, beware of unrealistic claims, and look for credentials and ask questions when soliciting practitioners. Remember that the quickest fix may not be the best fix, and the most expensive treatment may be the worst of all.

To locate holistic therapy practitioners, see the book *The Alternative Medicine Yellow Pages*, published by Future Medicine Publishing and listing practitioners in both the US and Canada. Locating the closest homeopathic pharmacy and asking for a referral to a non-allopathic doctor may work. Also, in the *Research Resources* section of this book, see the headings: *Alternative and Holistic Healthcare; Aromatherapy; Chiropractic; Herbal and Plant-based Medicines/Therapies; Massage, Rolfing, Reflexology & Yoga;* and *Oriental Medicine.*

6 • EATING AND HEALTH

Nutrition

Let your medicine be your food, and your food be your medicine.
— Hippocrates, often referred to as the father of modern medicine

The average American eats more protein and calories than his body needs and along with this he consumes a diet that is high in fat grams, concentrated sugars, and salt, is saturated with synthetic flavors and dyes, is very low in fiber, is often overcooked and over processed, and is lacking in nutritional caliber.

Nutrition has an effect on all areas of a person's well-being — from the way he feels mentally, to the way each cell in his body functions. For the body and brain to be in the best of health they need to be supplied with the right nutrients.

•

The combined medical costs of America's eating and smoking habits are greater than the estimated costs of insuring all currently uninsured Americans.
— Physicians Committee for Responsible Medicine, *Good Medicine*, Winter 1996

•

Not only are vitamins, minerals, trace elements, essential fatty acids, amino acids, enzymes, and other nutrients necessary for the brain and nerve systems to function properly, nutrients are needed by a fetus to form normally. During life nutrition plays a part in the ability of the body to develop, grow, and stay healthy, and in healing after becoming sick or suffering an injury.

Nutrition also influences the way the immune system functions. The immune system is of immense importance to the health of an individual because it is essential to the ability to resist disease. For instance, we can see how the weakened immune system of an AIDS patient can no longer fight off simple infections and makes the patient more vulnerable to germs in his environment.

Providing the body with the right nutrients makes the immune system stronger and more likely to fight off infectious diseases and a wide variety of ailments and illnesses, such as arthritis, allergies, and cancer. It is also important to keep the immune system strong because many of the microbes than can make a human sick always exist within the body. If the immune system is weakened, the microbes can take hold and this results in illness.

Vitamin and nutrition therapy has been proven beneficial in treating such diverse conditions as alcoholism by helping to decrease the urge to drink; retinitis pigmentosa by delaying the progression of that degenerative eye disease; Alzheimer's disease by helping to relieve symptoms; AIDS by strengthening the immune system; and a wide assortment of other ailments including hypoglycemia, diabetes, anemia, morning sickness, bulimia and anorexia, allergies, and many skin conditions.

As allopathic doctors and nurses are not required to take classes that provide thorough training in nutrition (have you ever had to eat hospital food?), they pay little if any attention to the diets of their patients, and many doctors and nurses are overweight, unfit, and do not eat healthfully. Though some allopaths might say they did study nutrition in college, they probably were limited to studying the chemical reactions of vitamins. Even the hospital cafeterias where many doctors and nurses eat regularly serve typical disease-inducing junk food.

Because many of the workers in the healthcare field have an insufficient knowledge of nutrition, their patients are left to educate themselves on what is and is not good to put into the body. This holds true even though most major surgeries are the result of diseases caused by people's eating habits. It is absurd but true that most of the medical workers who spend their days treating patients with arteries and hearts that have become diseased from high-cholesterol diets continue to maintain the same type of diets that cause the health problems the patients are experiencing.

The Recommended Daily Allowances (RDA) for nutrients established in 1941 at the request of the War Department leaders and promoted by the US Department of Agriculture (USDA) is also a trustless source for dietary guidance. The RDAs are used to set nutrition policy in the US and are based on outdated research. Many people believe the recommended doses are not high enough for maximum health. The doses are not expected to change because some people may suffer from iron overload or take too much of certain nutrients after obtaining a sufficient amount from their food. People of different age groups tend to metabolize vitamins at different rates, and therefore creating a standard dose of nutrients would not fit the needs of all people.

The USDA acts as a type of trade organization for the meat and dairy industries. The USDA also came up with the concept of the "Basic Four Food Groups." The Basic Four Food Groups were designed to promote the products of the animal-farming industries by telling people they should regularly consume meat, milk, and eggs. In fact flesh foods are not good sources for many nutrients, lack needed fiber, and contain cholesterol and saturated fat. Following a diet based on the food choices suggested by the USDA would induce ailments such as heart disease, strokes, osteoporosis, diabetes, high blood pressure, arthritis, gallstones, kidney stones, obesity, asthma, breast cancer, prostate cancer, colon cancer, possibly diseases of dementia, and other health problems associated with diets that are high in animal products.

> *Cancers of the prostate, kidneys, testicles, uterus, lung, colon, and breast and lymphomas are all more common in populations that consume diets high in fat.*
>
> — John Robbins, in his book *May All Be Fed: Diet for a New World*; William Morrow and Company, 1992

Even when doctors or nurses do understand the importance of nutrition, they do not have the time to sit around and educate every patient about exercise and nutrition and tell each patient to turn the TV off, get off the fanny, and get healthy. Doctors and nurses are too busy spending time with all the other patients who are unhealthy because all the other patients have also spent decades eating junk food and staring at the TV instead of eating healthfully and exercising.

The relationship between eating and health is rock solid. Luckily there are many good books on the subject of nutrition and natural foods. A person can start to educate himself on nutrition by checking out the bookshelves at his local library and healthfood store. Excellent books on eating and health have been written by such authors as Frances Moore Lappe, Michio Kushi, Dean Ornish, John Robbins, Edward Suguel, John Finnegan, Nathan Pritikin, and John and Mary McDougall.

People's absorption and utilization of nutrients vary. Before a person starts taking vitamin or other dietary supplements, it would be wise to understand what the various nutrients do and how they may benefit health. It may be wise to consult with someone, such as a nutritionist, read a variety of dietary reference books that are available in many healthfood stores and libraries, read the various magazines focused on nutrition and health, and otherwise become educated as to what combination of dietary supplements may be helpful and healthful. Taking some supplements too often or at high dosages may cause skin reactions, upset stomach, and other inconveniences. There are also some serious consequences of taking too high a dosage of certain vitamins. For instance, pregnant women who consume too much vitamin A may increase the risk of fetal birth defects (*Science News*, October 14, 1995). When in doubt, consult with a nutritionist.

Nutrients are powerful medicines. Without proper nutrients a person withers. Continued lack of proper nutrients can cause permanent damage to the human body. Consider the scenario of a houseplant that looks unhealthy because its owner has not taken care of it. To make the plant healthy its owner will change the soil, possibly replace the pot, feed the plant clean water, and supply it with the right kind of light. Eventually, if the owner continues to give the plant what it needs to become healthy, the plant will begin to restore itself and grow. Signs of the nutritional deficiencies the plant experienced may always be apparent in damaged structures of the plant, but as long as it continues to receive the proper nutrients it will continue to build healthy cells. The human body is no different from the houseplant in that if the human body is neglected through a junk diet and lack of stimulus, it will become ill — and may die an early death. If a human body that is unwell is provided with the right balance of nutrients and healthful surroundings it will often begin to restore itself both physically and mentally.

•

Essential fatty acids (EFAs) cannot be synthesized in the human body and must be obtained through the diet. Humans require EFAs for the proper development and function of numerous tissues, including the brain, retina, and sperm.

• • •

In 1982 the National Research Council identified fats as the single dietary component most strongly related to carcinogenesis. There is a strong correlation between fat consumption and incidence of gastrointestinal, prostate, and breast cancers. A correlation also exists with cancers of the testis, ovary, and uterus.

— John Boik, in his book *Cancer & Natural Medicine: A Textbook of Basic Research and Clinical Research;* Oregon Medical Publishing, 1996

•

To become healthier, learn which oils are bad and which oils are beneficial to health.

Everyone needs fat in the diet. Probably everyone knows that too much fat is bad for health. What many people do not know is why some fats are bad and some fats are good.

Some types of oil are unhealthful because they contain destructive disease-causing trans-fatty acids. Other oils are good to include in the diet because they contain omega-3 and omega-6 essential fatty acids.

Essential fatty acids are sometimes referred to as vitamin F. They are called essential fatty acids because they are essential to life. They cannot be made by the body and they must be obtained through diet.

Essential fatty acids contain antioxidants, assist proper cellular function, and help build a strong immune system. These fats help transport the fat-soluble vitamins A, D, E, and K. Omega-3 fatty acids form eicosanoids, chemical messengers that influence immune response, blood clotting, inflammation, insulin secretion, and early retina and brain development. Omega-3 may also protect against stroke because the fatty acid reduces the stickiness of blood platelets (*Stroke*, May 1995).

Even the good oils can be bad if a person consumes too much of them. Oils also become toxic when they are heated to high temperatures, such as in frying, because the heat changes the chemical composition of the oils. Refined oils have been robbed of their beneficial phyto chemicals and vitamins. Oils are best when they have been cold pressed and kept in dark bottles.

Oils to avoid and keep out of your diet: Saturated fats include hydrogenated palm and coconut oil, margarine, shortening, and all fats derived from animals, such as lard and butter.

A diet high in saturated fat can cause a person to have low energy. Saturated fats interfere with and slow down the function of body cells, including brain cells. Saturated fats also delay the elimination of waste products from the body.

If you want to experience maximum health, you should eliminate saturated fat from your diet.

Oils that are healthy, in reasonable amounts, to include in your diet (preferably cold- or expeller-pressed, sold in dark bottles, and refrigerated after opening): borage seed oil, brazilnut oil, canola oil, flaxseed oil, hazelnut oil, hemp seed oil, olive oil, pistachio oil, pumpkin seed oil, rice bran oil, sunflower oil, safflower oil, sesame oil, and wheat germ oil.

Also, in pill form, as dietary supplements: black currant seed oil, borage seed oil, grape seed oil, flaxseed oil, and evening primrose oil.

Flaxseed oil is the most common omega-3 essential fatty acid supplement. Flaxseed oil also contains lignan precursors, plant chemicals that have been found to reduce cancer cell formation. Bacteria in the colon convert lignan precursors into animal lignans and in this state the compounds are used by the body. Australian researchers found that flaxseed also has the ability to slow the progression of atherosclerosis and rheumatoid arthritis by causing a decline in the production of two proteins associated with those ailments (*American Journal of Clinical Nutrition*, January 1996). Flaxseeds, flaxseed flour, and flaxseed supplements, as well as other essential fatty acid supplements can be purchased at most healthfood stores.

Meat, Dairy, Eggs, and Human Disease

The meat, dairy, and egg industries work very hard to promote the products they sell. They hire top celebrities to star in funny little slick commercials promoting the consumption of meat, eggs, and dairy products. Everyone is familiar with one or more of the phrases, "Got milk?" "Milk does a body good," "Everybody needs milk," "The other white meat," and, "The incredible edible egg." More recently we have been bombarded with a slew of ads from the National Fluid Milk Processor Promotion Board featuring models, such as Naomi

Campbell and Christie Brinkley, singer Tony Bennett, sports stars, Broadway stars, and cast members of the *Friends* TV show wearing milk mustaches. The animal-farming industry also spends millions of dollars every year to influence government and industrial nutrition programs, and to produce and distribute free school materials to misinform children that eating meat, dairy products, and eggs is a good thing to do for the body.

What the commercials and promotional materials do not tell you is that the more meat, dairy products, and eggs a person consumes, the more likely he is to get cancer and experience other degenerative diseases. The foods that contain heart-choking cholesterol — meats, dairy, and eggs — also contain the worst kind of fat — saturated fat. Saturated fat and cholesterol clog the blood systems in the body and this causes heart disease and strokes. Heart attacks and strokes are leading causes of death in the US and Finland and both countries are the world's top consumers of meats. A person's risk of experiencing heart attacks, strokes, and cancers of the breasts, colon, prostate, and other cancers correspond with the amount of meat, eggs, and milk products that person consumes.

> The conservative estimate is that bad chicken kills at least 1,000 people each year and costs several billion dollars annually in medical costs and lost productivity.
> — *Time Magazine*, October 17, 1994

In 1993 many people were shocked to hear E. coli bacteria-contaminated beef sold in California, Idaho, Nevada, and Washington killed five people, sickened more than 500, sent 144 to the hospital, and caused thirty to experience kidney failure.

The occurrence of food poisoning is not rare. The Centers for Disease Control reports there are 6.5 million cases of illnesses and 9,000 deaths caused by food poisoning every year. Most of these cases of food poisoning are from contaminated meat, eggs, milk, and seafood products. In July 1996, when President Clinton announced sweeping changes in the government's meat and poultry inspection system, it was reported that salmonella bacteria kills more than 4,000 people a year and meat and poultry containing pathogens (microorganisms that cause disease) sickens as many as ten million (Centers for Disease Control statistics).

The US government began its USDA meat inspection program in 1907 after the filthy and hazardous conditions of Chicago stockyards and slaughterhouses were exposed in Upton Sinclair's book titled *The Jungle*.

Though the Department of Agriculture would like the public to think otherwise, meat inspectors do not inspect every nook and cranny of every dead hog, cow, chicken, turkey, lamb, and other farm animal to find diseases and contaminants before the meats from these animals are sold in markets. The dead animals pass by the inspectors at high rates of speed.

The inspectors, who are supposed to rely on touch, smell, and visual inspection of meats are hardly likely to detect some of the most obvious meat contaminants.

In his book, *Beyond Beef,* Jeremy Rifkin explains, "Under the new FSIS (Food Safety Inspection Service) program, federal inspectors no longer have the authority to even stop the line if they spot a problem . . . Unless the company itself agrees that a problem exists or a violation of law occurred, the federal inspector is helpless to take a remedial action." Stopping the inspection line to pull a carcass slows down the packaging plants, and slowing down the work costs money. Regulators have suggested making inspectors use microscopes to detect bacteria on the dead animals, but the industry has opposed such measures..

•

The inspection system is only marginally better today at protecting the public from harmful bacteria than it was a year ago, or even 87 years ago when it was first put into place. FSIS' recent efforts have neither dealt with the inspection system's inherent weaknesses nor fundamentally changed the system's predominant reliance on sensory inspection methods. These methods cannot identify microbial contamination, such as harmful bacteria, which is the most serious health risk from meat and poultry. Although FSIS has known about this problem for fifteen years or more, its major initiative in response — creating a new inspection system — is still years away.

— US General Accounting Office assessment of meat inspection in the US, presented to the Senate, May 24, 1994

•

The changes being made to the meat inspection process starting in 1996 will take years to implement. They may reduce the risk of becoming sick from contaminated meat, but no matter how many changes are made in the inspection process meat will continue to make people sick.

•

People see the juicy meat on their plates but are not exposed to the sight of the heart-stopping cholesterol and saturated fat that gets slathered through their veins and arteries when they eat that meat. The unhealthful animal flesh-based American diet contributes to many of the ailments people experience and for which they seek medical help. Beside being major risk factors in the most common types of heart diseases and strokes, meats are a major source of destructive free radicals that damage body tissues (*Tufts University Diet & Nutrition Newsletter,* September 1993). Eating animal products introduces prostaglandin-2 into the body and increases the uric acid level and these both promote arthritic conditions.

While many people believe they need to eat animal flesh to get protein and drink milk to get calcium, they would be better off getting their protein and calcium from plant sources. Trying to get calcium from milk to prevent osteoporosis actually does the opposite. The protein in meats, dairy, and egg products is concentrated and eating these animal products actually leads to bone calcium depletion. After the concentrated protein from animal products is consumed, it makes its way into the blood where it produces an acid condition. The blood then takes calcium out of the bones where the body stores calcium and uses the calcium to neutralize the acidity level of the blood. This calcium and excess protein is then excreted by the kidneys and this scenario (protein-induced hypercalcuria) leads to osteoporosis (bones lacking in calcium) and some types of kidney stones. Eliminating animal protein from the diet can cut urinary calcium loss in half (*American Journal of Clinical Nutrition*, 1994; 59:1356-1361). Osteoporosis and hip fractures are much less common in countries where meat, dairy, and egg consumption is low (The China Diet and Health Study, Colin Campbell, MS, PhD., director).

A high-protein diet is also not recommended for such ailments as Parkinson's disease (*Nutritional Considerations of Parkinson's Disease*, National Parkinson Foundation, 1995), and for kidney dialysis patients (*Journal of the American Society of Nephrology*, December 1995). For these and other reasons, the last thing people need to do is eat more animal-based foods. The more healthful way would be to consume fewer or eliminate animal-based foods — and instead, eat a more plant-based diet.

•

After heart disease, the second-leading cause death in the US is cancer. An estimated 1.3 million Americans will be stricken with cancer in 1996 and it will be the cause of 554,740 deaths — one-fourth of all deaths.

•

The second-leading cause of cancer-related deaths in the US is colorectal cancer. The American Cancer Society estimated that there would be 134,500 cases of colorectal cancer diagnosed in 1996.

•

Women ages fifty-five to sixty-nine who eat more than thirty-six servings of red meat a month appear to have a 70% greater risk of developing non-Hodgkin's lymphoma than those who consume less than twenty-two servings.
— *Time* Magazine, May 13, 1996

•

A considerable body of scientific data suggests positive relationships between vegetarian diets and risk reduction for several chronic degenerative diseases and conditions, including obesity, coronary artery disease, hypertension, diabetes mellitus, and some types of cancer.
— The American Dietetic Association

•

The US Public Health Service has said that there is consistent evidence between the intake of saturated fat with the incidence of higher blood cholesterol, and increased risk of colon cancer, breast cancer, and coronary heart disease.
— The Surgeon General's Report on Nutrition and Health, 1989

•

A 1995 study of 2,000 people published in the *Archives of Ophthalmology* suggested that eating a diet high in saturated fat and cholesterol increases the risk of age-related macular degeneration — the leading cause of irreversible blindness among persons older than sixty-five.

•

Advertising produced by the animal-farming industry can give a person the idea that meat, dairy, and eggs are healthfoods. The commercials mention the protein content of the products and say this is good. They tell us that "milk is a natural." This advertising is very inaccurate. Beef is not a healthfood. Cow milk is not a healthfood for humans. Cow milk is best consumed by baby cows. Chicken is not a healthfood. Chickens, hogs, lambs, cows, turkeys, deer, ducks, and other animal that humans eat have the fat and cholesterol that cause human disease.

•

On March 20th, 1996 British Health Minister Stephen Dorrell conceded that the incurable and deadly Creutzfeldt-Jakob brain disease, (CJD) which killed at least ten people in that country, was being linked to bovine spongiform encephalopathy (BSE) — now more popularly known as "mad cow disease."

Though cattle in Britain had been dying of the disease for more than a decade, and CJD was linked to meat consumption in the July 7, 1990 issue of the *Lancet* (British Medical Journal), the news from the British prime minister that BSE could cause humans to die was the first time many people heard of the disease. The news alarmed consumers, shut down the beef industry in Britain, and damaged the world beef industry. In April 1996, Britain began killing and incinerating nearly five million older cows at a rate of approximately 15,000 per week.

Scientists believe BSE in cattle is linked to ground-up sheep parts, ingredients cryptically referred to as "sheep offal," such as brains and spinal cords that were infected with scrapie and that had been blended into cattle feed to increase its protein content — a practice that was banned in Britain in 1989 — though some slaughterhouses have violated the ban. Because BSE hides in the central nervous system, the British ban on using sheep offal in cattle feed also included a ban on the use of brains and spinal cords in human food.

Dr. Stanley Prusner, of San Francisco State University, believes CJD is caused by a malfunctioning infectious protein called a prion (pronounced PREE-ahn). It is similar to a disease called "kuro" that was found in the 1950s in women and children who were members of the cannibalistic Fore tribe in New Guinea. It is also believed to be related to an ailment noticed in sheep and goats that causes the animals to lose their motor functions. The ailment in sheep and goats was given the name "scrapie" because the ailing farm animals often rubbed against trees and other objects. (*The Prion Diseases, Scientific American*, January 1995. *Mad cow disease: Is It a Prion or a Virus? Los Angeles Times*, May 26, 1996.)

Both CJD and BSE eat away at the brain causing microscopic holes and giving it a spongelike appearance. Cows with BSE lose weight, walk crookedly, become uncoordinated and aggressive, begin to shake and stare — essentially they go "mad." People with CJD become visually impaired, suffer from dementia, experience limb paralysis, lose the ability to formulate words, their thought processes become blurred, their memory fails them — and they eventually die.

The CJD cases among younger people in Britain rose from 18 cases in 1990 to 56 cases in 1994 and dropped to 42 cases in 1995. The average age of previous victims of CJD was 63 years. It is now believed that 10 or more years may pass after infection before physical symptoms of the disease become apparent.

The US Centers for Disease Control estimates that there are 250 cases of CJD in the US every year. Many people believe the number is much higher and that the CJD rate of infection will start to expose itself much in the same way that HIV has in the last 20 years.

•

Along with the cholesterol that is contained in meat, there are contaminants that can cause illness. Most people associate the salmonella and Escherichia coli (E. coli) bacterias only with flesh foods. The reality is those are only two types of contamination found in flesh foods. Other bacterias include clostridia, campylobacter, staphylococci, and listeria. Other than a variety of bacteria, some of the more common contaminants found in beef include urine, dirt, feces, bovine immunodeficiency virus, bovine leukemia virus, pus, rodent contaminants, insects, and parasites. Pork and poultry also contain some of these and other contaminants. Some of the carcinogens that meat eaters are exposed to are the residues of the toxic pesticides, insecticides, and other chemicals that are used on and around the livestock, and on the grains fed to them. Additionally, the antibiotics, breeding drugs, and other drugs fed to and injected into farm animals, and the fertilizers in the feed remain in the flesh and dairy foods that humans consume. According to the EarthSave Foundation, 55% of the antibiotics used in the US are given to livestock.

•

We prefer to numb ourselves physically to the fact of the slaughterhouse. We don't like to remember that a hamburger is a ground up cow.

— John Robbins, in his book *Diet for a New America*; Stillpoint, 1987

•

Most of the animals that are raised for human consumption in the US today live sad lives and are treated horribly. The unnatural conditions prevent the animals from natural patterns of behavior and they are fed an unnatural diet. (Some countries, such as Sweden, have passed laws preventing farm animals from being treated as badly as the US farm industry treats its animals.)

The open prairie type animal-farming is quickly disappearing in the US. Factory farms where thousands of animals are kept in steel confinement buildings as long as football fields are corporate investors' way of making money by producing as much meat, eggs, and milk in the quickest and cheapest way. Under factory farming arrangements, the corporations supply the animals, feed, drugs, and insecticides, and farmers working under contract provide the land, buildings, and labor. A few powerful companies now control the majority of animal-farming in the US.

Many people think that factory farming is used only to raise veal cows. In 1980 Jim Mason and Peter Singer came out with their book titled *Animal Factories*. The book exposed conditions of the US animal factories of the 1970s. Since that book was published, factory farming continues to take over more and more of the US livestock industry. It is becoming the standard way to raise dairy cows as well as chickens, turkeys, ducks, sheep, and pigs.

Other than egg hens, the animals in factory farms spend most of their lives in the dark or in very dim lighting. Most are confined to areas so small they cannot take a single step or turn around. Those that are not confined to single small cages are kept in crowded cages. The smaller farm animals, such as chickens, turkeys, and hogs, are kept in cages two or three stories high — this is known as "vertical integration farming" — where the animals on the lower levels spend their days covered with excrement.

Factory farm animals spend their lives on slated cement or grated steel flooring that injures their feet, which are designed to stand on Earth. The injuries affect the alignment of their bones, causing further physical pain. The animals are not allowed to exercise and are bred to become as heavy as they can. This unnatural weight creates more pain for their feet and legs.

•

The greatness of a nation and its moral progress can be judged by the way its animals are treated.
  — Mahatma Gandhi

•

As soon as the animals are large enough, or when the egg output of the chickens has decreased and the cows have slowed their milk production, they are sent off to the slaughterhouses.

Anyone who has spent time with an animal knows how sensitive animals are to discomfort and to emotions, such as anger, fright, and danger. Animals are also intelligent, experience joy and sadness, and continue to amaze us by proving over and over that the level of their intelligence is much higher than we have thought. The compassion of animals is displayed when they care for their young. Many animals have saved the lives of humans.

What happens to farm animals when they are taken to the slaughterhouses is a far cry from the happy, fun commercials the meat industry uses to sell the meat products.

Farm animals spend their last days without sufficient food or water. They are crowded into hauling trucks and rail cars where they become covered with urine and feces. Many of the animals are injured and some die from injuries, illnesses, or suffocation during the long, bumpy, and exhausting trip to the slaughterhouse. The animals that are too sick to walk, are suffering from exposure to extreme temperatures, or have injuries that prevent them from walking off the hauling trucks and rail cars are often beaten, electrically shocked, or dragged by chains. In the slaughterhouses cows are often hung upside down by one leg, which fractures from the strain, and they twist in fright and anger next to one another before they are killed. Chickens, turkeys, hogs, lambs, and other animals are treated with equal disdain, spending the last moments of their sad lives in the worst imaginable way.

Livestock and the Health of the Planet

In addition to the incapacitating degenerative diseases, the food poisoning, and the animal-suffering issues of raising, killing, and eating them, there are also those of the ecological damage to the planet caused by the livestock industry.

The livestock industry and companies that exist to service it use up more land and resources and create more pollution and ecological damage than any industry. There are tens of billions of chickens and turkeys, billions of pigs, over a billion cattle, and hundreds of millions of lambs and other farm animals being raised on millions of acres of land all over the world and this is ravaging the biodiversity (the full spectrum of living things including plants, insects, birds, and other land and water life) of the planet.

In his book *Beyond Beef*, Jeremy Rifkin explains that the raising of livestock for human consumption and all the ecologically destructive chemicals used by the animal-farming industry cause massive damage to the delicate ecosystems throughout the world. As more people around the world are converting to an American diet style, expansive stretches of virgin land and land that had been used to grow food for human consumption are being converted to provide space for cattle grazing and growing feed for livestock.

Anyone who studies the story of a Brazilian rubber tapper named Chico Mendez will begin to get an idea of how much corruption and damage the cattle industry has caused to the life-sustaining rain forests.

The main reason millions of acres of rain forests in South and Central America continue to be destroyed by cutting and burning is to clear new land for cattle grazing. This kills off many kinds of plants, insects, animals, and birds, and also destroys natural water filtration systems within the rain forests that have existed for millions of years. The cattle that are raised on the defiled rainforest land are used to supply beef to the Orient, to the Middle East, to North America, and to Europe where millions of acres of land are already being ruined to raise, feed, and grow feed for hundreds of millions of cattle and billions of other livestock.

> *The livestock population of the United States today consumes enough grain and soybeans to feed over five times the entire human population of the country. We feed these animals over 80% of the corn we grow, and over 95% of the oats. . . Less than half the harvested agricultural acreage in the United States is used to grow food for people. Most of it is used to grow livestock feed. This is a drastically inefficient use of our acreage. For every sixteen pounds of grain and soybeans fed to beef cattle, we get back only one pound as meat on our plates. The other fifteen are inaccessible to us. Most of it is turned into manure.*
> — John Robbins, in his book *Diet for a New America*; Stillpoint, 1987

Raising livestock and growing grains to feed livestock is not energy efficient. It takes significantly larger amounts of land, water, and other resources to produce cattle, poultry, and hog meat than it does to produce fruits, vegetables, legumes, and grains for human consumption. A large portion of the water used in the US goes to grow feed crop and provide water for livestock. Those uses of water have been blamed for the droughts in California, where water consumption by the livestock industry exceeds that of the state's human population. Much government money in the US and other countries is spent to help irrigate livestock grain fields and to build and manage water systems for the cattle industry. This water is then polluted by the chemicals used to grow the feed for the farm animals and by the farm animals themselves. This pollution and the soil erosion caused by livestock poisons streams, rivers, ponds, lakes, and oceans.

> Livestock grazing on public lands accounts for less than one-tenth of one percent of employment in the eleven Western states, including in Colorado (according to a study by Thomas Powers, chairman of the University of Montana's Department of Economics). However, this activity costs taxpayers anywhere from three to five hundred million

dollars per year (according to the Cato Institute). More significantly, cows and sheep on public lands pollute streams and rivers, and jeopardize the continued survival of many rare wildlife species (according to the Congressional General Accounting Office).
— *Colorado Wolf Tracks*

Some people would like the public to believe that pollution is the only, and worst, offender to wildlife in the US. While pollution does take a toll, the reason populations of native animals in the US have dwindled is because the animals have been killed to provide grazing land for livestock, and to protect grazing livestock.

To make it possible for cattle and other livestock to graze in open fields there has to be a safe haven created for them. This means that native animals have to be killed off. These animals include wolves, coyotes, foxes, lynx, mountain lions, bobcats, bears, elk, bighorn sheep, deer, and antelope.

Eliminating the native animals is done with poisons, with steel jaw leghold traps, by shooting them from helicopters, and by damaging their food supplies. The government offices involved in these activities include the Bureau of Land Management (BLM) and the Animal Damage Control (ADC) program of the Department of Agriculture. According to *Wildlife Damage Review*, in 1994 the government spent over $56 million federal, state, and cooperative funds to kill 783,585 wild animals.

The land that has been cleared of native wildlife is then used as pasture for grazing livestock such as cattle, sheep, and goats. The ranchers lease the land at very low rates that do not make up for the money spent by the government to manage the land for the ranchers. The balance is made up by tax dollars.

Killing predator animals damages the natural cycle of native animal life. When the predator animals are killed off, the animals they feed on are able to reproduce in massive numbers. This has resulted in large populations of animals such as mice, rats, gophers, squirrels, badgers, prairie dogs, skunks, rabbits, chipmunks, deer, and raccoons. The ADC programs attempt to control the populations of the smaller animals by sending out trappers to eliminate them. They eliminate the smaller animals by burning them, by bludgeoning them, and by poisoning their young. Many smaller native animals are also killed to prevent them from eating the crops that are being grown to feed livestock, and to prevent them from creating nesting and dwelling holes in the ground where livestock may injure their legs. To help control the population of some animals, such as deer, hunters are allowed to enter into controlled areas to kill a certain number of animals every year.

The techniques used to kill off smaller animals, and to eliminate brush and other native plants used by larger animals, also harms the bird populations. Not only do birds die when they get caught in traps and when they eat poison meant for other animals, large birds die after eating animals that have been poisoned. The ADC has targeted certain types of birds (including raven, magpies, and vultures) for population reduction by killing them. A decrease in the bird populations allows more insects to populate the land. To kill off the insects, the government and farmers use more chemical poisons. The pesticides then do even more damage to the bird populations, create insects that are resistant to pesticides, destroy beneficial insects, and pollute the land and water. And so forth, in a cycle that would naturally take care of itself if man would not interfere.

> The ADC program, created by the Animal Damage Control Act of 1931, is greatly responsible for the virtual extinction of the grizzly and wolf in the lower 48 states as well as for putting the black-footed ferret, jaguar, black-tailed prairie dog, bald eagle, and other wild animals in, or close to, the endangered category. ADC reported it poisoned 1.8 million animals in 1991 and distributed thousands of pounds of restricted-use pesticides to private individuals who poisoned untold numbers more. The US Agency for International Development works with ADC to export ADC pest control practices and chemicals, including those banned in the US, to developing countries.
> — *Wildlife Damage Review*

Ranchers and BLM workers eliminate shrubs that are used for food and shelter by native animals, and then plant grasses to feed grazing cattle. By eliminating native plants that provide food and shelter for wild animals, by eliminating small animals that provide food for predator animals, and by killing all kinds of native animals the government has had an enormous negative impact on the populations, life cycles, migrating patterns, and social structures of native animals of the North American continent. And this is done at great cost to taxpayers to provide grazing land for livestock ranchers. It is welfare farming and it is destroying the biodiversity and ecosystems of the continent. As more and more cattle are being raised on other continents, it is only a matter of time before these practices become the standard in other countries.

> Next to an all-out nuclear war, today's intensive animal agriculture represents the greatest threat to human welfare in the history of mankind.
> — Farm Animal Reform Movement

A vegetarian diet uses substantially less land and other resources than a wasteful and unhealthful meat-based diet. A plant-based diet is not only healthier for humans, but also for farm workers, for the land, for plant life, for the water, for the air, for the animals, and for the Earth.

Organic Foods

While many people know of the adverse effects that a tiny mosquito bite or bee sting may have on the health of a person, even to the point where he may die, they do not take into consideration what illnesses may be related to the hundreds of millions of pounds of various chemicals used to farm and process food. Toxic chemicals in human foods cause distress in humans similar to the allergic responses humans have to tiny bits of dust or pollen. On a long-term basis, chemicals used in food assault the human immune system and contribute to disease.

As billions of dollars are poured into research to try to find a cure for human diseases, most of the money may be spent more wisely on finding what man-made chemicals in the food and water supply may be causing the very same diseases these individuals are seeking to cure, and then banning the manufacture of those chemicals that poison the food supply and damage the ecosystems and seasonal rhythms of the Earth.

Chemical companies started funding research at agricultural colleges several decades ago. Since then there has been a huge increase in the amount of chemicals used on farms and a strong relationship between industrial farming and the chemical companies. There are now over 400 pesticides licensed for use on foods in the US alone.

It is known that pesticides and insecticides are toxic, many can cause cancer, and they are generally a risk to the health of humans, animals, and helpful bugs and ground organisms. One study found a four-fold increase in the risk of soft tissue sarcomas in children exposed to household pesticides in the first fourteen years of life (*Journal of Public Health*, February 1995). In the last forty years the incidence of cancer in the US has increased at a rate of about 1% a year. This corresponds with the growing use of chemicals for growing foods, killing household bugs, spraying yard plants, and preserving wood.

Because of their exposure to farming chemicals, farm workers have higher rates of cancer than the general population. For instance, non-Hodgkin's lymphoma is one type of cancer that is more common among farmers who work on farms where chemicals are used. Farming chemicals are also suspected of causing an increase in cancers of the breasts and testicles, in reproductive organ disorders, such as endometriosis, and in birth defects of the reproductive organs. The farming community is aware of the problems the farming chemicals may cause. In 1994 midwestern farmers were urged to wash their clothes separately from other family members to avoid exposing their families to the toxic farming chemicals.

Research is showing evidence that some widely used pesticides, fungicides, manufacturing chemicals, and other chlorine-based substances imitate estrogen and others block testosterone. The chemicals, known as endocrine disrupters or "hormone modulating pollutants," are suspected of depleting human sperm counts, feminizing animals, and causing hormonally related cancers. Pesticides and industrial chemicals are believed to be the cause of wild animals being found with half-female, half-male sex organs. The animals also have abnormal testosterone and estrogen levels. Animals with those deformities include otters in the Pacific Northwest, trout in British rivers, alligators in Florida, and birds found in the Great Lakes area and on the coast of California. One study conducted by scientists at Tulane University found evidence that some pesticides may become hundreds of times more powerful when combined with other pesticides (*Science*, June 7, 1996).

Many people have recognized the dangers that man made chemicals in the food and water supply pose to health. This knowledge is motivating a growing number of people to turn to whole organic foods in what some are calling a "clean-food diet." This way of eating includes water that is free from additives, and foods that have been grown or farmed organically. To satisfy the demand for these types of foods, the organic food market nearly doubled in the five years from 1989 to 1994.

Clean foods are vegetables, fruits, grains, legumes (beans, peas, etc.) that are free from refined carbohydrates, unnatural food dyes, flavorings, sweeteners, pesticides, herbicides, insecticides, ripening agents, growth-promoting chemicals, preservatives, waxes, and other synthetic and unnatural food additives. Some people also consider clean foods to be dairy products and food from animals that have been farmed without the use of growth hormones, antibiotics, steroids, and other drugs, and that have been fed organically grown grains.

Under the Organic Foods Production Act of 1990, producers of organic foods must be certified by independent agents registered with state government agencies. The act established a 12-member volunteer board, the National Organics Standards Board, to set standards for how organic foods must be grown. Under the NOSB standards, if a product contains at least 95% organic ingredients by weight, then it can be labeled "organic." Organic foods must be grown on land that has not had non-organic farming substances applied to it for at least three years. The act allows for foods made with at least 50% organic ingredients to be labeled "made with organic ingredients."

The prime source of toxic pesticides and other chemicals for most Americans is in the consumption of food high in fat content, such as meat and dairy products. A vegetarian diet, or one that minimizes animal products, can substantially reduce one's exposure to most of these cancer-causing chemicals.

> — Lewis Regenstein, in his book *How to Survive in America the Poisoned;* Acropolis Books, 1982

Most farm animals are given drugs by mouth or injection from their first day to nearly their last. These drugs include hormones, antibiotics, milk stimulants, tranquilizers, and chemicals that influence the birth rates. The animals are also sprayed with toxic insecticides, fungicides, and pesticides. These drugs and chemicals along with the chemicals used to grow the feed accumulate in the fat cells of the animals and these residues are transferred into the humans who consume the meats, milk products, and eggs.

I believe that in the US up to 14% of cows are ground up and fed back to cows. I am very concerned that this will lead to the same sort of thing that is happening in the UK.

> — Howard Lyman, a former cattle rancher from Montana, referring to mad cow disease in his testimony at the McLibel Trial in London in April 1996. The McLibel trial is McDonald's Corp. vs. environmental activists Helen Steel and Dave Morris. This is the longest-running civil trial in British history. The McDonald's Corp. is suing these two environmental activists for distributing leaflets that say, among other things, that McDonald's sells unhealthful, disease-inducing foods, has questionable business practices, helps destroy the rain forests, and pollutes the Earth. McDonald's is represented by high-priced lawyers. Steel and Morris are representing themselves. For more information on this subject, see the Internet: http://www.McSpotlight.org/

Because farm animals eat high on the food chain, their fats contain residues of all the chemicals used to grow their food. Because the feed given to animals raised in factory farms often contains portions of ground-up farm animals that died prematurely, the amount of drug and chemical residue found in meats from these animals contains a larger dose of the residues.

As if giving the naturally vegetarian animals a cannibalistic diet was not bad enough, some farm animals are also fed their own excrement. Some pigs are fed their own urine, and poultry waste and feathers are mixed in with feed. Not only does this magnify the amount of chemical and drug residues in the fat of the animals, it also increases the likelihood that the animals are harboring infectious diseases. The farm animals that die are not tested for diseases. Grinding up the animals to increase the protein content of animal feed increases the likelihood that contagious diseases, such as mad cow disease, are becoming rampant within farm animals.

Because meat, dairy, and eggs are likely to contain chemical contaminants, many people who eat organic foods stay away from animal protein, and concentrate on having more of a plant-based diet. They also often try to avoid produce that has been grown in other countries because imported produce is likely to have higher quantities of farming chemicals.

> One of the longest-running boycotts of any product is the boycott of fresh table grapes that has been held and promoted by the United Farm Workers of America. The farm workers are upset because grape growers commonly use toxic chemical pesticides on the grapes that risk the health of the farm workers. The farm workers have encouraged people to avoid purchasing grapes that are not organic.

While it is true that some pesticides have been made illegal for use in the US, there are still companies in the US manufacturing the pesticides and selling them to other countries, such as Mexico and Chile. Many fruits and vegetables that have been sprayed with the illegal pesticides are then imported by the US and are sold in US markets.

The most ecologically responsible and most healthful way to grow food is to use organic methods. Some farms also use the low-input sustainable agriculture (LISA) and the integrated pest management (IPM) techniques. Some farms rotate their crops every other season to help maintain a healthy soil and do composting to build the soil base. These forms of farming are safer for the soil, for wildlife, for native plants, for the health of humans, and for farm workers.

A person can reduce his exposure to pesticides on imported produce by purchasing fruits and vegetables in season. Other ways to avoid exposure to food-processing and farming chemicals are to purchase produce from local farmers' markets; purchase unpackaged items from the bulk bins at the local healthfood store; choose organic produce at the market; eat animal products sparingly or, even better, not at all; buy foods with labels indicating they are certified organic; and grow a home vegetable garden and keep it organic.

The larger farming corporations have mostly stayed out of the organic farming movement. By choosing organic produce you are supporting smaller farmers and their families. You are also supporting food distributors who concentrate on the organic market.

By choosing to eat organic foods, you are saying "no" to the chemical companies that make pesticides, insecticides, fungicides, waxes, and other chemicals used on farms and that pollute the land and water, damage wildlife, and risk human health.

Plant-Based Foods and Health

Inadequate nutrition and the consumption of junk food contribute to everything from skin problems to heart disease, and from depression to birth defects. Eating whole foods, such as unprocessed fruits and vegetables and whole grains, provides the body with important nutrients, such as vitamins, minerals, enzymes, and phytochemicals, such as isoflavonoids and lignans.

The 1990s have seen a number of modern science's recent "discoveries" that show certain vegetables (broccoli, peppers, onions, garlic, carrots, cranberries, beans, spinach, soybeans, etc.) not only provide needed nutrients that are beneficial to health but also contain and provide properties, such as phytochemicals that prevent certain serious ailments, such as cancer and heart disease, and limit intestinal exposure to carcinogens.

A number of studies have shown that cancer risk is lower and immune competence is higher in individuals who consume a vegetarian diet. Epidemiological studies almost unanimously report a strong correlation between a diet high in fruits and vegetables and low cancer risk.
— John Boik, in his book *Cancer & Natural Medicine: A Textbook of Basic Research and Clinical Research*; Oregon Medical Publishing, 1996

Myths and truths about vegetarianism:

By the term "meat," I mean all kinds of meat — cow, hog, lamb, turkey, chicken, fish, and any other animals that people eat. Someone who calls himself a vegetarian is not truly a vegetarian if he eats fish or birds. Lacto-ovo vegetarians do not eat meat, but do consume milk and egg products. Pure vegetarians do not eat any kind of animal product including oils from animals. The purest type of vegetarian is a vegan (rhymes with begin). True vegans do not eat meat, eggs, or milk products, do not wear leather clothing, and avoid products that contain animal derivatives, such as some brands of soaps, some brands of cosmetics, and some types of medicine.

Myth: Vegetarians do not get enough protein.

Truth: Vegetarians, even strict vegetarians who do not eat dairy products, get enough protein. Protein is made up of chains of amino acids. It is not necessary to eat animal protein to get the essential amino acids of the protein molecule. The amino acids needed to make protein in the human body can be obtained through a balanced vegetarian diet. It is **not** necessary to combine rice with beans to get protein in a vegetarian diet.

The protein found in animal products is much more concentrated than the protein found in plants. A diet that contains a lot of concentrated protein is a burden on the body, especially the bones and kidneys.

Myth: Vegetarians often become anemic because they do not get enough iron in their diet.

Truth: Vegetables have a sufficient amount of iron. Many vegetables, such as broccoli, cucumbers, cauliflower, bell peppers, peas, tomatoes, and spinach have more iron than beef. Many types of fruits are also excellent sources of iron.

The body needs vitamin C to use iron. Meat, eggs, and dairy products do not contain vitamin C; vegetables and fruits do.

Milk is *not* a good source of iron.

The iron in meat is heme iron (blood iron). A study conducted by researchers at the Harvard University School of Public Health found that high levels of heme iron raised the risk of heart disease. The iron found in vegetables is nonheme iron and is utilized by the body differently from the iron found in meat. (*Circulation*, 1994; 89:969-74)

Myth: Vegetarians do not get enough B-12 from their food.

Truth: There is some truth in this. But the statement does not take into consideration the fact that the bacteria naturally living in the mouth, throat, and intestines supplies some B-12. Many foods found in healthfood stores where vegetarians often do their shopping are fortified with vitamin B-12.

In 1996 the US Department of Agriculture and the Department of Health and Human Services came out with a revised form of its Dietary Guidelines for America. The guidelines are revised every five years and are used to create federal nutrition programs, nutritional labeling, and the *Food Guide Pyramid*. For the first time the guidelines endorsed a vegetarian diet. But it included a message that vegetarians may need to supplement their diet with vitamin B-12.

Vegetarians often take vitamin B-12 supplements. These supplements are inexpensive and do not have to be derived from animal products. There are vegetarian vitamin supplements available in most health-food stores. A person desiring to avoid animal products should make sure the label of the B-12 supplement indicates that the vitamin is derived from vegetable bacteria and not from beef liver or cod-liver oil.

Vegetarians who do not eat a balanced diet can have nutritional deficiencies much the same as people who are not vegetarians. The key is to eat a variety of healthful foods, and not empty calorie, sugary, salty, oily, refined junk.

Some people believe that vitamin B-12 supplements are not needed when a person is following a healthy vegetarian diet.

Myth: Vegetarians do not get enough cholesterol.

Truth: Cholesterol is made by human body cells. There is no need for adults to obtain cholesterol through food.

Strict vegetarians have healthier cardiovascular systems than people who regularly eat animals, milk products, and eggs. The main reason meat eaters have heart attacks and strokes is that their cardiovascular system has been damaged by eating animals. The majority of the people waiting for heart transplants are doing so because their hearts have been damaged from years of eating meat, dairy, and egg products.

Switching to a vegetarian diet can reverse some of the damage an animal-based diet has done to the cardiovascular system. For more information on reversing heart disease, see books written by Dr. Dean Ornish or Dr. John McDougall.

Myth: Vegetarian diets are not healthful.

Truth: Meats, milk products, and eggs contain saturated fat, cholesterol, and concentrated protein, have no fiber, contain no vitamin C, and are not a source of complex carbohydrates. Saturated fat, cholesterol, and animal protein play a major part in many health problems, such as obesity, gallstones, kidney stones, arthritis, osteoporosis, high blood pressure, heart disease, strokes, certain eye diseases, and hormone-dependent cancers.

Diabetics are more likely to suffer the ravages of diabetes if they are on a diet high in meat and dairy content. According to the American Academy of Pediatrics, "the avoidance of cow's milk protein for the first several months of life may reduce the later development of IDDM (insulin-dependent diabetes) or delay its onset in susceptible individuals."

Vegetarians have lower rates of cancers of the breasts, lungs, colon, prostate, and the reproductive organs. Women who eat an abundance of vegetables have a 48% lower risk of breast cancer (*Journal of the National Cancer Institute*, January 18, 1995).

People who are heavy experience more health problems than those who are reasonably thin. Vegetarians are less likely to be overweight than the general population (*Another Reason for Vegetarianism — Reduced Health Care Costs, Vegetarian Journal*, July/August 1996).

It is true that a person can call himself a vegetarian and eat mostly junk food, but vegetarians are more likely to be nutritionally aware and to eat in a healthier way than people who eat meat, eggs, and dairy products.

Myth: You need to eat from the Basic Four Food Groups to be healthy.

Truth: The Basic Four Food Groups promoted by the animal-farming industry interests were designed by the United States Department of Agriculture in 1956. They came up with the Basic Four Food Groups idea to increase the profits of the animal-farming industry. The colorful posters, teaching materials, and coloring books that teach children to eat daily from the Basic Four Food Groups are supplied free to schoolteachers in America by the groups working to promote the products of the animal-farming industry. Eating the meat, egg, and dairy products promoted by the animal-farming industry increases the risks of osteoporosis, heart disease, cancers, etc.

Vegetarians have their own basic four food groups: Fruits, vegetables, legumes, and grains.

Myth: Humans are carnivores, therefore they need to eat meat.

Truth: The teeth and mouths of humans are very different from the teeth and mouths of carnivores, such as animals in the cat, dog, and lawyer families. Carnivores have sharp teeth and wide mouths that can bite, lock, and tear at meat. Some people say the omnivore shape of human teeth suggests that humans are meant for a diet of both plant and meat content. Other people say that because human teeth are short and smooth, the human jaw swivels in a grinding motion, and human mouths are small and relatively weak, humans are therefore more attuned to eating plants. (Animals that eat plants are known as herbivores.)

Carnivores eat meat when it is raw. Humans are not natural meat eaters. When humans do eat meat they do so only after it has been tenderized or ground, then softened even more by cooking under high temperatures and then, at last, sliced with a knife. Even after preparing, cooking, and cutting meat, humans often have a hard time chewing and swallowing the stuff — sometimes losing teeth and gagging to death during the process (the animals' revenge?).

The human mouth structures are just part of the picture. Those who say humans are meant to eat a plant-based diet may have their beliefs verified by taking the human digestive tract into consideration.

Human bowels are very different from the smooth and relatively straight bowels of meat-eating animals. The puckered, long, and curved structures of the human digestive tract indicate that humans are more attuned to eating a fiber-rich plant-based diet. The stomach acids of the human are also much weaker than those of carnivores and more in balance with the stomach acid levels of herbivores.

Humans need fiber to help digest food. Meat, milk, and egg products do not contain fiber. Humans who do not eat enough fiber have higher rates of cancer and other diseases.

A healthy vegetarian diet contains lots of fiber.

Unlike carnivore animals, humans do not have claws that can tear into another animal to kill it and rip it open.

Humans are not carnivores. They can barely be described as omnivores.

•

While allopathic doctors release their various reports and announce "recent discoveries" showing "scientific evidence" that prove diets low in salt, sugar, oil, and animal products, and high in unrefined plant content lead to better health and lower cancer risks, the "healthfood fanatics" have always taught that edible plants contain healing properties and properties that fight diseases.

•

There is overwhelming evidence that the consumption of a plant-based diet, which is high in fruits, vegetables, grains, and legumes, including soy, and possibly flaxseed, may reduce the risk of breast and other types of cancers.

— Clare M. Hasler, PhD, director, Functional Foods for Health Program, University of Illinois. *Y-Me Hotline* newsletter, March 1996

•

As the "scientific" studies supporting the role diet plays in the healing process appear more and more in allopathic medical journals, the results are being taken more seriously by the US allopathic establishment. Dietary changes are being incorporated into the way allopathic doctors treat such conditions as arthritis, cancer, and heart disease. Nutrition is being used as a way to boost the immune system in cancer patients, and strict vegetarian diets are being prescribed in combination with exercise and stress reduction techniques to reverse heart disease and help patients avoid undergoing invasive surgery and taking expensive and risky chemical drugs (*Journal of the American Medical Association*, September 30, 1995).

When one considers that it costs several thousand dollars to send a patient suffering from heart disease to a health retreat, and several times that to perform bypass surgery, it is not too difficult to understand why the health insurance companies are embracing the lower-cost holistic treatments.

Probably the most popular vegetarian diet and stress management programs designed to treat heart disease are those advocated by Dr. Dean Ornish in books he has written and in classes he helped design at the Preventative Medicine Research Institute in Sausalito; in books written by John McDougall who has a health center in Napa Valley; and programs taught at the Pritikin Centers in Santa Monica and Miami. (For more information see the *Heart* heading in the *Research Resources* section of this book.)

The "healthfood fanatics" may not have had the so-called "scientific proof" of what a nutritional plant-based diet can do for the human body, but they knew all along of the health and ecological benefits of eating pure unadulterated plant-based foods that are free of animal oils and flesh. The body that is supplied with the proper fuel is healthier, feels better, and performs better than a body that has been gunked up with empty calorie, overprocessed junk foods, and heavy, disease-causing animal-based foods.

•

Nothing will benefit health and increase the chances for survival of life on Earth as the evolution to a vegetarian diet.
— Albert Einstein

•

Those at the forefront of the natural living movement understand that all living things are connected and nature will provide us with all we need if we would work with nature. A strictly vegetarian lifestyle promotes a simplification of living and works toward a balance with nature by adopting activities that contribute to a sound and clean natural environment. This can be done by not using synthetic chemicals, promoting sustainable agriculture, eating only organically grown foods, using only what we need, using only what can be recycled, restoring what we have destroyed, and protecting the ecosystems and plant biodiversity of the planet. If we damage the planet, we damage ourselves.

For more information on nutrition, see the *Nutrition, Health, and Eating* heading in the *Research Resources* section of this book.

7 • DECIDING ON SURGERY

Finding an Allopathic Doctor

A smart car shopper does a lot of searching before he makes the decision to purchase a car. Like a smart shopper, a person looking for a surgeon should check out more than one of them before deciding who is best for his needs.

When considering a doctor's training, think of an athlete. Some athletes train very hard every day and are not so great. Another athlete can train the same amount of time and be world class. Just because a doctor went through the steps to become a doctor does not mean he practices his profession well.

It is all too common for a medical consumer to choose a physician on the basis of his personality and not on the basis of his training, professional history or curative skill. People seeking medical care should concentrate on finding a doctor who is well trained, familiar with the latest information in the field and able to recognize when a patient needs the attention of another doctor. Consumers should also select a doctor who listens to his patient's health concerns.

Basing the choice of a doctor on the appearance of his advertisement is also an inadequate way to select a doctor. Great-looking ads are created by advertising agencies, photographers, graphic artists or some combination of the three. Ads have nothing to do with the capabilities of the doctor other than that they may show the doctor's skill in selecting a good commercial artist.

Because people with medical licenses can practice in any area of medicine, including brain surgery, they can advertise themselves in the phone book under any specialty they choose. Many doctors who advertise themselves in the phone book under a specific specialty are not board certified by the American Board of Medical Specialties, are certified in a specialty other than the one they list, or have not received any specialized training in the area of medicine they have decided to practice. The phone book companies do not have the interest, time or resources to check the accuracy of the information in each advertisement. That is the consumer's job.

In recent years there have been television commercials that advertise 800 phone numbers that people can dial to get a list of specific doctors who practice near where the consumer lives. These phone numbers are paid for by doctors who join in on marketing costs and pay for this consumer service. This can be one way initially to find a certain type of doctor. However, it should not be used as the only step. Do not wholeheartedly trust that the information the 800 number supplies on a doctor is 100% accurate. Additional background research on the doctor should be done to make sure the doctor is licensed and is someone who has surgical skills that you can trust and depend on.

> *The average person has more information when buying a car than when choosing a doctor.*
> — Sidney M. Wolfe, MD, Director, Public Citizen's Health Research Group

Consumer access to doctors' professional histories is limited. It took an act of Congress by way of the Healthcare Quality-Improvement Act of 1986 and the Medicare and Medicaid Patient and Program Protection Act of 1987 to create the National Practitioner Data Bank (NPDB), which is overseen by the United States Department of Health and Human Services. This data bank contains information about several thousand doctors and other medical professionals who have patterns of malpractice. Thanks to the powerful medical lobbies' influence over lawmakers, this data bank, which because of budget cuts was not activated until September 1990, is not accessible to the public, even though it is funded with tax dollars. Releasing information from the data bank is also punishable by a fine.

> *I think it is an effective tool to provide information. Fundamentally, the National Practitioner Data Bank is a tool for collecting data. But a hospital that has to credential and privilege physicians is required to query that data bank when there is an application for referrals and every 2 years at least thereafter.*
> *It makes information available, but it fundamentally is not the entity that has the responsibility for excluding an individual from transferring across state lines. For example, it is not a licensing board.*
> — Susan D. Kladiva, Assistant Director, Health Finance Issues, US General Accounting Office, during Congressional subcommittee hearing on issues relating to medical malpractice, May 20, 1993

State licensing boards, hospitals, medical societies, health maintenance organizations, and some other professional groups have access to the NPDB. It lists medical malpractice claims paid by insurance companies, professional limitations placed on doctors, actions taken by hospitals and other institutions to deny or revoke clinical privileges of doctors, and disciplinary actions taken by state licensing boards against doctors. Hospitals are also supposed to consult with the NPDB when hiring a doctor and every two years thereafter as a peer review precautionary measure. Hospitals are supposed to report doctors to the NPDB when any doctor has had his hospital privileges suspended for 31 days or more. About three-fourths of all hospitals have never reported a doctor to the NPDB.

The AMA, which works to protect doctors and uphold their standing in society, would like to see the NPDB canceled and is actively working to do so. The consumers' rights organization Public Citizen's Health Research Group would like to change the access rules to the data bank so that the public is given access to it. (For information contact PCHRG at the phone number given in the Research Resources section of this book under the heading of Patients' and Consumers' Rights.)

Some of the actions a person can take to find a doctor:
(These are numbered only as a form of reference and not as a grade of importance.)

1. Look in the *Marquis Directory of Medical Specialists*. This reference book is available in many libraries and it lists, by specialty, in alphabetical and geographic order, every doctor certified by one of the 23 medical examining boards officially sanctioned by the American Board of Medical Specialties. Also, check the *Compendium of Certified Medical Specialists*.

2. Check the *American Medical Association Directory*, which is published by the AMA and is available in many libraries.

3. Write to the AMA to find whether a particular doctor you are interested in checking out is listed in the Physician Master File (AMA, 515 N. State St., Chicago, IL 60610).

4. Call your insurance company and find out what doctors are accepted by your plan.

5. Ask friends or relatives what doctors they go to. Then take measures to check up on the doctors' educations and professional histories.

6. Look in the latest special summer healthcare issue of the magazine *US News and World Reports* and see what hospitals and other medical facilities they consider to be the best in the country.

7. Call the closest university hospital and ask for referrals to doctors who are associated with that hospital. Find out who is head of the surgical department in which you are seeking treatment. If that doctor does not have time to perform your surgery, he will likely be able to refer you to another doctor who is familiar with the latest medical procedures.

8. Find a top-rated hospital and ask which doctors are connected with that hospital. Ask for the name of a doctor who is chief of his department in the area of medicine for which you are seeking attention. If that doctor cannot treat you, ask him for two or three names of doctors he thinks are good.

9. Ask the head nurse at a top-rated hospital for a referral to a doctor.

Nurses are often aware of the qualifications and curative skills of particular doctors. Nurses are also in the operating rooms while the doctors are performing the operations. They know the doctors who make mistakes and are not so good as well as those doctors who perform successful and responsible operations.

10. Call the doctor's office to ask whether the receptionist will mail you the doctor's resume, or curriculum vitae, which should list where the doctor received his education, where he served his residency, what he considers to be his specialty, the boards he is certified with, and where he has practiced.

11. Call the state medical licensing department or medical board to find out whether the doctor is licensed by the state (the phone numbers to every state medical board can be found in the *Research Resources* section of this book under the heading *State Medical Boards*).

A. Find out the doctor's birth date (for searching records).

B. Ask for the address of the doctor to see if he has more than one business address.

C. Ask for the doctor's state license number and ask when it was issued.

D. Find out the status of the license — if it is in good standing, if there are any limits or restraints that the state has placed on the doctor, if the doctor has been put on probation, or if the doctor's license has been suspended or revoked.

E. Ask if there is any information about felony convictions.

F. Ask if there is any information about any disciplinary actions taken against the doctor by another state. Call that state medical board and find out the information it has on the doctor.

G. Ask if the state has any information it can release about lawsuits that have been filed against the doctor. Ask if you can find out if the board has formally taken action against the doctor for misconduct, and if so, find out what the charges were.

At If the state has not taken any formal action against a doctor, this does not mean that he has never botched any surgeries or violated any patients. It may mean that the victim of the bad medical care did not know how to go about taking action against the doctor or was unsuccessful in getting action taken, or it may mean that the victim was left incapacitated or dead.

In California the state medical board decided in May 1993 to give the public access to information about physicians who have lost malpractice cases in jury trials or who have had disciplinary action taken against them by the board for unprofessional behavior, incompetence, or for other reasons. Information is not given about malpractice cases where out-of-court settlements were made, where the award was less than $30,000, or where the malpractice case was heard before an arbitration panel. The available records start at January 1, 1993. The board relies on court clerks in each county to report malpractice judgments over $30,000. State law requires this reporting to be done within 10 days of the judgments. Records show that this is not always done.

12. Many doctors have been sued. This does not mean that the doctor is a bad doctor. You have to look at the situation and decide for yourself. Some areas of medicine attract more malpractice suits than others. If there are a number of lawsuits or criminal charges against a doctor, this is probably not a doctor you should trust with your health.

Pending lawsuits and legal judgments against a doctor are public record. These records and all sorts of other legal action documents, which are available at the district attorney's office at the county courthouse, include information on lawsuits that are currently pending and lawsuits that have gone to verdict in the county and the details of the verdicts.

Using the doctor's birthdate from the state board, search the criminal case index at the county courthouse of the city or county where the doctor practices to see if you can find any criminal information about the doctor. Search the index of civil cases for lawsuits against the doctor. You can also search for the lawsuit by using the type of lawsuit, or the type of surgery. Other information might be found in the court's minutes book.

If the doctor was sued along with a hospital, medical center, group practice, or other institution, the lawsuit might be filed under the name of the institution and not under the doctor's name. (You may also want to check and see if the doctor is suing someone else, and especially if he is suing one of his former patients.)

Some files may have been sealed by court order.

Some lawsuits may have been settled out of court as a way to avoid a lengthy and expensive court case, and so that the doctor would not have any record of a court case against him or any recorded admittance of negligence.

If the doctor was sued in an arbitration process, there is no public record, even if the patient won. The arbitration proceedings take place in private, are less formal than the courtroom process, and are heard in front of three panelists who are usually retired judges or attorneys — as opposed to a jury trial that is heard in court in front of a jury of from six to twelve people selected from the local population.

If the actions taken against a doctor were enough to attract attention from the media (a doctor's career nightmare), you may be able to find copies of these newspaper or magazine articles in your local library's periodical files.

13. Call the state board of medical examiners and have them send you a copy of the file on the doctor.

14. Call the county medical board and society and ask for a list of board certified doctors who practice in the area of medicine in which you are seeking treatment.

15. Call the professional boards the doctor claims that he is certified with to see if he is in fact certified by them. Ask if he is in good standing with the board (this might only mean that he has paid his dues) and ask what the requirements are for a doctor to be a member of the organization.

If you call 1-800-776-2378, the American Board of Medical Specialties will tell you if a particular doctor is board certified through them.

16. Contact the Public Citizen's Health Research Group and order their compilation of questionable doctors for the state you live in. The address and phone number of Public Citizen is in the *Research Resources* section of this book under the heading *Patients' and Consumers' Rights.*

Visiting with the Doctor

The local auto mechanic at the corner garage may have to have more training in his field to get a state license than some of these cosmetic surgeons need to start rearranging a person's appearance.

The public needs to start asking some tough questions about qualifications. The public also needs better information about the types of surgery that are appropriate for their medical needs and who is qualified to perform that surgery.

— Congressman Norman Sisisky, during Congressional subcommittee hearings on plastic surgery industry, 1989

When communicating with the doctor:
- Do not take advantage of the doctor's time.
- Respect his office hours.
- If you are going to call him, make some notes beforehand about what you want to ask.
- Be honest and address your concerns.
- Know that if you communicate well with the doctor you are more likely to receive the care that is best for you.
- Avoid producing unnecessary tension in the relationship with the doctor or within his office.

Consulting with a professional about performing some operation on your one and only body is not a time to be concerned about making new friends and being entertaining, nor is it a time to be unquestioning and docile. This is a time for you to be assertive and do whatever it takes to find out all your options and have those options explained, get the best information available, seek the best level of communication with the people you speak with, and, if you elect to undergo surgery, seek the best medical care you can get.

Doctors are not mind readers. Do not assume that the doctor knows what you do and do not want. What you tell the doctor will influence his actions. Make sure there are no mixed signals. The more research you do and the more questions you ask and get answers to, the lower your chances are of making the wrong decision and of being surprised by the results if surgery does take place. Any good doctor would not feel attacked by a patient who has made the effort to inform himself by doing his own research. If anything, it will increase the chances that, if surgery does take place, the doctor will perform a successful operation.

Be wary of a doctor who becomes defensive. A doctor who does not cooperate with you and is unresponsive to your need for information may be hiding something in his history or may be afraid you will find something out that will discourage you from the operation. Remember that the doctor may not make money unless he treats you for something. No sense in divulging the negative things about the surgery, such as the risks, when there is money to be made. If the doctor is offended by your need for information, find another doctor.

You should not settle for a doctor who tries to make surgery look secretive and magical as if only those with a medical education are capable of understanding the procedures. A doctor with this type of attitude may tell you that it is not in your best interest to know the details — that it might upset you or interfere with your rest and healing. If you are going to give your informed consent, he should do his part and inform you. No surgery is so complicated that it cannot be explained to you. The doctor should be willing to explain the procedures in words you will understand. If it would help you understand, have the doctor use medical models, drawings, and photographs to explain the procedure.

Some doctors dance around certain questions and give answers that may be what a patient wants to hear, but may be misleading, or are not exactly the truth. While there are some patients who become illogical and nervous when dealing with medical decisions, they should not settle for deceptive answers that are meant simply to calm them down and pacify their fears. A doctor who treats surgery lightly and talks to a patient as if the patient should not be so concerned about making sure the surgery goes well may not be the doctor the patient needs.

For the money a patient pays the doctor, the patient should get the answers he needs and in a respectable manner. A patient should not be afraid to walk out on a doctor if the patient does not get the service he feels he is paying for. A patient should not be concerned if the doctor seems disappointed that the patient chose another doctor. The doctor's disappointment may stem from the fact that he, as a person who may make money only when he operates, lost out on a sale. On the other hand, if he is giving the patient a strong warning to stay away from a certain doctor because of that doctor's lack of ethics, questionable skill, and history of negligence and incompetence, the patient may want to seriously consider this viewpoint.

One should avoid any marketing campaigns put out by a surgeon promising to transform a patient into physical perfection. A patient should also be skeptical of newly developed "medical breakthrough" operations, as the patient may find himself more of a guinea pig than anything else.

The doctor to abandon is the one who tries to talk a patient into unneeded or unwanted procedures. A doctor with a hard-sell tactic is also aiming for that hard cash. If the patient is insecure in the first place, he may end up going for the whole game and be stuck thousands of dollars poorer, leaving the doctor that much richer.

What matters is that whatever is done should be in the best interest of the patient, and that if surgery does take place, the patient is satisfied with the results.

The Consultation and Physical Exam

The initial meeting with a doctor is the consultation. At that time the patient talks with the doctor and asks questions while the doctor talks with and asks questions of the patient, considers the patient's health history, examines the area of concern, and evaluates the situation.

Doctors are used to a wide variety of patients, from those who have blown a small health concern out of proportion to those who show up with a serious injury but with not much concern; from those who think they know everything to those who think doctors can do just about anything.

Rather than assuming an attitude of distrust when you visit the doctor, it would probably be more productive and beneficial to both you and the doctor if you approached the consultation with a receptive frame of mind. Remember that the doctor may provide information that will contribute to your making a decision that is in your best interest if you provide the right information and ask the right questions.

Before going to the consultation:
- Find out if there is a charge for the consultation.
- Find out what you should bring — paperwork you have from other doctors, a list of medications you are taking, insurance forms, or anything else the doctor may find helpful. (Do not leave your personal

medical files that you have brought with you. Let the staff make copies of anything they may need.)

- Find out how long you should expect to be in consult (if you know you are going to need more time, let the doctor's office know ahead of time so they can adjust their schedule).
- Write down your symptoms so you do not forget to tell the doctor anything that may be important.
- Make a list of all the medications you are taking. Include prescription and nonprescription drugs.
- Bring this book with you so you have something to read while you are in the waiting room. Review the parts of the book that pertain to your medical concern.

If you expect the doctor to treat you in a professional manner then you should give him the same respect. Be on time or be in contact. If you make an appointment with a doctor and you are going to be late, call his office as soon as you can and let them know you are running late so they can use their time wisely. If you have to cancel the appointment, let the doctor's office know as soon as you can. Do not just not show up.

When you are in the consultation, be prepared to explain your feelings regarding your health concern:

- When did you first notice that you may have a condition needing medical attention?
- What made you notice the condition?
- What kind of changes have you noticed about your condition?
- Does the condition make you feel ill or dizzy?
- Does it make you feel hungry or cause you to lose your appetite?
- Is there anything that makes the condition worse, or is there a time of day when it is more intense?
- Have you noticed anything that helps the condition?
- Does eating certain foods seem to make the condition better or worse?
- Is there pain involved and what kind of pain is it?
- Have you had the condition in the past — either in the same area you are having it now or in another area?
- Does the condition prevent you from any activities?

A consultation may include some type of physical exam. During the exam, the doctor may perform one or more of the following exam techniques:

- **Auscultation**. This is done by listening, such as through a stethoscope.
- **Palpation**. This is done by feeling various parts of the body to find abnormalities.
- **Percussion**. This is done by tapping on various parts of the body, such as the back or chest, to listen to what type of sound the area of the body makes.

The exam may include:

- Questions about any aches, pains, or abnormalities you may be experiencing.

- Examination of various body parts from head to toe to look, feel, and listen for unusual growths or abnormalities in textures, shapes, colors, movements, and sounds.

You should not feel any pressure to undergo a non-emergency surgery. It is not the kind of decision that should be made under pressure. It should be your own decision after you have been sufficiently informed rather than a decision you felt you had to make after going through a process of manipulation.

The motivations a doctor might have to pressure you into undergoing surgery may not line up with your best interests. The doctor may think that he can do a great job on you, but his idea of a great job and your idea of how you would want the result of the surgery to be may not be in sync.

The doctor is the one you should be communicating with, and all your concerns and expectations should be very clear. Many patients who have had a bad experience with surgery later found that they were misinformed, misguided, or lied to by the doctor or the doctor's staff.

Ignore promises made by the doctor's staff. They may be receiving a bonus for bringing in business. The staff might not have any medical training, and no special training is required for a person to work in the front office of a medical center or doctor's office. It is inappropriate for any office staffperson to try to diagnose the doctor's patients.

At best, the office manager may have attended seminars given by the Medical Group Management Association, but these seminars teach how to manage a medical office, not how to diagnose patients. A person working in a doctor's office may hold a certificate showing that he is a Certified Medical Assistant. This is a certification program that is conducted by the American Association of Medical Assistants in conjunction with the Committee on Allied Health Education and Accreditation of the American Medical Association. The AAMA was founded in 1956. The membership consists of doctor assistants, secretaries, receptionists, bookkeepers, nurses, laboratory personnel, and other individuals who work in medical facilities. Only a very small percentage of medical workers are members of the AAMA.

You may come across a doctor who wants total control, is not interested enough in what you have to say, thinks he knows what is best for you, and gives everyone the same alteration regardless of the patient's individual needs.

Is the doctor listening to what you say, or his he trying to get you to say what he wants to hear so that he may diagnose you with the health problem with which he is most familiar?

Are you telling the doctor what you want him to hear so he may diagnose you with the medical problem you think you have, or are you telling him the truth?

•

Your reason for consulting with a surgeon may be that you want him to advise you on what you want done. And you may be hoping to find one that has a good idea of what surgical change, if any, will and will not be right for you. But if a doctor takes control and immediately starts taking snapshots of you and examining you here and there without asking you what your concerns and ideas are, the doctor may have his own ideas of what should be done to you or is in a hurry to get from patient to patient so he can attain his financial goals. This doctor may end up doing things to you other than what you had in mind and may try to talk you into other procedures or a more involved operation than you originally wanted — simply so that he can make more money.

Suggestions from a doctor that you also have a second procedure done during an operation "while we are in there" can sometimes be translated into, "Hey, I don't have enough experience doing this particular procedure, so why don't you let me try it out on you?" If you realize you are in the presence of this type of ambitious doctor, the best thing that you can do for yourself is to leave.

You should be comfortable while you are having your discussion with the doctor and he should not have you lying on your back or situated in some uncomfortable position when he is not examining you. You might feel vulnerable if you are sitting disrobed or in some flimsy medical gown. If the exam is obviously over and you need to speak with the doctor further, tell him you would like to get dressed and would like to speak to him afterward. This will also give you a couple of minutes alone to think of anything you need to speak to the doctor about.

•

Before doctors or nurses touch you, they should wash their hands — preferably while you are in the room so that you can see them do it. Medical people dealing with ailing patients handle such things as wound dressing, urine samples, syringes, needles, and other people. To help prevent the spread of germs, doctors and nurses should wash their hands after every patient visit and wear gloves to protect both themselves and the patients.

•

If you are undergoing a physical exam, you have the right to have a third person present with you in the room. This may be someone you bring with you or a nurse or other employee of the doctor.

During the consultation or at any time when you are being examined and you do not understand what he is doing, ask the doctor or nurse. Not to be rude, but to be sure that nothing is done to you that you do not want done and that you do not want to be billed for. If he seems to be busy or is not interested in answering you, stop him from doing what he is doing; if you have to, tell him to take his hands off you and remind him that you want an explanation of what is being done. His explanation may tell you that he was doing something or planning to do something to you that is not in your best interest.

Some doctors have autographed "grip 'n' grin" (shake hands and smile for the camera) photographs of celebrities hanging on their office walls. This does not mean that the doctor has operated on the celebrity. The doctor may be implying that he operated on the celebrity so that you are brought to believe that if the celebrity has trusted his or her body or face to the surgeon, the surgeon must be good. However, anyone with the right connections can get autographed photos of celebrities. If the photo is of the doctor standing with the celebrity, it may have been taken at some social event and the doctor paid the photographer for a copy of the photograph, or the doctor received the photo in appreciation for a donation he made to a charity in which the celebrity is involved. Do not base your decision to employ the doctor on the impressiveness of his connections. Even some celebrities have had careless surgery performed on them.

Second Opinions

While physicians usually agree on whether surgery is unwarranted, they do not always agree on whether surgery is the best course of action when there are effective alternative treatments available. In all cases, you, as a patient, are entitled to know the range of choices available to you, to have those choices objectively considered by more than one professional, and to have your own preferences considered before undergoing an elective surgical procedure.

You should feel free to ask . . . questions. Once you have the answers, you will be better prepared to make a decision. Do not be hesitant to seek a second opinion. It is an acceptable medical practice. Most doctors want their patients to be as informed as possible about their condition.

You should consider getting a second opinion whenever the surgery is not required for an emergency condition, and it is up to you to decide when and if you will have it.

A second opinion generally is not appropriate when the surgery is required on an emergency basis and to delay it could be life-threatening. For example, cases of acute appendicitis or injuries from an accident are considered emergencies.
> — From the US Department of Health and Human Services Healthcare Financing Administration pamphlet *Medicare: Coverage For Second Surgical Opinions*

Just because a doctor agrees to operate on you does not always mean that you need an operation, or that you will benefit from one.

A good doctor will not be insulted if you go to another doctor and ask for a second opinion. Getting a second opinion protects both you and the doctor. Some doctors will give you a list of doctors practicing the same specialty. Beware that he may send you to his friend, possibly already set up to give certain advice. It is better to pick the doctor yourself, or ask your family physician or insurance plan to refer you to a doctor for a second opinion.

Evidence suggests that when medical practitioners are aware that their surgical recommendations will be reviewed fewer surgical procedures are recommended.
> — *Second Opinion Elective Surgery*, by Eugene G. McCarthy, Madelon Lubin Finkel, and Hirsch S. Ruchlin; Auburn House Publishing, 1981

Before undergoing elective surgery, remember these seven things:
1. Get a second opinion even if you like and trust the doctor.
2. Get a second opinion even if you agree with the doctor.
3. Get a second opinion from a doctor who is financially unconnected to the first doctor.
4. Get a second opinion from a doctor who may not be a surgeon but who is knowledgeable in the area of your health concern.
   Surgeons are taught to perform surgery. If you go to another surgeon, he may also recommend surgery. Getting a second opinion from a nonsurgeon doctor may be helpful.
5. Get a second opinion even if you have to pay for it out of your own pocket.
6. Do not forget to get a second opinion.
7. If you are not satisfied after the second opinion, get a third opinion.

There are at least three sides to every story. Many people recommend that you get not only a second opinion, but also a third, and even a fourth opinion — especially if the first two doctors have disagreed with each other and if you are dealing with a major medical decision. A second opinion can help you feel confident about your final decision.

Many insurance plans will cover second surgical opinions as long as it is for the treatment of a condition covered by the insurance. Your insurance carrier may also require you to get a second surgical opinion. They also may pay for a third opinion if the first two opinions differ. Contact your health insurance representative for details.

•

Some people do not feel comfortable letting the doctor know that they want a second opinion. However, by informing your doctor that you want to get a second opinion, you can then also ask that your medical records be sent to the physician providing the second opinion. In this way, you may be able to avoid the time, costs and discomfort of having to repeat medical tests. [emphasis added]

When getting a second opinion, you should tell the second doctor the name of the surgical procedure recommended and the types of medical tests you have already had. Even if the second doctor disagrees with the first, you will have information that will help you make a decision. If you are confused by different opinions, you may wish to go back to the first doctor to further discuss your case. Or, you may wish to talk to a third physician.

Second opinions are your right as a patient, and can help you make a better informed decision about non-emergency surgery.

— From the US Department of Health and Human Services Healthcare Financing Administration pamphlet *Medicare: Coverage For Second Surgical Opinions*

•

If it is more timely, convenient, and less costly to transport your medical records, or copies of them, from doctor to doctor yourself, request to do so. Expect the second opinion doctor to review these records and perform some type of physical examination with respect to the health condition that is being talked about.

Talk with Former Patients

It may be helpful to talk with some of the doctor's former patients who have gone through the same operation you are considering. This does not include the office staff, who may have had surgery performed on them by the doctor. The doctor or one of his staff may be able to connect you with a few former patients who are willing to talk freely about their surgery. This can give you an idea of what you are in for and an idea of the possible results. If the surgery was performed on a non-private area, you can see the type of scar caused by the surgical wound. (One cosmetic surgeon in Los Angeles was paying his wife's friends to pose as former patients even though he had never operated on them.)

For a list of organizations that can connect you with other people who are experiencing the same health problem you have, see the *Self-Help Groups* heading in the *Research Resources* section of this book.

Medical Tests

There are thousands of different tests, and new ones are always being developed and becoming available. Doctors and the facilities they own or work for make a lot of money by ordering and performing x-rays, scans, other imaging procedures, and lab tests. Medical testing in the United States is a $430 billion side industry (1993 figure).

The Rand Corporation of Santa Monica, a non-profit research group, believes that as many as one in three medical tests can be considered inappropriate. Many tests are overused. Some are done to prevent lawsuits against doctors or to pay for equipment purchased by the medical group to which the doctor belongs.

Doctors are bombarded with advertising and marketing literature from medical testing equipment manufacturers. Many of the ads allude to the financial benefits a doctor may gain by having the medical testing equipment in his office, where he is more likely to use it and therefore can charge patients more money than if the tests were done elsewhere (*New England Journal of Medicine*, December 6, 1990).

Many testing facilities are doctor-owned. Even when a doctor refers a patient to a separate medical facility, the doctor may receive a commission from the other doctor or facility in a "fee-splitting arrangement" as the referring doctor. A 1991 study by the state of Florida reported that within that state, the number of tests per patient is almost twice as great in doctor-owned labs as in those not owned by doctors.

Laboratory companies compete for business from doctors' offices. This is an area where kickbacks come into play. It is not uncommon for a lab company to purchase some of the equipment used in the doctor's office if it means the doctor will commit to sending his lab specimens to that company. Doctors are often given incentives to order tests. The more money the doctor makes for the lab, the more favors the lab does for the doctor. The favors can come in the form of office supplies, tickets to events, travel, having bills paid, and various gifts.

Though a patient may think it is kind of neat to have some of the high-tech medical gadgets and gizmos used on him, the tests may not be of any benefit to him and the reason he undergoes the test may be so that the person operating the doodad can get more practice. Many of the tests may also be incorrectly interpreted and this can result in unnecessary treatment.

Before a test is done, you should find out:

- What is the test meant to reveal?
- How accurate is the test?

    Accuracy in medical screening tests is important because a test result may inspire the doctor to prescribe medication or recommend surgery. In the case of a patient receiving a drug prescription, the test results prompt the doctor to prescribe a certain type and amount of medication.

- What happens if the test does show that you have a problem?
- Are there other ways to find what the doctor is looking for?

    Many tests may be avoided if the doctor conducts a more thorough physical exam of the patient.

- Does the test require your presence, or are you supposed to supply a specimen (urine, blood, mucus, or tissue)?

    Any tissues removed from the body will go through a preparation and examination that may take several days. If the tissues are removed while the patient is undergoing surgery, the tissues may be frozen and examined by a pathologist in a matter of minutes to determine what may need to be done during the surgery, such as when cancer may be present.

- If the test is invasive, is there a less invasive test that may be helpful?
- Where is the lab work performed?
- Who owns the test equipment?
- Is the test equipment operated by someone who has had special training in operating it properly?

    If the test is performed outside the doctor's office, do not call the lab to try to find out the test results. They cannot legally give you the results. The only person you should rely on to give you your test results is the doctor.

    Patients should always question the accuracy of medical screening tests, especially when the test is performed by an employee of the doctor who may have had no special training to conduct the test, as opposed to a person who is a certified laboratory technician.

- If you need to be present for the test, what should you wear, how long does it take, and what will you be doing during the test?
- Do you need to avoid a certain type of food, or all food, before the test is given or before a specimen is taken?
- Will you have to take any medications before the test?
- Are there any injections given before or during the test?
- Will these medications interfere with your ability to drive yourself home from the test?
- Are there any medications that you are currently taking that could interfere with the test results?
- What are the risks of the test?
- How much does the test cost?
- Does your insurance cover the cost of the test?

Medical tests are not always accurate even when they are positive. For example, a blood test, developed at the Dana Farber Cancer Institute in Boston, which shows elevated levels of a protein called CA-125 is used to detect ovarian cancer, but endometriosis and pregnancy are also associated with CA-125. Additionally, some lab tests are inaccurate because some of the people working in the labs are overworked, sick or not trained properly, or because the equipment they are using is defective.

If a nurse who works for the doctor proceeds to take blood from you or, even worse, arranges for you to get an x-ray before the doctor even sees you, put the breaks on. Ask why the nurse thinks these are necessary. The answer may be that "we do this with all our patients." You are not just another patient. You have your specific health concerns, and others have theirs. You or someone will have to pay for these tests.

One reason you may be told you need an x-ray is that an x-ray is less expensive than another imaging procedure, such as an MRI. Even though the MRI may provide a better picture and does not expose the patient to radiation, the patient is given x-rays, and this decision is based on cost. With more and more patients being covered under HMO programs, the less money spent on the patient, the more money the insurance companies get to keep and the larger the doctors' bonuses for keeping costs to a minimum.

Besides the financial concerns, undergoing an x-ray exposes you to radiation and radiation is cumulative, so it is good to keep exposure to a minimum. Though new technology has reduced the dose of radiation that is needed to obtain x-rays, they should be taken only when they are absolutely necessary and limited to as few exposures as possible. A patient's decision to undergo an x-ray or not should depend on the benefits of the information that may be gained about the patient's condition.

Do not let anyone try to sweet-talk you into the x-ray room. This is true especially for women who have a reason to believe they may be pregnant. X-ray radiation can injure a developing fetus. Many medical offices have x-ray machines that are outdated and may give off more radiation than they should. Those taking the x-rays may not have any special training to operate the equipment. The patient may be getting the x-ray because the doctor makes extra money by giving each patient an x-ray whether the patient needs it or not.

Another reason to avoid this type of situation is that many x-ray machines are old and do not provide a good quality exposure. In this case, even when an x-ray may provide important information, the x-rays will have to be done over on a newer and better quality x-ray machine to obtain a clearer image.

Avoid unnecessary x-rays.

Avoid rushing to get some form of treatment that you know nothing about, that may not be necessary, and that may do more harm than good — especially when the decision to undergo the treatment is based on one set of lab tests, or the opinion of one doctor.

Unless it would be a health threat to delay treatment, when test results come in that the doctor believes indicate that you need some form of treatment, take time to find out what your options are. When possible, especially if the diagnosis shows a serious health problem or the suggested treatment is very invasive, request more tests from a separate lab to lower the chance that the treatment the doctor is suggesting is not based on a false positive. Take these test results with you when you obtain your second opinion.

Whenever you are undergoing a test, avoid talking to the person conducting the test about anything other than the testing procedure being performed. They may be occupied with watching monitors and circuit boards and listening for prompts from the medical machines. If you take his mind away from the procedure he may forget a step and you will end up with an inaccurate test result or the test may have to be repeated.

•

In December 1995, five doctors and one medical testing clinic in Southern California agreed to pay more than $1 million in penalties and restitution for marking up patient lab test bills by as much as 100% and failing to inform patients where tests were performed. The action was the result of an ongoing investigation of illegal medical business practices being conducted by prosecutors in San Diego and Los Angeles counties. The action did not affect the licenses of the doctors.

A 1993 California state law prohibits doctors from marking up the cost of lab testing to justify the costs when no service had been performed. The law also requires doctors to disclose the name and address of the labs where tests were conducted and the cost of the lab tests.

•

Whenever you get a medical test, you should get a copy of the results for your own records.

Medical Records

The forever advancing technology available to government and private companies to collect, store, and use information has brought about the ability to keep personal, consumer, financial, and medical history files on every individual. Various companies and research groups are involved in finding statistics on who uses what products, goes where, when, why, how much, how often, for how long, and for what price. Some of these companies also like to know where you live and your marital status, age, height, weight, race, religion, and even your hair and eye colors.

Some of the computer data collected on you may be inaccurate because your file was mixed with that of another person who has a similar name, address, or Social Security or credit card number. Much of the information, as accurate or inaccurate as it may be with intentional or unintentional errors, can be kept by the company that collected it or sold to another company for a reason other than what you had believed it was for.

Such information storage is legal, and it is used by many organizations to do everything from creating marketing and advertising campaigns to financial, medical, and other types of research, planning, and studies. In addition, law enforcement and other government agencies may use the information for their own needs. Most people would be surprised to see the details such records can include and would probably question how this can affect their privacy. Because these records are in computer memories, this raises the issue of security, as anyone with access to these computers and the codes to operate them may gain access to and alter the records.

It has been the general practice in the medical industry to keep medical files on paper, and much of it in handwritten form. One of the problems with this is that some of the written material may be indecipherable because some doctors have unclear handwriting. Another problem is that this paperwork takes up a large part of the doctors' and nurses' workday.

Computers are now being introduced into more and more hospitals to store clinical data and other patient records. This is expected to cut down on operating costs as it streamlines menial tasks, does away with illegible handwriting, and prevents unnecessary and repetitive testing and medical procedures. It will also make it easier to store medical files in an off-site or out-of-state location in case of a disaster. And it may make patient confidentiality harder to control as the electronic records containing sensitive personal information become accessible to more researchers, government statisticians, drug companies, marketers, and insurance companies.

The largest computerized health information network as of this writing has been developed by Los Angeles-based Healthcare Data Information Corporation and Pacific Bell. It allows health care providers, insurers, and others to electronically exchange information on more than half of all state residents covered by health insurance. HDIC plans to expand the system nationwide and eventually on a global basis sometime after 2000.

Nationally there is a data bank called the Medical Information Bureau (MIB) that is used by hundreds of insurance companies with the belief that it helps guard against fraud. The information is also used to decide whether you are at high risk of having serious (expensive) health problems and therefore not financially desirable to insure. Lawyers also can gain access to this information to be used for or against you in a lawsuit. The data bank includes both medical and non-medical information about you that is gathered when you apply for individual life, health, or disability insurance or file an insurance claim. The MIB may keep a coded report on each individual who has significant underwriting risks that could affect health or longevity. Depending on the information source and the translation of the records, your MIB file may contain inaccuracies, and this could interfere with your insurance eligibility.

Some information from your MIB report may be obtained by writing the bureau. Under a Federal Trade Commission agreement with the MIB, if you have been turned down for insurance, or if your insurance premium has been raised based on information from the MIB, you have thirty days to obtain a free copy of your MIB records. If the originating insurance company believes there is sensitive medical information in your file, the company may require the MIB to send your medical file only to your doctor. The MIB has a set process by which you can correct errors or dispute inconsistencies. (The MIB address is in the *Research Resources* section of this book under the heading *Records*.)

•

> *In my work I have spoken to many, many victims who have brought malpractice cases as well as product liability cases and other lawsuits. I have never heard them complain about the amount of money their lawyer took from their award. I do, however, hear them complain ferociously about the person they are suing and the fact that they delay that case sometimes for years and years and years. Every time they want another document, they have to go back into court to litigate to get that document. It is pulling teeth to go through a lawsuit, generally, against these big corporations or large defense insurance firms.*
> — Pamela Gilbert of Public Citizen's Congress Watch, testifying before subcommittee hearing on issues relating to medical malpractice, May 20, 1993

•

Because physicians and hospitals do not necessarily keep records indefinitely (in Los Angeles some medical centers sell old medical records to companies that provide props to movie and television sets), and there is always the chance of records being lost during office moves and disasters, anyone wanting a copy of his medical records should seek to get his own copies as soon as possible.

Some doctors might require you to send a letter of request before they will supply you with copies of your files. Although most doctors will provide you with your records, some records can be legally kept from you. Obtaining your records may be difficult because each state has its own set of medical records disclosure laws. Some doctors may tell you that you do not need to keep records and this could be because the doctor is trying to protect himself. He may also feel that you are doubting his diagnosis and suggested therapies. If you request a copy of your records from a doctor with whom you are disappointed, the doctor may have his staff tell you they misplaced your file because he may think you are going to sue him, or they may only provide a select portion of the records. Some doctors might delay giving you copies of your records so they have time to alter any information that could be used in a malpractice lawsuit.

Contact the file clerk or medical record librarian of each institution (hospital, ambulatory surgery center, or doctor's office) where you have received treatment (for some good reasons, separate laws govern those records kept for mental health purposes and may not be available to you).

Medical records can include:
- Your medical history form including information on
  - Injuries you suffered and how they were treated.
  - Major illnesses and how they were treated.
  - Inherited disorders.
  - Health problems of your parents and siblings.
  - Medications you have taken.
  - The names of doctors who have treated you and the names of medical facilities where you have received treatment.
  - Your age, weight, height, and other physical characteristics.
- Consultation forms.
- Doctors' notes and order sheets.
- Diagnostic images of the bones, organs, tissues, and blood vessels.
    These images may be made by using various image-producing machinery, such as X-rays made with the use of ionizing radiation, MRIs made with the use of magnetic pulse sequences, and ultrasound images made with the use of sound waves.
- Videos of your tests or actual surgery.
  - Some diagnostic imaging tests are performed with the use of radiopharmaceuticals. This radioactive matter is injected, inhaled, or taken through the mouth. Imaging devices are then used to follow the matter and record the distribution, flow, and concentration of the material in the body. The image of the material in the body can be projected onto a screen and recorded on a videotape.
    Radiopharmaceuticals are often used to help diagnose diseases in, and injuries to, such organs as the kidneys, heart, pancreas, liver, brain, thyroid, gastrointestinal system, lungs, and spleen.
  - Fiber optic cameras can be used to film the inside of the body during diagnostic tests or surgery.

- Sonography (ultrasound) uses high-frequency soundwaves to create images on a screen and this can be recorded on film or videotape.
- Lab results and pathology reports.
- Hospital admission and discharge paperwork.
- Nursing care records/nursing documentation and flow sheets/progress notes.
- Operating room reports that tell
  - What anesthetic agents were used.
  - What procedure was performed on you.
  - What techniques were used.
  - The length of time it took to complete the surgery.
  - Information about the success of each step of the surgery.
- Prescription records.
- Letters among doctors, lawyers, and medical facilities.

    Even if you are successful in obtaining your records, you may not be able to read everything on them. Besides the common abbreviations, the doctor may have his own set of abbreviations that only he and his office staff understand. Some doctors use a variety of colored stickers on patient records. These might be used to protect your privacy. One colored sticker may mean that you are pregnant and you do not want anyone to know. Another colored sticker may mean that the file contains information regarding the sex of your unborn child that you do not want revealed to you. Another colored sticker may signal that you have a contagious disease. Various other stickers, markings, and "office esoterics" may mean that you are a problem patient, or that you have a tendency to talk too much. But do not be offended if you see the abbreviation "SOB" on your record. That simply means that you experienced some "shortness of breath."

    Keep personal copies of your health records in a safe place where they have little chance of being damaged or misplaced. Keeping track of your health history is good not only for you; it also can be valuable to people who are related to you as there may be a genetic link to your health problems.

    For more on medical records, order the book *Medical Records: Getting Yours,* by Bruce Samuels and Sidney Wolfe, published by Public Citizen's Health Research Group. See the *Records* heading in the *Research Resources* section of this book for ordering information.

Price

The price of each surgery depends on the amount of money the doctor wants for his time and service (doctors set their own prices — if the treatment is done in agreement with a health plan, the insurance company may have a pre-set price agreement with the doctor), the type of procedure being performed, the amount and complexity of work being done, the surgical team needed to perform the surgery, the complexity of the operation, where the surgery is performed, the type of drugs and anesthesia and other medical supplies and care needed for the recovery.

Methods of payment for healthcare

- The way the doctor is paid may dictate what kind of treatment you receive.
- If you carry health insurance, the doctor may be receiving a set amount of money for each patient he treats, for each procedure he performs, a set salary, or some combination of these. Some doctors enjoy getting paid on salary because they believe it allows them to have a more normal life. On the other hand, many doctors do not like the situation that HMOs have introduced in which medicine is run in a manner of a tightly controlled business and patients are limited to a closed network of doctors and hospitals. The particular gripe many doctors have has to do with the doctors being paid a salary and being second-guessed by the insurance companies whenever they prescribe a special treatment to a patient or want to keep a patient in a hospital for longer than the insurance company says is necessary.
- You may be going to a primary (gatekeeper) doctor for all your health needs unless you need care from a medical specialist. To see a specialist and get the insurance company to pay its share of the cost, you will have to get the approval of the insurance company.
- The doctor who receives a flat fee from an insurance company for each patient may do fewer procedures, because he does not get paid extra for performing more procedures since the incentive is to do less. If you need a procedure that the insurance refuses to pay for, you and your doctor may have to fight the insurance company to try to get the insurance company to pay for it. A doctor also may not spend as much time with each patient conducting interviews and examinations because he does not get paid any more to spend extra time with the patients.
- The doctor who gets paid by the insurance company may be encouraged by the insurance company to keep costs down and be rewarded for doing so at the end of the year by receiving a financial bonus. This bonus may come from a "shared risk pool" of money the insurance company has established for special testing and specialist care patients under the insurance plan may need. At the end of the year, the remaining money in the pool is split up and distributed as bonuses to the doctors under contract with the insurance plan.
- There are many insurance plans and each one has its own set of rules and payment plans.
- If you are paying the doctor out of your own pocket, then you are getting charged for each procedure — and the more procedures the doctor performs and the more time you spend with him, the more money he makes.

Although the doctor who charges the highest price is not necessarily the best, a patient should be very cautious about trusting his body to the lowest bidder. The doctor who charges the least may be cutting corners to offer the lowest price, which may mean a certain level of the safety and quality is also being sacrificed. The medical team, if there is one, that works with the doctor may also lack the quality of education necessary to provide the care the patient needs. On the other hand, the doctor who charges the most may be interested in nothing other than making a profit.

If there is more than one procedure done at once, or even at a different date, the doctor — or the person in his office who handles the financial arrangements — will usually give the patient a lower package price than what he would have charged for two operations that are done separately. Because the person is already under anesthesia and needs no extra preparation, two procedures done at the same time are usually less expensive.

> *After I was in a car accident that ruptured my spleen, I spent a week in the hospital trying to get better while my doctor fended off this other doctor who wanted to remove my spleen. He was there with one hand out ready to take money and a scalpel in the other hand ready to operate. When they sent me the bill, I couldn't believe how much it was padded. There were charges for tests that were never taken and charges for equipment that was never used. Out of a $6,000 or $7,000 bill there were hundreds of dollars in charges for stuff that was never done. Even though my insurance paid for everything but $2 of the bill I didn't want to screw my insurance company out of their money. Through my church, I knew one of the men who was on the hospital's board of directors and I asked him what was going on. He said, "We have to make up for the people who don't pay."*
> — A Los Angeles woman

Some doctors will perform additional procedures during an operation without the patient's consent, and then charge the patient for it.

Many doctors would rather have nothing to do with discussing fees with patients and leave financial arrangements up to the office staff. If you have questions about the price you are going to pay for the surgery or other financial matters, talk to the person in the doctor's office who handles the financial arrangements. They may know more about the payments you will make than the doctor does.

Call the insurance company to tell them what surgery you are considering, and they will tell you what portion, if any, of the operation they might cover. Depending on the type of operation, the expense might be eligible to be taken as an itemized tax deduction.

See the *Billing Problems* heading in the Research Resources section of this book for more information on billing problems.

Payment

> *STARK: Can I give you one little bit of testimony we had once not so long ago. Guess who are the biggest users by half, more than all the other people combined of collection attorneys? Guess who uses collection attorneys more than any other group in the country combined? I don't want to lead you, just guess. Would you guess it was doctors or hospitals?*
>
> *GILBERT: Either one.*
>
> *STARK: More lawsuits for collection are brought by doctors and hospitals than any other group of people combined in this country. So when it comes to suing a patient, to provide the money, they don't wait a minute. But when it comes to the reverse, they are in here pleading poverty and crying all over the place. Very interesting.*
>
> — Dialogue between Congressman Pete Stark and Pamela Gilbert, Public Citizen's Congress Watch, during Congressional subcommittee hearing on issues relating to medical malpractice, May 20, 1993

Payment is nearly always required in advance of the surgery by way of insurance, cash, credit, or other payment arrangements with the doctor. Some insurance plans will cover part or all of certain elective surgery procedures, depending on what they are and why they are being done.

8 • PROCEEDING WITH SURGERY

Blood

The doctor should be made aware of your blood type. It should be written in all your medical records. Receiving the wrong blood type can kill you. Transplanted organs and tissues also need to originate from a person with the same blood type as the receiver.

Several days before you undergo surgery you will have some of your blood taken and tests will be performed on this. These tests will be done to determine the blood count, chemistry, sugar level, liver and kidney function, cholesterol level, lipid content, and clotting ability. The tests can identify abnormalities, such as diabetes, liver and kidney disease, anemia, thyroid or parathyroid problems, heart disease risk factors, and nutritional deficiencies. Most blood is now tested for 24 results using a machine called a Sequential Multi-Analysis Computer.

Emergency surgery and some medical conditions account for the majority of transfusions. For this, a public blood supply is maintained. Most types of planned surgery patients generally lose so little blood that they do not need blood transfusions. Few plastic surgery procedures require any type of blood donation. If a blood donation is needed, there are questions that should be asked and precautions to take.

A "team approach" with your doctor, the blood collection facility, and you, the patient, is needed to determine what the safest transfusion procedure is that may be taken.

Seven Important Questions to Ask Your Doctor (before undergoing surgery):
1. *Will I need blood for my operation?*
2. *Can I give blood in advance in case I need it?*
3. *Is there enough time before the operation to give the blood I will need?*
4. *Where should I go to give blood for my operation?*
5. *Can my blood be saved during the operation and given back to me if I need it?*
6. *What are the risks in giving or receiving my own blood?*
7. *Will I have to pay extra if I use my own blood?*
   — From the publication *Your Operation — Your Blood,* by the National Heart, Lung, and Blood Institute, a branch of the National Institutes of Health

Some of the more common operations in which enough blood will be lost to require transfusing are orthopedic, cardiac, chest, gynecological, and blood vessel surgery. Under rare circumstances blood transfusion may also be needed during pregnancy and delivery.

The procedure where a person donates blood before getting an operation is called "autologous" blood donation (blood intended for use by someone other than the donor is known as "homologous"). It is based on the fact that donating before surgery, and receiving your own blood during and after surgery, is better and safer than receiving someone else's blood.

Some advantages to donating one's own blood for later use are
- Reduced risk of infectious disease transmission.
- Reduced risk of transfusion reactions related to differences between donor and recipient, such as blood type.
- More rapid replacement by your body of blood lost during surgery, since the bone marrow where blood cells form has already been activated by the process of donating blood.
- Less demand on the community blood supply.

In autologous donation, a person can often give one unit of blood a week for up to six weeks, depending on the anticipated need. Each unit is just under a pint and is about 10% of the total blood supply of an average-size adult. The last donation is usually made no closer than three days before the scheduled surgery. This allows the body time to replenish the fluid that has been removed. It is possible that iron supplements may be prescribed to build up the number of red blood cells to avoid anemia.

As public interest in blood donations has increased, a number of entrepreneurs have entered the market. These facilities will — at their locations around the country — collect, freeze, and store your blood, and then deliver it to you — thawed and ready to use — when and if your physician calls for it.

Costs can be high, and shipping charges may be added. There is no guarantee the blood would be available when needed or that there would be time to thaw and ship it. (Under present FDA regulations, frozen blood may be kept for only 10 years and cannot be shipped between states.) In addition, frozen blood contains only red blood cells. If you need blood platelets or plasma, you may have to turn to the public blood supply. (As liquid blood, the donated units can be kept for up to 42 days, depending on the preservative used.)

— From *Who Donates Better Blood for You Than You? FDA Consumer Magazine*

About 2,500 gallons of blood pass through the heart every day. An average size man has about 5.5 quarts of blood and an average size woman has about 3.5 quarts. During surgery the volume of blood in the body must be maintained.

Hematocrit level is a measure of red blood cells. During surgery if the level falls below a certain mark, a transfusion is needed.

A depletion in the volume of blood in the circulatory system can lower blood pressure and threaten the delivery of oxygen and the removal of waste products from the vital organs. A sustained flow of minimal blood flow, called shock, can lead to infection, irreversible organ damage — including damage to the brain, and death.

Losing one quart of blood is usually enough to send an average size man into shock.

If blood pressure is too high, blood clots can be dislodged and this can contribute to more bleeding.

When an operation is being performed that causes a large amount of blood loss, autotransfusion devices can sometimes be used to collect the patient's own blood shed during surgery and return it back into his body. This is called "blood salvage" or "intraoperative blood collection and reinfusion," and is often done during heart, vascular, and orthopedic surgeries, solid organ transplants, and other very complicated operations. The amount of blood recovered during surgery varies with the operative procedure, but may amount to 50% or more of the blood lost. Blood salvage is not done with patients who have infections (because there is no existing system that can effectively clean the blood), cancer (because of a risk of transferring malignant cells to another location), or other risk factors.

Two ways of salvaging blood and reinfusing it into the body exist. The first is to reinfuse the blood after mixing it with an anticoagulant. The second is to clean the blood with special equipment before reinfusing it. The fastest of these models processes a unit of salvaged blood in just a few minutes. The process that cleans the blood may be safer than the one where the blood is not cleaned because cleaning the blood can remove tiny bits of tissue and other debris introduced into the blood during the surgical procedure. When blood is salvaged during surgery, a specially trained person whose job is to run the machinery that treats the salvaged blood is required to be present, with no other responsibilities during the surgery.

Sometimes blood is collected after surgery through the use of drains located at the surgical sites and reinfused without being processed.

Another form of self-donation is called "acute normovolemic hemodilution." This is done by drawing blood from the patient before surgery and immediately infusing the patient with fluids to compensate for the blood that has been removed. The blood is collected into labeled blood bags and mixed with an anticoagulant. It can then be stored at room temperature for up to four hours or refrigerated if more time is needed. After the surgery the patient is reinfused with the blood that was drawn. This preserves red blood cells by preventing them from being lost through bleeding during surgery. The procedure is usually performed by the attending anesthesiologist. Some in the medical community question the safety of this procedure.

Some items to consider if you are going to need to receive blood during a surgery and you are going to donate your own blood:

- You may not be able to donate blood if you are on certain medications, you have an infection, you have abnormal blood pressure, you have cardiovascular disease, or you are otherwise weak or ill.
- You may need more blood than the doctor predicts.
- One surgery might not be enough to correct what the surgery is meant to correct.
- You might have complications that could require further surgery.
- The blood you donate might be contaminated after you donated it because of a lab accident or neglect.
- The blood you donate might be mislabeled.
- Some relatively rare cases have occurred wherein people have contracted blood-related illnesses from donated blood when they received donated blood after autologous donations were used up.
- Those seeking to avoid a blood transfusion may opt for injections of erythropoetin to stimulate the bone marrow to produce more red blood cells. The injections may start a few weeks before the surgery. Vitamins and iron supplements will be given to help build a strong blood base.
- If you are having blood tests to help diagnose your condition, each time blood is taken from you in the week before you undergo surgery, the greater your chance of becoming anemic and requiring a blood transfusion during surgery.
- A doctor may not operate on you if you become anemic, unless you receive a blood transfusion to raise your blood counts.
- Depending on the facility where your blood is stored, unused autologous donations may be discarded upon your release from the hospital, or may be stored until the blood is expired. Your interests might best be served if the blood is kept until it expires in case you need it. Find out what the policy is at the facility you are dealing with. Extended storage can usually be arranged.

Hepatitis

There are at least eight types of viral hepatitis. These include hepatitis A, hepatitis B, hepatitis C, hepatitis D, and hepatitis E. Symptoms of hepatitis infection include flu-like illnesses, such as mild fever, aches, vomiting, nausea, and fatigue. Jaundice may develop, but most people with hepatitis do not develop jaundice.

Before blood is transfused, it is tested for viruses of hepatitis B and C, and for signs of abnormal liver function. The presence of the hepatitis B virus can be identified with a simple blood test. Because hepatitis D is only present when hepatitis B is present, a blood test for an antibody to hepatitis D, along with a positive test for the hepatitis B virus, must be positive to show that hepatitis D is present. According to the American Liver Foundation, this testing has reduced transfusion of hepatitis C to

.5%. According to the Centers for Disease Control, testing has reduced the risk of contracting hepatitis B to 1 in 200,000. These blood tests are not usually included in routine blood tests done when a person is having a physical exam but are performed when a person donates blood.

- The hepatitis A and hepatitis E viruses are excreted in feces. Direct or indirect contact with the contaminant through unsanitary conditions spreads the virus. According to the American Liver Foundation, hepatitis A is rarely transmitted through blood transfusion. The vaccine for hepatitis A may be effective for more than four years.

- Hepatitis B is the most common strain of hepatitis. There are believed to be over one million people infected with it in the US, and 300 million carriers worldwide. The hepatitis B virus is more infectious than HIV (though more people die of AIDS), and is transmitted through infected blood and other body fluids. The hepatitis B vaccine provides immunity from hepatitis B for most people for at least five years. When the anti Hbs (antibody to hepatitis B surface antigen)test is positive or reactive, it means the person has recovered from past infection, will not get it again, and therefore cannot pass it on to others. The only treatment for hepatitis B is interferon, which may permanently eliminate the virus in about one-third of patients.

- Hepatitis C was discovered in 1987. It is spread through blood and is more likely to be transferred in a blood transfusion than other types of hepatitis. There is a very low risk of transmitting the hepatitis C through sexual contact. The hepatitis C virus is most common in underdeveloped countries, in Africa, and the area around the Indian Ocean. Alcoholics may be at a greater risk of becoming infected with the hepatitis C virus and of progressing to chronic liver disease than non-alcoholics.

- The hepatitis D virus is spread through blood and is often found in intravenous drug users. The hepatitis B virus must be present for the hepatitis D virus to spread.

- At the time of this writing, a test for the hepatitis E virus had not been developed. There is also no vaccine for hepatitis E.

- Those with hepatitis should not donate blood, plasma, body organs, tissue, or sperm.

- The viruses of hepatitis B, hepatitis C, and hepatitis D may remain in the body forever. According to the American Liver Foundation, about 90% of adults recover from hepatitis B in a few months, clearing the virus from their systems and developing an immunity. They will never get hepatitis B again; however, their blood test will always show that they had been infected and blood centers will not accept their blood. This is because there is a very small chance that the test results are "false positive" for the immunity and the person might still be infected. A carrier is infectious even though he has no signs or symptoms and should never have unprotected sex unless the other person is immune to hepatitis B, or has been vaccinated. Those who do not clear the infection from their bodies become carriers or are chronically infected with hepatitis. Chronic carriers of hepatitis B or hepatitis C may progress to chronic liver disease, cirrhosis, and possibly liver cancer.

There are currently more ways to test blood than ever before. This has made today's blood supply safer than at any time in the past. But blood reinfusion (receiving your own blood) remains the safest option.

- The FDA has said that an allergic reaction to transfusion is as high as 1 in 25.
- Most Americans and many doctors think that the risk of transferring the AIDS virus is much higher than it actually is.
- The FDA has said that blood harboring HIV sometimes gets through the testing system — 1 in 61,000 to 1 in 225,000 transfusions. The American Red Cross has said it may be 1 in 500,000 units of blood.
- According to the FDA, blood with the hepatitis C virus is believed to still be a risk in about 1 in 900 transfusions.
- Blood taken from people who are infected with dangerous viruses can test clean because the tests actually screen for antibodies and not for the actual virus, and the body can take weeks or months to start producing antibodies after a person is infected.
- Not all viruses have been discovered.
- There is no solid screening test for a toxic bacterium called yersinia which can cause massive blood clots.
- Most blood banks are not required to be federally licensed and are not required to report mistakes to the FDA.
- The FDA records several thousand blood bank errors every year, including mislabeling of blood with the wrong blood type, inaccurate or inadequate blood testing, and improper storage.
- Some blood products used in America are imported from other countries where testing procedures may not have been performed properly.
- The possibility of lawsuits being filed against them is a serious consideration, when blood banks and medical facilities learn that a patient may have received tainted blood; they do not always notify the patients even if they know who the patients are and how to contact them.

Other blood facts:
- The process of donating blood stimulates the bone marrow to produce more blood cells.
- It takes the body about 24 hours to replace the fluid lost during donation of one unit of blood, but up to two months to replenish the supply of red blood cells contained in that unit. Taking iron supplements can assist the body in replacing blood cells faster.
- Red blood cells survive for about 110 days.
- Liquid blood can be stored for 42 days.
- Frozen blood can be stored for ten years.
- A unit of blood is just under a pint.

- The average person carries about ten units of blood and a healthy person can quickly recover from the loss of 10% of his blood volume.
- When donating for autologous collection, the last donation is usually collected no later than 72 hours before surgery.
- Many patients can give blood as frequently as every three days, although once a week is most common when donating for autologous purposes.
- Some patients, such as those needing cardiovascular surgery, may risk deterioration of their condition if they delay surgery in order to donate autologous blood. The risk of contracting a contagious disease through America's donated blood is generally very slim. In cases where a patient is delaying needed surgery where the health condition is deteriorating, a greater risk is created than any presented by receiving blood from another person.

The only blood substitute currently approved by the FDA is Flousol-DA 20%. It carries only a fourth of the oxygen that real blood carries. Researchers are trying to develop a blood substitute that carries a higher amount of oxygen.

Consent Forms

Some patients are rudely surprised when they end up with much more done to them than they ever desired and the doctor thinks he did them a "favor." To prevent such surprises a patient should make sure he knows what the doctor plans to do to him, and everything agreed to and things not agreed to should be detailed in the consent form. Give them an inch and they may take a foot (or too much bone, cartilage, organs, or skin).

> *Once they sign those consent forms we can do whatever we want to them. We have all power.*
>
> — Said by a Beverly Hills plastic surgeon when he was asked what he thought of some plastic surgeons who do more than the patient wanted done

The influence of lawyers is seen throughout the medical world — especially with consent forms. Consent forms are designed by lawyers to protect doctors. The consent form may have been supplied to the doctor by his malpractice insurance company, the hospital, the HMO he works for, or by one of the associations he belongs to. If you are going to be operated on at a medical facility that is not owned by the doctor, the facility will likely have a separate consent form to release the facility from any liability caused by the medical professionals who are treating you.

The reasoning for the existence of consent forms is simple: Doctors and medical facilities want to protect themselves. This reasoning should also be held by the patient — a patient should make sure he is not signing something that may allow room for harm, or provide a way for doctors to do whatever they want to the patient.

•

The consent forms most doctors use are pretty standard and include spaces for the name of the patient, the name of the doctor, the date, the address of the facility where the procedure is being done, and the type of procedure being performed. The form may also ask for the patient's permission to let the doctor use any photos or videos taken during the surgery for educational or promotional purposes.

•

A doctor should never override a decision you made about your health. If he does something to you that you told him not to do, he is violating your basic human rights.

•

Some doctors will tell their patients that the consent form is not negotiable and the wording cannot be changed. This is untrue. Consent forms are well thought out and written in the interest of the doctor. They are not what some patients think: Forms that provide a way for the patient to be involved with his medical decisions. A patient can turn the tables and make a few changes that will ensure the consent form also protects him. It is the legal right of the patient to cross out anything he wants on any informed consent document he is asked to sign. For this reason, a consent form should not be shoved under a patient's nose minutes before he is to walk into a surgery room to undergo elective surgery.

•

Signing the consent form:
- If you do not clearly understand what it is the doctor intends to do to you, do not sign the consent form.
- Never sign a blank consent form.
- Do not sign anything you are not comfortable with and never sign anything that you do not understand.
- Always ask questions about what you do not understand.
- Look for risks listed on the consent form that your doctor did not mention.
- Do not sign a consent form if you are under the influence of mind-altering drugs.
- Being ill can interfere with your state of mind and judgment. It is best to have a relative or close friend with you who can help evaluate the consequences of the consent form.
- You are under no obligation to undergo the surgery, even if you have already put the money down and signed the consent form. Money can be returned; surgically removed body parts cannot.

Because the use of consent forms has been abused and because elective surgery is planned and scheduled days, weeks, or months in advance, a person planning to undergo elective surgery can obtain an unsigned copy of the consent form from the doctor's office days, or weeks, before the surgery. This will give the patient time to read it over, clear up any questions he has about the wording used on the consent form, and make sure that the operation described on the consent form is in fact the operation that the patient was planning on having, and nothing more. It may be helpful to seek the advice of a separate doctor who will not make money if the patient does undergo the operation, or a lawyer can help compose the consent form to suit the desires and needs of the patient.

The actions you take concerning the consent form all depend on how safe you want to be. You may want to have the consent form re-typed to include any of the changes you request, and, within reason, you should state what it is you do and do not want done.

Most doctors are nowhere to be found when it is time for a patient to sign the consent form, as getting the signature of the patient is a chore the doctor usually leaves this chore up to the office staff. When the patient has questions about the consent form, he should speak to the doctor, not the office staff, and should have the doctor explain anything and everything on the consent form that the patient does not understand. The doctor must know about and agree to the modifications before the patient signs the consent from. A patient should never settle for a verbal modification to the consent form.

Doubts about surgery should be cleared up before surgery. Afterward is too late.

You do not want the doctor to have the freedom to do whatever he feels like doing. Do not sign a consent form that contains any type of wording that gives the doctor and his staff freedom to make additional changes to your body above and beyond what you agreed to.

A consent form should never be signed by a patient who has taken a mind-altering drug, such as a pain killer, muscle relaxer, or sedative.

A patient who is under the age of eighteen will need to have a parent or legal guardian sign the consent form, unless the patient is married or is a parent. The family may also give consent for a patient who is incapacitated.

Where the Surgery Is Performed

No hospital review board verifies the quality of these surgeons' work. No one guarantees whether the "operating room" has even basic life support equipment. No one ensures that the doctor has good, qualified staff to give anesthetic, to monitor the patient, and to respond quickly should complications arise.

• • •

Even normal Government and private audit systems are absent, since, in most instances, these surgeries are covered neither by Medicare nor private health insurance.

— Congressman Ron Wyden, during Congressional subcommittee hearings on plastic surgery industry, speaking about surgery done in doctors' offices, 1989

Surgery is normally performed in one of these three locations:
1. A hospital.
2. An ambulatory surgical care center.
3. An office surgery room.

Elective surgery often takes place outside of hospitals, such as a doctor's office operating room. Therefore, these surgeries are not supervised by anyone other than the doctor, and are performed to his standards. This leaves the doctor to determine what will serve as an operating room. There is also no one required to check up on the quality of the doctor's office staff and surgical team, and no one to see if the equipment is properly sterilized, or if the operating room is a safe place to perform the surgeries.

Some doctors voluntarily pay a fee to have their surgery sites accredited by the Association for Ambulatory Healthcare, or the American Association for Accreditation of Ambulatory Plastic Surgery Facilities. This can show that the doctor has taken some steps to protect your safety, and that the operating room meets certain standards.

Requirements for standards where surgery takes place vary from state to state. For instance, in California, legislation (Assembly Bill 595) was signed into law on September 30, 1994 and requires accreditation for any setting in that state where surgery is performed with sedation or general anesthesia. The law gave facilities until July 1, 1996 to comply with the accreditation process. Accreditation certificates will be valid for three years. By calling the state Division of Medical Quality of the Medical Board of California, patients in California may find out if a surgery setting is accredited, certified, or licensed, or whether the setting's accreditation, certification, or license has been revoked.

Before you decide to undergo elective surgery, check up on the location of the surgery, and see if this site has been approved by one of the associations listed above. If the surgery is to take place in a hospital, check to see if the hospital has been accredited by Medicare, or the Joint Commission on Accreditation of Healthcare Organizations — see the *Accrediting Healthcare Facilities* heading in the *Research Resources* section of this book.

When outpatient surgery takes place, the doctor should have an emergency transfer agreement with a local hospital in case there is a complication during the surgery. There should also be well-maintained medical equipment, including a pulse oximeter to monitor the patient's vital signs during the surgery. The patient should also make sure there will be a nurse present during the operation — no doctor should perform elective surgery unassisted. If anesthesia is needed, an anesthesiologist or an anesthetist should be present before, during, and after the surgery.

If your surgery is to be performed in a teaching hospital, there may be students involved in the procedure and involved in other parts of your care at the hospital. Make sure the doctor you approve of is the one performing the procedure — or at least present and very involved in and closely supervising the procedure (who treats you is your decision). A teaching hospital will likely have the most recent medical equipment, and the staff is more likely to have up-to-date medical training. A non-teaching hospital may also have updated equipment, and there you are less likely to have students involved in your care.

Even if the surgery is to be done in the doctor's office or other independent operating facility, make sure the doctor has permission to perform the operation in a nearby hospital. To operate in a hospital, a doctor's credentials are reviewed by a credentials committee. A doctor who has gone through the credential and training background check is a safer bet than one who has not.

For more information on preparing for surgery, see the *Strategic Planning* section in this book.

Informing the Surgery Team

Before undergoing surgery, the surgery team should be made aware of the following:
- Your past and present drug use. This includes recreational drugs, drugs prescribed by a doctor, and over-the-counter medications.

  The doctor should also be told of any vitamin or nutritional supplements and herbs you are taking.

  Some drugs and supplements may have to be stopped before surgery. Others may need to be changed.
- If you know that you have an allergy to a specific drug.

- All your past and present health problems including
  - If you have had surgery before, what it was for, when it was done, and if there were any complications.
  - Any heart conditions, such as heart failure, heart attack, heart murmur, or mitral valve prolapse.
  - If you have kidney disease.
  - If you have a history of fainting.
  - If you have a hiatal hernia.
  - If you have ulcers.
  - If you have a history of bleeding problems.
  - If you have recently donated blood.
  - If you have had a blood transfusion, and if you had an allergic reaction to it.
  - If you know that you have antibodies against red blood corpuscles or red cells.
  - If you are a diabetic.
  - If you, or anyone in your family, has sickle-cell trait.
  - If there is any possibility of pregnancy, and the date of the last menstrual period.
  - If you have been pregnant within the last several months.
  - If you have ever experienced a seizure, and if you have epilepsy.
  - If you have Rh disease.
  - If you have had rheumatic fever.
  - If you have had tuberculosis.
  - If you have bronchitis.
  - If you have asthma, and if you have ever been treated at an emergency room for asthma.
  - If you currently have, or recently experienced, a cold or flu.
  - If you have back or neck problems, pain, or injuries.
  - If you have ever experienced an allergy to latex. If you have, latex-free gloves will need to be used during your surgery.

    Patients may develop latex sensitization after undergoing multiple medical procedures. Being exposed to latex can trigger the body to produce an antibody called IgE, which causes the allergy symptoms. Patients with latex allergy can experience mild symptoms, such as irritated skin or itchy eyes. The most severe latex allergy reactions are anaphylactic shock and death. Latex allergy can be detected through a skin-prick test.
- Whether your family members have had significant unfavorable reactions to anesthesia.
- If you smoke.
- How often you consume alcohol, and especially if you have within the past twenty-four hours.
- If you have recently lost or gained a significant amount of weight.
- If you wear contact lenses.
- If you have loose teeth, false teeth, or if you have veneers or caps on your teeth.

- If you have any artificial body parts or implants.
- When you last ate and when you last drank any fluids.

Anesthesia

Although anesthesia mishaps are relatively few in number, when they occur, they generally result in injuries more catastrophic than those experienced in other specialties, and may, therefore, be quite costly in terms of personal and financial loss.
— Lawrence H. Thompson, Assistant Comptroller General, Human Resources Division, US General Accounting Office. Presented at a subcommittee hearing on issues relating to malpractice, May 20, 1993.

According to the American Association of Nurse Anesthetists, every year, more than 26 million people undergo some form of medical treatment requiring anesthesia.

Over a hundred years ago surgery was performed only when it was thought to be absolutely necessary. Unfortunately stories of people gulping booze before and biting something hard while undergoing surgery are true. Patients also were held down, screamed, went into shock, and sometimes died during these early attempts at surgery. In the 1800s this all changed when a Georgia doctor named Crawford Long experimented with ether vapor by first using it on himself and then in 1842 performing surgery with it. In 1844, an American dentist named Horace Wells used laughing gas (nitrous oxide) on himself while undergoing a procedure to pull a tooth. A dentist named William Thomas Green Morton brought the use of ether vapor as an anesthetic into common medical knowledge by demonstrating the process before a group of his peers in an amphitheater at the Massachusetts General Hospital in Boston in 1846. In 1847, a Scottish doctor named James Young Simpson used chloroform as an anesthetic agent on women undergoing labor, including Queen Victoria of England.

Anesthesia means "absence of sensation" and was given the name by William Morton at the suggestion of Oliver Wendell Holmes. Anesthesia works by blocking or greatly inhibiting pain, touch, heat, and cold sensor nerve cells from sending information to the brain.

The specialty of anesthesiology did not become a separate medical specialty until the middle of the 20th century. Before this time many mistakes were made that resulted in injuries and deaths of both patients and doctors who were exposed to too much anesthesia, or were burned or killed when anesthetic substances exploded in surgery rooms.

Anesthesia is safer today than ever before. This is because measurements of anesthesia have become more precise and can be balanced against a patient's height, weight, and health conditions. New medical machinery can also monitor the heart, lung, brain, liver, and kidney functions of a patient during surgery. Having a person such as an anesthesiologist or anesthetist present during the surgery to focus attention on the anesthetic and monitoring needs of the patient has also greatly improved the safety of the patients.

There are now a variety of anesthetic agents and sedatives that can be used to reduce pain, get a patient to relax, prevent voluntary movements, help reduce bleeding, and make a patient feel little if anything (analgesia) during surgery. These agents may be taken in pill form, by way of a skin patch, through intravenous injection, or delivered in a gas form that the patient breathes in (inspired gases) — or some combination of these. Children may be given a lollipop laced with pain medication.

The type of anesthesia a patient receives depends on the type of surgery to be performed, the patient's health status, and the training and preferences of the anesthesia specialist. Because different patients respond to pain in different ways, the tolerance of the patient is taken into consideration when the decisions are made about what type of anesthesia is to be used for the surgery, and what type of pain medication will be prescribed after the surgery.

Most surgeries today are performed with local or regional anesthesia while the patient remains awake and somewhat aware of what is going on without feeling pain in the area of the body that has been "blocked" from sensation by the anesthesia. Other surgeries are performed under general anesthesia — which is what people think of when they hear the term "going under."

The kind of procedure being done determines what type of help is needed to perform the surgery. A patient undergoing a simple skin procedure may be given an injection by the doctor to numb the skin before the procedure is performed by the doctor, who is assisted by a nurse. A patient undergoing a more invasive procedure will need a complete surgical team including an anesthetist or anesthesiologist.

What a patient remembers about his surgery depends on what kind of anesthetic agents are used. Patients who undergo some surgeries receive anesthesia that only affects one part of their body and this allows them to be awake and able to communicate during the surgery while feeling no pain. Other anesthetics allow a person to become very relaxed and to be in a state similar to a light sleep. The patient may be able to hear what is going on in the surgery room but, because of muscle relaxants, is unable to move or respond while feeling no pain. Patients undergoing general anesthesia are most likely not to feel or remember the surgery.

•

There have been cases where patients who were improperly anesthetized were able to feel pain, but because of muscle relaxers, were not able to move, speak, or open their eyes. This left them unable to communicate with the surgery team. This is considered to be very rare but can be extremely traumatic for those who have experienced this type of situation. This has led some patients to experience posttraumatic stress disorder that may last for many years. The overwhelming and intrusive memory of the traumatic event allows depression, anxiety, restlessness, fear, sadness, and anger to invade normal expressions and prevent the person from being able to cope with normal life situations. (For information on posttraumatic stress disorder, contact the organization called Gift From Within as it is listed in the *Research Resources* section of this book under the heading *Mental Health*.)

•

Patients are able to hear during all surgeries, even under general anesthesia. How they react to what they hear and what they remember about what they heard depends on the patient. Most patients who undergo general anesthesia do not seem to remember anything about the actual surgery.

Even when a patient is under general anesthesia he is able to hear noises and conversations that take place in the operating room. It is unknown why some general anesthesia patients are able to remember details about what they heard during surgery while other patients seem unable to remember anything about their surgery. Some patients remember details about the surgery but think that it was some type of dream before realizing that it was real. Some drugs used during surgery seem to affect the ability to recall the events of the surgery. Some patients are able to repeat conversations that took place among the surgery team that was performing the operation. Other patients are able only to recall surgery room conversations when they are placed under hypnosis.

Many patients wear headphones and listen to music or positive suggestion tapes during surgery. This may help a patient relax. Because pain is part emotion, it is important that the patient be relaxed.

Listening to a headset may also prevent the patient from hearing any unpleasant sounds or conversations that take place in the surgery room, such as the sounds of drilling or sawing, or discussions the surgery team may be having about other patients with more serious conditions than the patient who is being operated on.

•

- Topical anesthesia is applied directly to the wet mucus surfaces such as the eyes, nose, throat, or mouth. No needles are used and it affects only the areas where it is applied.

- Local anesthesia numbs a small area of the body by directly influencing receptors in nerve membranes after it is injected into the area of the surgery or along the major nerve bundle that serves the area being operated on. Local anesthesia carries significantly less risk than general anesthesia and is the simplest form of anesthesia. Dentists most often use local anesthesia to numb a part of the mouth before performing dental work.

  Local anesthesia with a vasoconstrictor (such as epinephrine) can help prevent fluid loss since it constricts blood vessels and keeps the anesthetic in the desired area much longer. Epinephrine (adrenaline) can make a patient more nervous, but this can be avoided by giving the patient a sedative. It is important for a surgical patient to be relaxed so that his blood pressure does not rise during the surgery.

- Regional anesthesia is done to numb a specific area of the body by administering anesthesia to the group of nerves controlling that area. The patient is awake but does not feel any pain in the area where the cutting is being done because the transmission of pain sensation is blocked from reaching the brain. This type of anesthesia is commonly used in obstetrical procedures, and in prostate surgery and joint replacement surgery.

  A person undergoing regional anesthesia may also elect to receive medications to make him drowsy and relaxed.

  Epidural and spinal anesthesia is preferred over general anesthesia in cases of pregnancy and delivery because general anesthesia is likely to enter the blood stream of the baby.

  Epidural anesthesia is a type of regional anesthesia where a needle is positioned just outside the spinal chord in the epidural space. Epidurals are given to numb a patient from the waist down. This needle may be replaced with an epidural catheter (a little plastic tube) that is left in place after the operation to deliver pain medication into the epidural space.

  A spinal is an injection of an anesthetic agent into the cerebral spinal fluid that surrounds the spinal cord in the lower part of the back.

  A patient who has received spinal anesthesia may experience a headache afterward.

- Anesthesia is often delivered through an intravenous line in combination with local or regional anesthesia together with pain relievers and sedatives. The intravenous line is put in place and the medications are delivered through this line before the local or regional anesthesia is administered. The line remains in place during the procedure so that medications may be given as needed to keep the patient sedated and free of pain.

  An intravenous medicine, such as Valium, may be given through the line to relax and induce amnesia in a patient who does not necessarily need general anesthesia. For instance, a patient undergoing facial cosmetic surgery, such as a nose job, under local anesthesia and intravenous medicines may be fully aware of all that goes on around him or he may drift in and out of sleep. Sounds may seem to be distant, as if they are coming from another room. The patient may hear what is going on in the operating room but may feel nothing other than a light touching of the area being operated on. There is usually no pain during this time.

This combination of anesthesia can make the patient lose the ability to track time. The patient may be able to talk a little to the doctor while the operation is being performed or might be unable to formulate words. Memory of the surgical events may be altered or distorted, but often a patient may be able to remember all the conversations that were said during the surgery by the surgical team.

- General anesthesia almost always leads to complete unconsciousness. Sensation throughout the entire body is suppressed and reflexes are largely absent.

The unconscious patient who is under general anesthesia has an endotracheal tube placed into his trachea to control breathing, deliver anesthetic gases, and protect the lungs from stomach fluids.

Monitoring equipment must be used to track all the patient's vital signs while he is under general anesthesia.

A patient who undergoes general anesthesia is often given four types of medications. These include a mild tranquilizer, narcotics to block pain, an anesthetic, such as sodium pentothal or propofol, to make him unconscious, and another agent to paralyze the muscles. The medication is administered in liquid form through a vein, or vapors are mixed with oxygen and inhaled through a mask.

It is rare to have a patient emerge from unconsciousness while under general anesthesia. Patients under general anesthesia often show some type of physical reaction to the surgery, such as increased pulse rate, facial tension, tears, and sweating. If a patient who is under general anesthesia does become aware of what is going on, he will likely feel no pain and almost always will drift back into unconsciousness.

General anesthesia carries the greatest amount of risk. Invasive procedures, such as heart operations, necessitate the use of general anesthesia. Some surgeons prefer to use general anesthesia during certain less invasive operations. General anesthesia can be used if the patient feels that he would rather not be aware of what is going on.

Many doctors recommend that general anesthesia be used only within the walls of a well-equipped hospital where major surgeries are commonly performed so that if there is a significant complication (such as trouble bringing the patient back out of anesthesia), needed equipment and an experienced staff will be immediately available.

•

No anesthesia is totally risk-free. Adverse reactions can include nausea, shivering, low blood pressure, and shallow breathing. Anesthesia can cause a patient to vomit, which may cause him to choke, and if any of this stomach content gets into the lungs (aspirated) it can cause an infection (aspiration pneumonia). Most patients do not experience any of these reactions.

To protect the lungs from stomach contents and to control breathing, an endotracheal tube may be placed into the mouth and down the trachea. The placement of this endotracheal tube may irritate the throat, and this is why some patients wake up with a sore throat after surgery.

Allergic reactions to anesthesia are also possible. These can lead to complications including hives, convulsions, shock, and cardiac arrest. Reactions may be related to the epinephrine (adrenaline) that is sometimes used to constrict the blood vessels. If the oxygen level becomes limited, the brain can be damaged. In the worst case, death can occur. Serious complications, such as convulsions and problems with the heart, can also arise if there is an overdose of anesthetic.

Reactions similar to an overdose can occur when a normal amount of anesthetic is given but the patient's organs are not working in a way that would normally metabolize and eliminate the drug from the body. For instance, if the heart is not working properly, the drug may not travel to the liver fast enough to be metabolized, and this can result in a toxic reaction. An overdose can also occur if the drug is injected too rapidly. Too much anesthesia can interfere with blood circulation and delay the recovery process.

Less serious side effects from anesthesia include forgetfulness, lack of concentration, a bad taste in the mouth, nausea, dizziness, lack of sleep, constipation and difficulty in urinating, and lack of appetite.

Your Anesthesiologist

One young Los Angeles woman who went in to get a chemical peel on her face was told that an anesthesiologist would be present. She agreed to have the operation after the anesthesiologist did not show up. The doctor administered the anesthetic and placed his office assistant in charge of monitoring the vital signs. The young woman died.

A 41-year-old mother who was in the recovery room after a radical hysterectomy stopped breathing. No one noticed because nurses failed to monitor her vital signs after surgery. She was left severely brain-damaged. A court in San Jose, California, awarded her $1.44 million. Under the terms of the settlement, the medical center where the surgery took place did not admit guilt or liability.

Your surgeon should be focusing his full attention on you while someone else administers the anesthesia and monitors your vital signs (including blood pressure, temperature, pulse, and respiration) and your oxygen level.

Although anesthesia is safer now than it has ever been, a minor mistake can be devastating or even fatal. While you are undergoing a surgical procedure, the second most important person in the operating room, along with the surgeon, is the person who is administering the anesthesia. Anesthesia is given throughout surgery, and is not just a single shot that knocks the patient out.

The anesthesia will be administered by one of these three people:
- An anesthesiologist which is a physician who is trained in the area of anesthesia. He or she administers the anesthesia and monitors your vital signs during and after the surgery.
- A certified registered nurse anesthetist (CRNA), which is a nurse with some extra training and has a minimum of a bachelor's degree in science. The anesthetist may be supervised by an anesthesiologist, but may also work without an anesthesiologist present. CRNAs perform more than half the surgeries in the US.
- The surgeon.

There are no laws that require an anesthesiologist to be present during an operation. Because anesthesia carries serious risks, you should request to have an anesthesiologist or an anesthetist present during the operation along with the proper monitoring equipment. This person should also be with you after the operation until you have safely recovered and your vital signs are stable.

It is best that one anesthesiologist be present for each patient. Many in the medical community believe that a nurse anesthetist has sufficient training to administer anesthesia and monitor the patient, but this also depends on the type of surgery that is being performed.

Often when a surgery takes place in a hospital, the anesthesiologist is supervising more than one operation at a time as surgeries take place in different operating rooms. In this scenario the anesthesiologist is not always present in the room but is "supervising" the person who is monitoring the patient during the operation — usually a nurse anesthetist. This is called "medically directed anesthesiology."

If you are undergoing a surgery where the anesthesiologist is not always present in the room, you should at least request that he be present when the anesthesia is initially administered, present when you awake from the surgery and until your vital signs have stabilized. You should also request that the anesthesiologist be immediately physically accessible during the operation. This means that he should remain in the general vicinity of the operating room and not on another floor of the facility, or outside. If an emergency arises, you will want a specialist near you and not have to depend on the surgeon to handle everything.

The possibility of an emergency during the operation is also the reason you want to have a doctor who has up-to-date emergency equipment immediately available in the operating room, and an emergency transfer agreement with a local hospital if the surgery is not taking place in a hospital.

If the anesthesiologist is a member of the American Association of Anesthesiologists, he is supposed to meet with you before the surgery to assess any potential risks and to determine what type of anesthesia is best for you.

In any case, it may be a good idea to meet the person giving the anesthesia a day or more before the surgery, either in person or by phone. When and how you meet him depends on the type of surgery and where the surgery is taking place. Patients often meet the anesthesiologist when they go in for the preoperative testing. Other times the anesthesiologist may call the patient at home, or the patient may be instructed to call the anesthesiologist at a certain time.

Get answers to any questions you may have about the anesthesia and the person who is administering it.
- Find out what school he attended, what year he graduated, and what year he became board certified.
- If you choose a nurse anesthetist, check to see if he is certified by the American Association of Nurse Anesthetists.
- Find out what type of anesthesia he recommends for your procedure and if he is comfortable with and experienced in administering that type of anesthesia.
- Find out if the surgeon's choice for anesthesia differs from that of the anesthesiologist's or anesthetist's.
- Find out what options you may have with the anesthesia, such as if you would like to stay aware or if you would like to be "put out."
- Find out what the risks are for each option.
- Find out if there is anything you should do to prepare for the anesthesia, such as avoiding certain foods, food supplements, or medications in the days before surgery.
- Find out what you should expect in regard to what you will feel during and after surgery.
- Find out if he believes that the surgery room has all the equipment that will keep you safe if an emergency should arise during the surgery.

If the doctor who is performing the surgery uses the same anesthesia specialist all the time, the doctor's office may have a copy of the anesthetist's or anesthesiologist's resume. Ask for a copy to learn about his education, training, and experience.

If you have insurance, find out whether part of or all the cost of the anesthesia specialist is covered. It is possible that you may get a separate bill from the anesthesia department.

The Surgery

The preparation of a patient in the operating room usually goes very fast. The staff has probably done this routine hundreds of times. They each have a job to do and will probably spend little time talking to you. It is typical of the surgery team to be carrying on conversations totally unrelated to the surgery, such as what they saw on TV the night before.

You will either walk right into the surgery room after you have changed into a gown, or you may be taken to the surgery room from your hospital bed in a wheelchair or on a gurney (a bed with wheels). Before you are taken into the actual surgery room you may spend time in a hallway or a preoperative holding room.

When you are finally in the surgery room you may be surprised to see the doctor and the other team members dressed in what may appear to be space suits. They will be wearing gloves, masks, caps, special shoes, and, depending on the type of surgery you are having, may be breathing through filtered air tubes.

You may also be surprised to see people you have not met. Except for the most simple procedures, there may be more than one surgeon and a team of other workers who will be involved in the surgery. The surgical team may consist of the surgeon, the assistant surgeon, the scrub nurse, the circulating nurse, the anesthesiologist, and other assistants and technicians as needed. In uncomplicated procedures the surgical team may consist only of your doctor, the anesthetist or anesthesiologist, and a nurse.

•

The patient can feel lost in the operating room shuffle. If you have any concerns, be sure to speak up, especially if you are in pain or uncomfortable. Your well-being is more important than anything else in the operating room. Do not expect them to read your mind. If you have a question, speak up!

•

Once you are on the operating table, you will then be "draped" in sterile sheets so the area to be operated on is exposed while the rest of your body is covered. The area of your body that will be operated on will be cleansed with an antiseptic solution either before you are draped, after you are draped, or after you are under anesthesia.

A tourniquet will be tied around your arm by the person who will be administering the anesthesia. You will be asked to make a fist to help locate a suitable vein in your hand or arm where intravenous lines may be placed to provide avenues for anesthetic agents, intravenous nourishment, or blood. You may feel some pain as the needle is pushed through your skin and into the vein (a numbing cream applied to the skin before the needle is inserted may prevent this pain). The needle will be taped in place and attached at the other end to an IV tube, bottle, or bag containing fluid. In a child this process of placing an IV line needle may be performed after the child has been given anesthesia gasses by way of a face mask.

Some of the monitoring and other machinery that may be used on you during the surgery may include (not all these are used during every type of surgery):
- EKG electrodes taped to the skin of the chest or other areas to monitor the rate and rhythm of the heart.
- A blood pressure cuff for the blood pressure monitor (sphygmomanometer) placed on your arm or leg, which will put a tight squeeze on your limb and then release as it inflates and deflates automatically over and over again before, during, and after the surgery.
- A pulse oximeter clip placed on your finger, toe, or ear to measure the oxygen level in your blood.
- An oxygen monitor to measure the oxygen you are given.
- An expiratory gas monitor (capnograph or end-tidal carbon dioxide monitor) to record the gases you exhale.
- A respiratory rate monitor to record the breathing pattern.
- A body temperature monitor with a probe that is taped to your skin or, after you are under anesthesia, placed in your esophagus.
- An intravenous pump to measure the rate of fluids being delivered through the intravenous line.
- A Swan Ganz catheter to measure the pressure inside the heart.
- An ultrasonic monitor (echocardiogram) to follow the movements of the heart.
- An EEG (electroencephalogram) to monitor brain activity.

Some adjustments to the table or pillows may be made to make you comfortable, especially if you have a sore back or other physical problem. Heated water or gel pads may be placed beneath you. Your arms, legs, torso, and head may be immobilized by using straps or braces. A safety belt may be strapped across your torso. You will notice that the lights are very bright and they may be adjusted so they do not bother your eyes.

The anesthesiologist will administer the anesthesia. Then he will check the vital signs and allow the anesthesia to take effect. The surgery will begin only after the anesthesiologist has given the go-ahead.

If you are receiving a type of anesthesia that does not cause you to be unconscious, you will be awake during the surgery. If you are receiving general anesthesia, or if the drugs cause you to fall asleep during the surgery, the next thing you may notice is that you are no longer in the operating room. Instead, you will have already been transferred to the recovery room. The surgery is over.

You may still have the pulse oximeter, blood pressure cuff, oxygen mask, and other monitoring equipment attached to you. You may also have bandages, or a cast, covering the surgical wound and intravenous lines, catheters, and drains attached to you. You may notice that a catheter tube has been placed into your urethra to access your bladder to eliminate your urine. A tube may be in your nose or the endotracheal tube may still be in place. An ointment used on your eyes during surgery may make them sticky. You may feel chilly since the operating room is kept cool (extra blankets can keep you warm).

In the recovery room you may feel confused and very drowsy. You may notice workers walking by you and ignoring you, but they are busy with other chores. One of them should be keeping an eye on you and the monitoring equipment that is attached to you. This will usually be a nurse who has had training in recovery room care. Depending on your situation, the doctor and the anesthesiologist may be in the room, or very close by, as you recover from the anesthesia.

As soon as you are starting to wake up from the surgery you may be coached to breathe deeply and to cough. You may be given water or ice chips. You may be asked to sit up. Depending on the surgery, you may be helped out of bed and assisted as you walk around. These are ways to help you recover from the anesthesia, clear your lungs of any collected fluids, and wake up your system.

The amount of time it takes you to recover from anesthesia depends on the amount you received and your sensitivity to it. How long you are attached to the monitoring equipment and where you go — to your hospital room, to the intensive care or critical care area, or to your home — depends on what type of surgery you had and how your body reacted to it.

Intravenous (IV) Lines

Not everyone who undergoes surgery will have an IV line attached to him. Some simple skin surgeries may include only an injection of anesthetic that lasts long enough for an abnormality on the skin to be excised. Others who undergo surgery will need to have an IV line placed so they can receive the anesthesia or other fluids as their condition dictates. Patients who have had to fast before surgery will need the fluids that are delivered through the IV line.

Fluids delivered through an IV line may include:
- Blood, or a blood content, such as packed cells, plasma, or platelets.
- Anesthesia, or medication.
- Saline. This is a solution consisting of sterile water and salt (sodium chloride)used to replace the fluids that are lost through sweating, breathing, and digestion.
- Ringer's lactate. This solution contains sterile water, salt, and minerals.
- Other types of fluids as needed.

Problems with IV lines may include:
- Infection. The IV and the area of the skin where the IV line enters the skin must be kept clean. The insertion point will likely be covered with tape to keep the IV in place with bandaging for further protection. IV lines that are left in for a long period of time are more likely to cause problems.
- Extravasation. This is when the fluid from the IV is not making its way into the vein, and instead is leaking into the area beneath the skin, or is coming out of the insertion point. The doctor or nurse should be notified as soon as this complication appears.
- Irritation from medications. There are times when a medication may irritate the IV area. The medication may need to be diluted, or a less irritating medication may be used. The IV site can to be switched to another area.
- Patient discomfort. Do not scratch the skin around, or pull on the IV.
- Phlebitis. This is when the vein becomes inflamed. It is often caused by an IV line that has been left in one place too long, usually more than 48 hours. The inflammation may be the veins' response to the catheter, the medication, or to an infection. The time and date that the IV line was placed may be noted on a piece of tape that is placed on the IV line to keep track of how long the IV has been in place.
- Sclerosed veins. A patient who has had to rely on IV lines for months or years may have veins that have closed down. This makes it hard for a nurse to find a usable vein in the arm. If this has occurred, the patient may undergo a surgical procedure to place a long-term indwelling catheter into one of the large veins located in the neck or chest area.
- Other complications. If you notice that the IV is becoming loose, appears to be falling out, is causing pain, or the skin around the IV looks infected, notify the nurse or doctor immediately.

Avoid the use of any lotions, creams, oils, cosmetics, medications, cleaning solutions, or any type of solution on or near the IV unless you have the approval of your doctor.

9 • RECOVERY

It is not possible to discuss all risks, but this chapter discusses those that are common.

Healing

There is no telling how long anyone is going to take to heal until it actually happens. It may take more time or less time than the doctor estimates. A patient should not "try" to recover so fast that he endangers his health. Surgery, even when it is done through small incisions, is a shock to the system. The body will need a day or more to rid itself of the anesthesia and to begin repairing the surgical wound that was created. Some surgery patients may need physical therapy to assist in their healing. Other patients, especially if cancer is involved, may benefit from group therapy to help them cope with their situation.

Many elective surgery patients recover at home. If the surgery is more involved, you may spend a day or more in the hospital. It is important for you to know that you may need to take days, weeks, or even months off from work to recover. You may also need someone to drive you home from the hospital and to and from the doctor's office for checkups. You may also need someone to care for you and perform your chores while you recover.

If you have the resources, choose to hire a private duty nurse to care for you while you recover at home. The hospital or doctor's office should be able to connect you with one. Some people also hire private duty nurses to care from them while they are in the hospital.

Another option, for people with money, is to use recovery center facilities. These are set up like little hotels staffed by nurses. If you want to be pampered, and can afford the extra expense, spend a day or more at a center during the initial stages of recovery. These hideaways usually offer transportation along with room and board at a much lower rate than what hospitals charge. They can also be well worth the extra money to assure that your initial recovery period goes well.

Carefully follow any instruction you are given to guide you through healing. During this period you should let the doctor know whether you have any excess bleeding, fever, pain, or any change that concerns you.

It may be wise to avoid physical contact with animals and small children for a week or more if there is the possibility that they may bump your surgical wound. But some studies show that having supportive friends and family around helps patients recover faster. One study done by researchers at Yale University School of Medicine concluded that elderly patients are more likely to survive a heart attack if they have emotional support from family and friends. (*Annals of Internal Medicine,* December 15, 1992)

Some activities, such as going for walks, may help your body recover. Find out what you can and cannot do during recovery and how the surgical wound will affect your mobility. Various movements may have to be avoided so there will be no strain to the incisions or the surgical wound — especially during sleep. Any action that would cause you to lower your head may need to be avoided — especially if surgery had been performed anywhere on the head or neck. Facial surgery patients may have to avoid foods that require hard chewing, and any conversation that would cause any more than very casual facial movements. You may also need help getting dressed. Bending, heavy lifting, and any action that would elevate blood pressure or result in increased body heat might need to be limited for a number of days or weeks. When you sneeze or cough you should do so with your mouth wide open to avoid a pressure burst within your body. You may have stitches or surgical tape and scabbing that cannot get wet, which means you will not be able to shower or bathe for a certain number of days.

Stitches:
- Stitches hold the skin and other tissues together so they can adhere to each other and heal.
- When a large incision was made, metal staple-type stitches may have been used.
- To avoid "zipper" or "railroad-track" scars, subcuticular stitches may be used. This is done by closing the wound using dissolvable stitches in a criss-cross pattern under the skin rather than on top of the wound.
- When recovering from surgery, keep your hands away from the surgical wounds to avoid contamination with bacteria.
- Do not let anyone other than the doctor or nurses touch the sutures, and they should do so only while wearing surgical gloves.
- Do not scratch the sutured area, or pull the sutures that seem to be loose.
- If you notice that the stitches are becoming loose and the incision is opening up, notify the doctor.
- Avoid the use of any lotions, creams, oils, cosmetics, medications, cleaning solutions, or any type of solution on or near the wound unless you have your doctor's approval.

Smoking should be avoided for at least two weeks before surgery and two weeks after surgery. Nicotine inhibits the healing process because it impairs blood flow to the tissues, increasing the chance of necrosis (tissue death). Infections are more common in patients who smoke. Researchers at the University of Texas Southwestern Medical School found that bones take nearly twice as long to heal in people who smoke. Researchers at Emory University School of Medicine found that nicotine interferes with bone fusion. Nicotine is in all tobacco products. Smoker's gum also contains nicotine and should be avoided by anyone who is to undergo surgery.

Alcoholic beverages, certain foods, and possibly drinks with caffeine, such as coffee, may need to be avoided for a couple of days before surgery and for four to seven days after surgery — or for as long as the doctor advises. Drinks that contain alcohol can interfere with medication, intensify the effect of the medication, may be dangerous when combined with certain medications, and may cause you to become lax in caring for yourself during the recovery period.

Some medications interfere with blood clotting and will need to be avoided. This is one of the reasons why the doctor must know of all prescription, over-the-counter medications, and food supplements you are taking. Products that might need to be avoided or limited before and after surgery include aspirin and aspirin substitutes, such as Motrin and Advil; ibuprofen, and other nonsteroidal anti-inflammatory agents. You may also be told to avoid cough medicine; Alka Seltzer; vitamin B supplements; Darvon and Darvon-related medications; vitamin E supplements; fish oil in both pill and liquid form; garlic supplements; Pepto-Bismol, and other medicine or diet supplements as your doctor advises.

Water-based cosmetics should be used in place of oil-based cosmetics around the operation site during the month after surgery because they are easier to wash off. Oil-based cosmetics can cause infections. Any makeup used should be new, clean, and hypoallergenic (be cautious when using products labeled hypoallergenic because not all companies follow the same standards). Avoid products with dyes that can stain, and even tattoo, the fresh scar during the first few weeks after surgery. Cosmetics with alcohol or perfumes should be worn at a distance from the operative site, because they can irritate the incisions and cause dryness.

Limit direct, unprotected sun exposure to any surgical wound until the wound has healed for at least three months. Apply sunblock and wear protective clothing when you do go out in the sun.

When your body is healing from a surgical wound, it will need nutrients to heal properly. Eat a nutritious, low-fat, high fiber, plant-based diet. Avoid meats and dairy products because they contain saturated oils that may help cause post-surgical infections and slow wound healing. Avoid foods that are refined, fried, salty, or sugary. Avoid coffee and sodas. Concentrate more on fresh vegetable salads, fresh fruits, and whole grain foods. Drink raw fruit and vegetable juices – especially carrot juice — daily. The enzymes from the raw plants will help the body rid itself of dead cells from the wound. Drink echinacea tea three or four times per day to help boost the immune system. Get arnica flower, burdock root, and chaparral herb capsules from your healthfood store and take these to help the wound heal.

A list of recovery instructions detailing your specific needs may be available from your doctor. (See the *Strategic Planning* section for more information on preparing for and caring for yourself after surgery.)

Pain

Be sure to ask the doctor what kind of pain is associated with the surgery you are having. Ask how long you should expect to experience the pain, and what kind of discomfort you will most likely experience during and after the surgery.

Get prescriptions for the pain medication filled before surgery takes place. Bring the pain medication with you when you go in for the surgery.

The amount of pain after surgery depends on how the operation is done, the patient's pain tolerance, his expectations, his emotional state of mind, and other factors, such as fear and physical condition. Some pain or discomfort is expected after all surgery because surgery involves cutting into the body. One patient may feel little or no pain while another patient who underwent the same operation can experience a lot of pain. Pain can be related to the way the incisions were made and what was done to the body. Pain may also be related to the type of anesthesia used, the way the anesthesia was administered, and where the anesthesia was administered. For instance, some types of anesthesia may cause the person to experience a headache after surgery.

Unusual pain may indicate a complication. A pool of blood (hematoma) can place pressure on a nerve and cause pain, and may require surgery if the problem continues or if the hematoma becomes infected. Pain may also be caused by an infection where no hematoma is present. If you have any unusual pain or pain that concerns you, be sure to notify your doctor as soon as possible.

How would you describe the pain?
- Does it radiate to other areas?
- Does it throb as your heart beats?
- Does it interfere with your breathing?
- Does it happen only when you make a certain movement, or is it always present?
- Is it a dull or a sharp pain?
- On a scale of 1 to 10, with 10 being the worst, what rating would you give the pain?

Pain management has grown into a subspecialty of anesthesia. Managing a surgical patient's pain may involve placement of a line that delivers pain medication directly to nerves (patient-controlled analgesia, or PCA, where a patient presses a button to deliver pain medication as he desires), or by giving injections or pain pills at set times.

If you feel the prescribed pain medication is too strong, ask the doctor, the anesthesiologist, or the pain management department of the hospital if there is another type of drug that is not as strong, or if there is a weaker dose of the same drug available. Find out if cutting the individual pills in half with a knife would be a reasonable solution.

Becoming addicted to pain medication is considered a rare occurrence in relation to the number of people who undergo surgery, but is one risk of taking pain medication.

Do not hesitate to express your need for pain medication. If you think what you are taking is too weak, contact your nurse, doctor, anesthesiologist, or the pain management department of the hospital. Do not increase the amount of pain medication without first clearing this with your doctor. Unusual pain may be an indication of a problem with healing.

Do not mix the medication with another medication without first asking your doctor, and do not mix pain medication with alcohol.

Bleeding, Bruising, and Swelling

Complications from surgery can include hemorrhaging and hematomas. A hemorrhage occurs when clotting does not proceed properly. A hematoma is a collection of clotted blood beneath the skin. A hematoma can also occur inside the body. Both these complications may require additional surgery.

Some surgeries can cause intense bruising and swelling. Ask your doctor about the likelihood of this happening to you. The doctor may be able to show you photos of someone with surgical bruises and swelling who has had a similar operation — but remember that not everyone bruises or swells in the same manner.

Keeping the surgical wound elevated (when the surgery is on the arms, legs, or head) above the heart level for the first 24 hours after surgery can help minimize bruising.

Cold constricts blood vessels. Applying ice and cold compresses after surgery can help control the swelling. Ask the doctor if applying ice bags or other cold compresses to the surgical site will benefit you.

The swelling and bruising from surgery can last anywhere from a few days to more than a month. Bruising around the eyes can cause persistent dark areas under the eyes. Swelling can sometimes permanently stretch the skin and cause scarring — especially if the swelling causes stitches to break open, or tear the skin.

Bruising that occurs on the upper parts of the body can eventually fall to lower areas as healing progresses. An example of this is when someone undergoes nasal surgery that causes bruising on the eyes and cheeks. This bruising may fall down into the neck over the next several days as the healing takes place.

The body breaks down old coagulated blood and dissolves the dead cells. As the dead cells are diminished, the bruise becomes lighter in color and eventually disappears.

Bruises often appear their worst on the third day. If your bruising keeps increasing beyond what was expected, notify your doctor. A bruise that appears red and feels hot should also be reported because these are signs of infection.

Aspirin (acetylsalicylic acid) can increase bleeding and swelling because it interferes with the normal clotting ability of blood platelets. Some other medications, such as ibuprofen, and blood-thinning drugs, can also lead to increased bleeding.

Infection

I began to see many, many advertisements . . . and thought well, gee, with all this advertising this cannot be too unsafe.

The doctor who I chose after checking him out with the American Medical Association and the California Department of Health did the operation in his office.

[After complaining to her doctor that she was short of breath, her doctor told her she was experiencing the normal aftereffects of surgery. When her bandages were removed they revealed two black patches and a wide-open gap in her lower abdomen that was oozing pus.]

Four weeks after the surgery, I still had an open wound, and I had uncontrollable infections, three kinds of infections. . . . the infections spread through my bloodstream to my lungs and landed in the mitral valve of my heart. The mitral valve was destroyed by infection. I ended up in an emergency room hospital — very, very close to death.

I was in emergency for seven hours. . . . There was this green gel and pus in my incision . . . they removed suture [material] that the doctor left in my tummy and the infection was clinging to that . . . I was in and out of the hospital six times in a year and a half. Five times I went into heart failure. . . . I had a stroke. The defective valve threw a clot which landed in the right side of my brain . . . I had open heart surgery to replace the destroyed valve in my heart . . . I hear the sound of the fake valve in my heart . . . I will be on blood thinning medication and have to go to the doctor every month for the rest of my life.

Two months after he operated on me he did the same procedure on a 36-year-old RN. I am the lucky one because I am alive today and she is not. She died.

[She later found that for two years before she had her surgery the state had been trying to take the doctor's license away. The doctor was found murdered a few years later in a parking lot of a restaurant.]

— Joyce Palso, testifying in 1989 before Congressional subcommittee hearings on the plastic surgery industry and telling how a botched tummy tuck operation nearly killed her

Infection from surgery is potentially serious and fatal. Any time you undergo surgery, there is a chance of getting an infection. The risk of infection increases if you are a smoker. Infections are among the leading causes of post-operative death. One of the common causes of infection is improperly sterilized surgical tools or equipment. Infection can also be caused by a surgical site that was not cleaned properly, unsanitary medical workers, hair or sweat from the medical team falling into the incision during surgery, or unsanitary conditions during recovery.

It's safe to say that ten percent of all people admitted to a hospital will acquire an infection during their stay. That's about double what it was 15 years ago. The Centers for Disease Control and Prevention estimate that 80,000 people die from hospital-acquired infections each year. . . The number one reason they spread in hospitals is the failure of staff members to wash their hands between patient contacts, immediately upon removing their gloves, or after touching contaminated instruments and equipment.

— Charles Inlander, president of People's Medical Society, June 1996

A study presented to AMA policy makers in June 1995 showed that doctors wash their hands only 14% to 59% of the time before seeing patients. For nurses, the rates were 25% to 45%.

Some studies have shown that patients who receive antibiotics intravenously before certain surgeries will have a smaller chance of infection if the antibiotics are administered no more than two hours before surgery. Regardless of the antibiotic statistics, health workers should be washing their hands much more often than the study statistics indicate.

GRANDY: Let me ask you this and you might have said this, I didn't pick it up if you did. Did you draw any conclusions in your study as the incidence of negligence and adverse events as relates to age? In other words, are you more inclined to see incidence of negligence and malpractice claims in patients 65 and over?

THOMPSON: I think in the Harvard study (of New York hospitals) the answer is yes.

KLADIVA: What the study suggests is that the individuals who are most likely to sustain injuries in the healthcare system are the older individuals and they are less likely to file claims than are other citizens.

GRANDY: But they are also more likely to have accidents wherever they are, right. I mean to some extent the older and frailer and sicker you get, the more likely you are going to be at risk.

THOMPSON: Yes. And you should know that if you look at what these incidents are that are being reported out of the Harvard study you will see things like infections that are picked up in the hospital or drug reactions and, especially with infections, older people are probably more prone to pick up an infection.

— Congressman Fred Grandy; Lawrence H. Thompson, Assistant Comptroller General, Human Resources Division, US General Accounting Office; and Susan Kladiva, Assistant Director, Health Financing Issues, US General Accounting Office; during a Congressional subcommittee hearing on issues relating to medical malpractice, May 20, 1993

Depending on what is causing an infection, the type of surgery you had, and your body's ability to fight the infection along with the help of antibiotics, the infection could clear up easily, or it could prolong your recovery period and cause unwanted scarring and other complications that might necessitate further surgery.

If you had an implant put in during the surgery and an infection develops, the implant may have to be removed. If the implant cannot be removed right away, antibiotic therapy may be needed for four to six weeks, or until the implant can be removed safely. After the infection has completely cleared, the implant can be replaced, but this requires additional surgery with additional risks. All these scenarios can take their toll on your health and well-being, and certainly your bank account.

Scars

Whenever an incision is made, damage is done to skin tissue, blood vessels, and nerves. All incisions will produce some scarring. No scar is absolutely invisible, but many scars will become less noticeable with time. After several months, the scar may fade to a fine line. Sometimes the scars are larger and thicker than the person would care to have. Scars caused by facial surgery can usually be covered by makeup and hair. The most obvious surgical scars are caused by operations done on areas where there are no natural skin folds to hide them.

Your doctor may advise you to use an over-the-counter anti-bacterial lotion on your surgical wound. After the stitches are removed, some people use such things as vitamin-enriched skin lotions, aloe vera, and even olive oil to coat the scar. These may aid in healing and result in a less noticeable scar. Oil applied to a wound may cause infection. Ask your doctor before applying any lotion, cream, oil, or other product to your surgical wound.

Follow-up Appointments

The follow-up visit schedule will vary depending on what type of surgery you had and your reaction to it. There should be daily contact with the doctor or the doctor's office for at least the first few days after any significant surgery.

Depending on the surgery, you may have to see the doctor several times within the week following the surgery for operation wound checkups. There might be a follow-up schedule that includes a one-week visit, a two-week visit, a one-month visit, a three-month visit (which is when the "after" photos are usually taken), a six-month visit, and a one-year visit. These are done to make sure there are no problems with healing. You also may need to undergo physical therapy and rehabilitation. Patients who have undergone cancer surgery may be scheduled for chemotherapy or radiation, if that is the therapy they choose.

Follow-up appointments might be included in the price you pay the doctor for the operation. If you are paying for the surgery out-of-pocket, inquire whether follow-up appointments are included in the surgical fee, or whether they are additional.

Taking Drugs

Whenever a person takes a drug, he runs the risk of prescription errors, drug interactions, and potential side effects. Medications vary in strength. Everyone metabolizes drugs at different rates. Body weight along with age, kidney, liver, heart, and lung function play a part in how a person metabolizes and reacts to a particular drug. The temperature of a room, air conditioning, heating blankets, and heated water beds may cause some drugs to be metabolized differently than intended. The fluctuating cycles (circadian rhythms) of the body also affect the way a drug is metabolized. Many medications that are believed safe for adults can be lethal when given to infants and elderly patients because these groups respond to medications differently and experience more side effects than other patients not in these groups. Part of the reason for this is that older people take more drugs than younger people and have more drug residue flowing within their systems, and when two incompatible drugs match up with each other in the system, there can be an adverse reaction.

When a doctor prescribes a drug for a condition other than what the drug is meant to treat, the doctor is then prescribing the drug "off label." An example of this is the drug Prozac, which is sold to treat depression but is being prescribed "off label" by some doctors to treat patients who suffer from eating disorders. Off-label uses of drugs may account for as much as 60% of all prescriptions. In 1991 the FDA adopted a policy restricting drug companies from distributing information about off-label uses of drugs. The drug company is supposed to put the drug through the FDA approval process to get the drug approved for each use. Many doctors, drug companies, and patients feel that the policy is an unnecessary restriction.

Medication errors may occur when:
- A drug is taken at the wrong time.
- A drug is taken too often.
- A drug is taken with alcohol or when the patient has alcohol in his system.
- The drug is taken with another drug in a combination that can cause harm.
- The wrong amount of a drug is taken.
- The wrong drug is prescribed.
- A patient is allergic to a drug.

Much, if not all, of what the doctor knows about a drug is what he learned from the advertising put out by the drug company, from the pharmaceutical salesperson, or from another person who works for the drug manufacturer. Many of the allopathic medical journals would not exist without the money they receive from the drug companies that advertise in the journals.

The drug company representatives who are in contact with the doctors are known as "detailers" because they explain the details to the doctor about how the drug is to be prescribed. These detailers hand out samples of drugs to doctors, provide free office supplies with drug company logos, and may even bring food for the office staff or take the doctor out to lunch and give him gifts, such as tickets to sporting events.

The materials that the doctor reads about a drug may be overly enthusiastic and rely on statistics that are not exactly truthful, or at least present information in a way that makes the drug appear to be more reliable than it actually is. For instance, one drug may cause 1% of a study group to have a favorable result while 2% of the patients taking another drug have a favorable result. Therefore the drug company can say that the second drug is 100% more effective than the first drug. Truthful? Kind of. Misleading? You be the judge.

Many people feel cheated or as if their health concerns were not taken seriously if a doctor visit does not result in a prescription. Taking *no* medication may be just what the patient needs as many ailments, such as the common cold, heal without intervention.

Despite the healing capabilities of the human body, many patients seek, and too many doctors give in to, chemical drug interventions when there is a narrow chance that the drugs will be of any benefit to the patient getting better. What happens in many cases of a person seeking drug therapy for a common ailment is that the patient gets better after taking the medication when they would have gotten better regardless of whether or not they took the medication. As they say, a cold gets better in a week without antibiotics, or it gets better in seven days with antibiotics.

What many people do not know is that doctors often have a financial interest in independent pharmacies, especially when the pharmacy is located within a medical building. The lease agreement for the pharmacy may require the pharmacy to pay a percentage of its profits to the landlord. If the doctors who occupy the office space in the building also own the building, they are getting money from every prescription filled. Does this motivate doctors in this type of situation to hand out more prescriptions? Is it the reason many patients are guided to certain pharmacies, even to the extent that the doctor's receptionist will offer to call the pharmacy to have the prescription filled for a patient before the patient arrives at the pharmacy?

As Michael Schmidt's book *Beyond Antibiotics* makes clear, many doctors are still prescribing antibiotics to patients whose symptoms indicate a viral infection. Viruses do not respond to antibiotics, and prescribing them for viral infections helps promote resistance to antibiotics. This is one example where the overprescribing of a medication has become a serious risk to the general population.

Antibiotics penetrate the wall of a bacterium cell and destroy its protein. Scientists have found that bacterium can develop genetic mutations that strengthen the cell walls or protect the cell protein. When a bacterium gene becomes resistant to antibiotics, that gene can be transferred to a different type of bacterium.

While just a few decades ago patients with pneumonia were being successfully treated with penicillin, today, because of overuse of antibiotics in both people and farm animals, doctors are finding more and more patients who have strains of bacteria that have become resistant to antibiotics. A patient with a healthy immune system may be able to fight off the infection, but if the immune system is weak and there is no response to antibiotics, the patient dies. Bacteria that are resistant to antibiotics cause thousands of patient deaths in the US every year.

The large majority of the antibiotics prescribed in the US are used on farm animals. People who eat meat, eggs, and dairy products are ingesting antibiotic residues found in the animal products. The chronic overuse of antibiotics in both humans and farm animals not only make bacteria resilient to antibiotics, it also suppresses the human immune system by killing the gastrointestinal microflora (billions of organisms that live in the intestines and aid in digestion of food, vitamin production, and in intestinal immunity).

Eliminating the good "symbiotic" strains of bacteria, such as Lactobacillus acidophilus and Bifidobacteria bifidus, in the digestive tract makes the human body more susceptible to infections, such as Candida albicans (*Alternative Medicine Journal*, September/October 1995). A lack of intestinal bacteria interferes with nutritional intake. It also contributes to intestinal illnesses, such as diarrhea and constipation, and chronic conditions, such as colitis.

Some nutritional supplement companies now make "probiotics" that help restore intestinal bacteria and this strengthens the immune system. Check with your healthfood store for probiotic supplements (one such product is *Nutra Flora FOS*, made by KAL of Broomfield, Colorado) as well as immune-strengthening herbal remedies, such as echinacea tea, garlic tablets, and herbal supplements containing licorice, red clover, goldenseal, Irish moss, myrrh, and burdok root. In addition to beneficial bacteria, proper nutrition is important in maintaining a strong immune system. Nutrients, such as vitamin B-5 (pantothenic acid), zinc, the amino acid L-glutamine, and fiber ingredients inulin and fructooligosaccharides aid in the health and function of the gastrointestinal tract. Vitamin C has antiviral and antibiotic effects and intake of this vitamin should be increased at the time of illness.

To find out about non-antibiotic treatments for infection, visit with a homeopathic or natureopathic doctor.

Over one and a half billion prescriptions are filled in the US every year. This amounts to astronomical numbers of pills, yet few Americans know what it is they are taking and what potential side effects the drugs have. Besides the side effects of a medication, there is also the risk of being prescribed the incorrect dose, having an inappropriate medication prescribed, and risks of allergic reactions. Many patients receive medications to counterattack the side effects of another prescription.

A study released in 1994 by the National Council on Patient Information in Washington concluded that although people over age 60 comprise only 12% of the nation's population, they take one-fourth of the nation's prescriptions.

The FDA has said that 17% of the hospitalizations among seniors are caused by the side effects of prescriptions drugs. The General Accounting Office reported that nearly 6 million of the nation's 30 million Medicare patients take drugs that are considered unsafe for their age group or duplicate a drug already being taken (*Health After 50: Johns Hopkins Medical Letter*, November 1994 and January 1996).

The Healthcare Compliance Packaging Council has estimated that over 100,000 Americans die each year from using prescriptions incorrectly. The National Center for Health Statistics estimates 125,000 deaths a year are caused by adverse reactions to prescription drugs. Sometimes this can be the result of inaccurate information being given out by some pharmacists who are overworked, are hired by temp agencies, are drug abusers, or who simply make mistakes. Other times it can be caused by patients taking the wrong dosage , or a dangerous combination of medications. These deaths may also be the result of incompetent or uninformed doctors. They may rely too often on pills for treatment, or do not know what other medicines a patient is taking. Some physicians may simply not know the full effects of the medicines they prescribe.

We believe that at least half, probably two-thirds of older adults in this country are being prescribed a drug that is doing unnecessary harm to them and the toll is enormous.

— Dr. Sidney M. Wolfe, director of Public Citizen's Health Research Group

I had pills to go to sleep, pills to wake up, pills for pain, pills to counteract the reactions of all the other pills. And each of these, please note, was from a doctor's prescription.
— Former First Lady Betty Ford, speaking of her drug addictions, November 1995

A Harvard University study published in the *Journal of the American Medical Association* (July 1994) found that:

- Almost one-fourth of the United States senior citizens — 6.6 million people over age 65 — were being prescribed drugs that had been recognized as dangerous to their health.
- 23.5% of older Americans received at least one drug that, according to the conclusions of a panel of experts, should be prescribed to the elderly in only the rarest of circumstances.
- Some of the drugs prescribed to the elderly cause mental impairment that results in misdiagnosis, seizures, and heart problems. They also contribute to falls — which can lead to hip fractures.

Over-the-counter drugs, such as Tylenol, Anacin-3, Panadol, and other medications that contain acetaminophen are useful in treating certain ailments, but they can also damage kidneys and lead to kidney failure if taken daily over a long period of time (according to a researchers at Johns Hopkins University). Acetaminophen can cause liver damage and death if taken in high doses, especially by children.

Taking two over-the-counter medications at the same time that contain the same ingredient can also lead to overdose. When in doubt, ask your pharmacist.

When a doctor hands you a prescription and you cannot read what it says, turn the prescription over, ask the doctor how to spell the prescription and clearly write or print it on the back of the prescription. Ask the doctor if the prescription he is giving you is a brand name, a generic brand, or if the pharmacist will be compounding the prescription.

When you give the prescription to the pharmacist, let him know that the name is written clearly on the back. When you get the prescription back, check to see what it says on the bottle and ask the pharmacist (not the cashier) how you are to take the prescription.

Do not assume that the medication a doctor prescribes has no side effects simply because the doctor did not mention any. Doctors often do not know about all the side effects of drugs they prescribe, and many lack knowledge about significant risks that exist when patients combine drugs.

Medication risks may include:

- Interference with normal thought processes and this can effect work and social activities.
- Sleep disturbances.
- Upset stomach, irritation to digestive tract, or damage to the tissues of the digestive system.
- Loss of appetite or increased appetite.
- Sexual dysfunction.
- Interaction with other drugs.
- Interference with nutritional substance metabolism.
- Creation of stress.
- Skin irritation.
- Increased sensitivity to light or sun rays.
- Damage to organs, such as to the liver or kidneys.
- Addiction.
- Depletion of tissues, such as when a drug causes bone loss.
- Risk of causing disease, such as cancer.

Whenever you are given a prescription, unless delaying the intake of the medication would interfere with your health, take time to learn what the drug's side effects are, and what the drug is meant to do. Learn how long it works, and if it interferes with any other medications you are taking. Find out if it has any known long-term risks. Know how much medication you are supposed to get, and how often you are supposed to take the medication.

Under federal law, pharmacists must offer information on new prescriptions given to Medicaid patients. Some states have laws that require pharmacists to counsel all patients who ask questions at the time a prescription is filled.

Information on drugs can be obtained through the manufacturers; however, do not rely solely on literature put out by them. Try finding additional information on the drug at your local library or through the book *Worst Pills, Best Pills* that is published by Public Citizen's Health Research Group. Also, ask for a copy of the FDA-approval label. This should be available at the pharmacy.

10 • QUESTIONS

Questions to Ask the Doctor and Yourself

Many of the following questions are listed to present information so that you will not experience any surprises. Many others may be useful in determining the quality of care you may receive if you decide to undergo surgery.

Find out as many answers as you can that apply to your needs before you see the doctor. Be realistic about the amount of time you require of the doctor, or be prepared to pay extra for an extended consultation.

Turning the consultation into an FBI-type investigation is not the idea here. No doctor should be expected to sit and answer the abundance of questions in the following pages. Any questioning may make a doctor uncomfortable because he is essentially having his strengths and weaknesses evaluated by someone who has walked into his workspace.

Sugery may be beneficial or disastrous. The outcome of surgery depends on the doctor's talents and abilities, techniques used during surgery, and the motives of the medical team performing the operation. It also depends on the motives of the patient, the post-surgical care, and the patient's mental and physical response to the surgery.

Some surgeons will spend one or two hours talking to their prospective patients to get to know the patients' motives and expectations. Others will spend only a few minutes with the patients; dismiss the patients' concerns; schedule them for surgery; do a quick slice, cut and stitch; and be done with it. If one patient is dissatisfied, there is always another waiting at the door.

Before a person decides to undergo surgery, the operation should be put in to perspective. There are any number of factors that can determine whether proceeding with surgery is within responsible reasoning. Any personal difficulties or life changes the patient is currently experiencing that can affect the surgery should be put into consideration.

Because altering a body part can be a major decision, you may feel intimidated during the consultations, and forget what to ask. Set the stage to have a successful session with your doctor. Get past the technical terms and medical phrases. Take a notebook and a list of questions — or highlight the questions in this book that you want to find answers to. Some people bring tape recorders to the consultation

so they can listen to it later to determine whether there was
something they overlooked.

*There is no more dangerous activity than walking into a doctor's office,
clinic, or hospital unprepared.*

— Dr. Robert Mendelsohn, in his book *Confessions of a Medical Heretic*;
Contemporary Books, 1979

It is good to have a relative, friend, or spouse (and a copy of this
book) with you when you are talking to the doctor. Your friend may
remember what you may forget to ask. He also may ask questions
that you did not think of and notice something that the doctor said or
did that you did not notice. You are protecting yourself and you have
the right to have a third person of your choice in the room with you
whenever you are speaking with a doctor. If the doctor refuses your
request to have a third person with you, you may want to question
this, or simply leave.

Some people are so unfamiliar with and are so intimidated by
doctors and lost in the mystique of medicine that they treat medical
care with an unquestioning religious reverence. They are passive and
submissive rather than active and assertive in their own care, and
this is when harm can be done. These are the same people who do not
ask enough questions, do not do their own research, are afraid to
walk out on a doctor, do not realize that they are hiring the doctor
and can end up being, in a sense, used as human guinea pigs in the
doctor's "practice" of medicine.

Many people will go to a doctor who is a complete stranger, fill
out paperwork that includes very personal questions, go into the
examination room, take off their clothes, let the doctor come into the
room, be asked more personal questions, let the stranger put his hands
on all their private parts, and even let the doctor operate on them —
then still feel as if they are being too aggressive and will refrain
from asking the doctor a few questions that will determine whether
the doctor is competent and if his prescribed form of treatment is best.

These very same people, if they are in the position to have a
home built, may, when searching for their architect and builder, do
more background checking on these professionals than on the doctor
they are trusting with their life. Even after having their house
built, they may decide they do not like it. You may live in your house
temporarily, but your body is something you will be living in for the
rest of your life.

It is important that you make the right choice about whether to
have the surgery and, if so, how it is to be done and who is to do it.
The decision to undergo surgery can sometimes mean the difference
between life and death. Because of these risks, the last thing you

need when looking into surgery is some clever smarmy doctor whose talk is filled with medical euphemisms and who tosses you vague answers to your questions.

Do not tolerate incompetent medical care. Find the best caregiver you possibly can. You do not want to be one of the thousands of people who find themselves involved with a lawsuit against a doctor while hopping from doctor to doctor to try to find one who can correct messy surgical results.

You have the right to be informed about the operation you are going in for, and about the medical staff that is involved in your care. This means checking out the background of the doctor and his staff, and may involve researching in books found in bookstores and libraries, reading pamphlets, and possibly watching videotapes that will teach you about your treatment options.

Do not worry about offending the doctor or irritating the staff by asking questions or by letting them know that you are being very cautious. Just remember how offended and irritated you will be if, after you undergo the operation, you find yourself injured, disfigured, or handicapped by what the doctor did to you. Besides, if they see that you are serious about getting good medical care, they are more likely to give it to you. If a medical worker tells you that you have no right questioning his professional judgment, maybe you should take your business elsewhere.

Even with all your precautions there is still no guarantee that everything will go right. Doctors cannot always control everything in the operating room; some of what goes on depends on you and your reaction to the surgery, and therefore doctors cannot always be held accountable when things do not go as planned.

Aim to get a complete understanding of the procedure you are considering. Speak frankly with the doctor and do not be afraid to push him to explain things. The doctor went to medical school; you probably did not. It is you and not the doctor who might be getting on that operating table. The doctor may never have been a patient. If the doctor uses a term or phrase you do not understand when he is talking to you, or in any literature he or his staff give you, have him explain it to you in words you understand.

If there are questions that you think of after you leave the doctor's office, write them down and ask them later, but before you decide on having the surgery.

The numbers on the following questions are given only as a form of reference and not as a grade of importance.

Not all the questions listed here will apply to all operations. Additionally, there may be many questions unique to your specific health concern that are not listed here and that you will have to consider. Many of the questions are listed only to inform, and are not necessarily meant to be asked.

• EVALUATING THE DOCTOR

Q1: Does the doctor have a resume/professional biography/curriculum vitae that lists his schooling and other training, fellowships, and other credentials?

Some doctors will freely provide this printed material. You can sometimes get this mailed to you before you make an appointment to see the doctor. This way you can do some checking up on the doctor before you see him. Call the doctor's office and see if his staff will send, fax, or e-mail you a copy.

Q2: What boards is he certified by and what year did he receive his certification?

Call the boards and find out if the doctor is certified and how long the certification lasts. If you are having breast surgery, you probably do not want to go to someone who is board certified in ear, nose, and throat surgery.

Q3: Where did he attend medical school?

If he is an American and went to school in another country, you may want to question this. Medical schools in the Caribbean, Mexico, and some other foreign countries advertise themselves to American students who do not have the grades that would get them into an American-based medical school.

On the other hand, there are 125 allopathic medical schools in the US and these graduate 18,000 doctors per year. There are 25,000 residency positions available at the 400 US teaching hospitals. The remaining 7,000 residency positions are filled by foreign graduates.

Q4: What year did he graduate?

Staying current with changes in operative techniques and the increasingly sophisticated medical devices that are now being used requires continuing medical education (CME), and constant evaluation of medical knowledge. If he graduated decades ago, he should have updated his education to include the modern technological advances in his field of medicine. No matter how recently he completed his medical training, he should be reading the medical journals and other literature, such as textbooks, that cover his area of medicine.

Q5: Where did he serve his residency and internship?

Q6: How many years has he been in practice and what other areas of medicine, if any, has he practiced or specialized in?

Q7: Is the doctor a Fellow of the American College of Surgeons?

Beyond residency training, which trains physicians in a specialty, some physicians go on to train in fellowship programs.

Q8: What does the doctor consider to be his specialty? Does the doctor limit himself to the face and neck or another specific area of the body?

The programs for becoming a specialist include added training and supervised experience. It is best to go with a surgeon who specializes in a few procedures that include the surgery you are interested in and who has received his training in that area.

Q9: When did he last attend a continuing education class, what organization offered the class, and what was the subject of the class?

The Accreditation Council for Continuing Medical Education accredits sponsors of continuing medical education programs and is organized under the sponsorship of several organizations: the American Board of Medical Specialists, the American Medical Association, the American Hospital Association, the Association of American Medical

Colleges, the Council of Medical Specialty Societies, and the Federation of State Medical Boards.

Continuing education classes cost money and take time out of the doctor's schedule, but are well worth the investment to his career and curative skills, and to the safety of his patients. A doctor may be required to attend a certain class as a requirement of the hospital where he has admitting privileges, or the insurance company that insures him. A continuing education class may also be a requirement placed on the doctor by the State Medical Board to meet education purposes of a probation action that the board took against the doctor because of malpractice.

Simply because a particular doctor says that he attended a continuing education class does not mean that he actually stayed for the class. He may have signed in and gone elsewhere.

Q10: In what other states has he practiced medicine and why did he move?

Having a doctor who has moved a few times can be a bonus. He may have gained more experience than if he had stayed in the same region because he will have worked with different doctors, learned their techniques, and experienced a variety of patients. But if the doctor has had to move because of his involvement in criminal activity or negligent behavior, he may be a doctor you should avoid.

When a doctor loses his license in one state he can go to another state to get a license and not be subjected to any preclusions. Some crooked states medical boards used to sell licenses, but it is hoped that practice has ended.

For various legitimate reasons, some doctors maintain licenses in more than one state. If the doctor works for the federal government in the veteran's hospital system or for the armed services, all he needs is a license from any state in the union.

Q11: If the doctor was trained and licensed in another country, did he pass the Foreign Medical Graduate Examination?

About 20% of United States doctors are immigrants. Some of them received their training in the United States. Some doctors who were born in the United States received their training in other countries. If they have not passed the Foreign Medical Graduate Examination in the Medical Sciences, they should not be practicing medicine in the United States.

The Foreign Medical Graduate Examination in the Medical Sciences is a 1,000-question exam that screens the credentials, knowledge in medical matters, and English language ability of foreign medical school graduates who intend to practice medicine in the United States. Those who pass these criteria are eligible to apply for residencies in the United States. The exam is given in each state and has been overseen since the 1950s by the Educational Commission for Foreign Medical Graduates. The commission is a private group that is organized and supported by the nation's major medical associations. The commission's organizational members are the Federation of State Medical Boards of the United States, the American Medical Association, the American Hospital Association, the American Board of Medical Specialists, the Association of Medical Colleges, the National Medical Association, and the Association for Hospital Medical Education.

Q12: What is the doctor's state medical license number and in what year was it first issued?

Call the state medical board to find out this information. The phone numbers of each state medical board are listed in the *Research Resource* section of this book.

Q13: Is the doctor working out of an office all by himself where he is the only doctor and the office staff works only for him, or is he in a group practice?

A doctor who is practicing in an office with no other doctors may not be exposed to the discussions of his peers where he may learn more about the current changes in medicine — especially if he is not in a medical office building. If he also spends a day or more every week working at a hospital, this may make up for some of the solo practice.

Q14: Does he have a clinical faculty appointment at a medical school? Has he taught, or is he currently teaching at any of the local colleges, and what does he teach?

Call the college or check the college class directory to see if the doctor does currently teach there. It is a good sign if the doctor is so knowledgeable that he is teaching others to become doctors. Working or taking continuing education courses at a university can give him experience with state-of-the-art equipment, and keep him current on the latest advances in medicine.

Do not be fooled into thinking that a doctor is a university professor simply because he has an office on the grounds of a university. He may simply be renting office space from the university.

Q15: Does the doctor have an active staff membership at a local hospital that has been accredited by the Joint Commission on Accreditation of Healthcare Organizations?

Hospitals have credentials committees that are responsible for saying which physicians are qualified to practice there and what they are allowed to do — and for disciplining those who abuse the privilege.

Before the doctor is granted full privileges in the hospital, he may be subject to a probation period where he is supervised by another doctor. This probation period is more likely to occur in a larger hospital. Smaller hospitals are less rigid in their monitoring of doctors.

A doctor pays nothing for the use of the hospital facilities, equipment, and services. Doctors bring business to the hospital. The hospital bills the patients separately for hospital facilities, services, and use of equipment. This is why hospitals want to maintain relationships with doctors. The doctor-patient base is the lifeblood of the hospital. When there is a conflict between a hospital administrator and a doctor, the administrator is more likely to lose his job than the doctor is of being banned from the hospital. Doctors are more important to the hospital than the hospital administrators, nurses, or other hospital workers and doctors know this.

A doctor who is working for an HMO may be under salary and get paid by the HMO that owns the hospital.

A doctor who has been scrutinized by a hospital review board and been placed on staff at a local hospital is a safer choice than a doctor who has not. On the other hand, the hospital may not have checked into the doctor's background as thoroughly as may be considered safe. This may be because the doctor provided the hospital with inaccurate information on the application he submitted. Some hospitals also have a history of accepting doctors who have a record of negligence.

The doctor may also be practicing a legitimate form of what a group of allopathic doctors may consider to be "alternative medicine," in combination with his training as an allopathic medicine doctor. This situation may also keep a doctor from being given staff privileges at an "allopathic hospital" because the doctor may be considered to be a heretic.

•

THOMPSON: . . . in a hospital today, the care is provided not by one physician, but by a whole team and when the hospital itself then becomes the focus of responsibility, the hospital itself becomes responsible for making sure that the team functions as a team.

KLECZKA: But the hospital — I don't know. Who do we mean by the hospital, maybe the administrator or some overseer is not in every surgical suite where the possibility of a malpractice injury could occur. And playing the devil's advocate, I would liken that to blaming the car for the accident and not the driver and to shift that liability to the hospital where they don't have a direct hands-on overseeing ability for every surgeon who might be working under their roof.

THOMPSON: Well, hospitals are supposed to. Those hospitals are supposed to check what their [the doctors'] credentials are. You [the hospitals administrators] are not supposed to privilege a physician if you [the hospital] are not confident that physician can practice good medicine. You are supposed to have quality-assurance systems and risk management systems. This all has to be in place [within the hospital] in order [for the hospital] to be accredited by the Joint Commission.

KLECZKA: I am not sure when you have a situation where a physician is involved in repetitive medical practice-type incidents, but for the one slip of the knife and some examples, the wrong liver being taken out. The hospital just can't comprehend those before they happen, naturally.

THOMPSON: You are not going to reduce to zero the incidence of these things. Indicated in this Harvard study [of hospitals in New York], 1% of the people were victims of negligence and 4% had bad things happen to them. About three quarters of the unfortunate events were accidents — might even be a slip of the scalpel — and only one quarter seemed to involve physicians' negligence.

> — Lawrence H. Thompson, Assistant Comptroller General, Human Resources Division, US General Accounting Office and Congressman Gerald D. Kleczka, during Congressional subcommittee hearings on issues relating to medical malpractice, May 20, 1993

Q16: Has the doctor ever lost his privileges at any hospital because of unacceptable practices? What were the reasons?

Losing the privileges at the hospital means revoking the doctors' ability to treat patients within the hospital and is sometimes done because the doctor did something seriously wrong, has a history of negligence or of being sued for malpractice. The doctor may also lose his hospital privileges because he has failed to stay updated in his field of medicine, or because a utilization review showed that the way he practices medicine is too expensive for the hospital — even if his expensive actions were better for the patients he treated. Losing hospital privileges will restrict the doctor's access to medical equipment, severely restrict his ability to practice medicine, and have a negative effect on his income. He will then have to try to gain privileges at another hospital, or limit the procedures that he can do.

However, a doctor may also may lose privileges if the hospital signed on with a health maintenance organization and for some reason the doctor did not sign a contract with the HMO. If the doctor has a medical specialty in contraception or fertility and was once affiliated with a hospital that was taken over by the Catholic church, the doctor may have lost his privileges at the hospital because the Catholic church is against certain types of medically induced contraception and fertility procedures.

Q17: Is the doctor involved with any research in which he plans to include your records, photos, and test results? What kind of research? What is the purpose of the research? Through what organization? Will there be money made from this study?

Ask to see a copy of the information about the research.

Q18: Has a formal accusation ever been filed against the doctor by the county or state attorney general or has any disciplinary action been taken against the doctor?

Doctors can have their licenses revoked, be suspended from practicing for a period of time, be fined, or have restrictions placed upon them by the state licensing board. The insurance company through which he gets his malpractice insurance may place restrictions on the amount of money the doctor is insured for, or drop the doctor altogether.

You may have to write the state medical board or other governing body to find if a doctor has any record of misconduct, if he has ever been disciplined, or to find out what a doctor has been formally accused of by former patients. Thanks to the medical lobbies' ability to influence lawmakers, some state boards are not permitted to tell you if a doctor has lost multi million-dollar lawsuits, has had multiple complaints filed against him, has had a history of drug abuse, has sexually molested a patient, or has caused a patient's death.

Q19: Does he carry malpractice insurance?

If he does not, it is time for you to leave the office.

Some doctors say they cannot afford malpractice insurance. Others claim that carrying malpractice insurance increases their chances of being sued, whereas some doctors cannot get insurance because no insurance company will cover them. "Going bare" is the term used to describe doctors who are practicing without malpractice insurance.

Q20: What is the company he has the insurance with and what is the policy number? The insurance company may be listed on his resume.

Also find out how much he is insured for. You can call the insurance company to confirm this. In a newsletter put out by one medical malpractice insurance company in the fall of 1995, doctors were advised to carry at least $1 million in malpractice insurance and preferably $2 million. If a doctor is limited to only $100,000 or so in malpractice coverage, he may have restrictions put on him by the insurance company because of a history of being sued, or because of a negligent background.

Even if he does have malpractice insurance, it may not cover the operation you are having. Check to see if the insurance plan covers the specific surgery you are considering.

Q21: Has the doctor ever been sued by a former patient? What were the consequences?

Having had a malpractice lawsuit brought against him does not mean a doctor is a poor physician. The determination of whether the doctor is dangerous depends on the consequences of the situation that led to the malpractice suit. He may treat high-risk patients who have a greater chance of complications, or he may specialize in a rare but necessary type of treatment that is also high risk. About 20% of malpractice suits result in serious settlements and judgments against doctors. About 1% of all doctors account for 50% of the malpractice awards.

Q22: How many times has he performed the operation you are considering, how often does he perform it, and when was the last time he performed it?

The doctor may have learned the procedure by watching other doctors perform it and assisting them; watching a video that shows the operation being done; reading about the procedure in medical manuals or other literature; attending a seminar or class that teaches how to perform the surgery; performing the procedure on cadavers; performing the operation on animals; practicing on realistic models; using audio-visual equipment; developing the procedure himself; or some combination of these.

Remember that the doctors "perform" operations and that some of the performances do not turn out as well as others. Though it is not ethically wrong for a doctor to perform an operation that he has not performed in the past, he should know what his limitations are, and refrain from reaching beyond his practiced skills. A responsible doctor will admit when it is time to refer a patient to another doctor who has more experience in a particular area. The risks of surgery are reduced if the patient is being operated on by a doctor who is experienced in the type of surgery that is being done.

Q23: Is the doctor, his office, and his staff clean and organized?

Q24: Has the doctor written any articles that have been published in any journals or magazines?

Many doctors have written articles for various magazines and have appeared on television. A doctor who has a research article printed in certain professional publications, such as the *New England Journal of Medicine*, exhibits his expertise in a certain area of medicine, can become a medical celebrity, and be sought after to give lectures to audiences of medical professionals. Having an article published does not guarantee that the doctor is a good doctor.

• COMMUNICATION WITH THE DOCTOR

Q25: Are you difficult to communicate with? Is your own lack of communication skills having a negative influence on your relationship with the doctor?

Is this because you are nervous, or uncomfortable, or is it caused by medication or your health condition?

Having a relative or friend present when you visit the doctor might be of help in this situation.

Q26: Did the doctor give you his undivided attention or was he carrying on unrelated conversations with his employees during the time you were paying him to give you his attention?

Q27: Has the doctor treated you as an individual, or do you feel he is running his office more like a factory where he does the same thing to everyone?

Q28: Do you feel comfortable with the doctor? Do you have doubts about the doctor's abilities? Do you feel the doctor has lied to you or misled you? Did you feel as if you were being manipulated? Has the doctor or the staff made you feel as if you will miss out on something if you do not undergo the surgery?

Often when a person is in a doctor's office the doctor is standing while the patient is sitting down. That arrangement invites dominance. If you are talking with the doctor and he is standing, he is not examining you, and there is no reason for you to be sitting down, if you are able to stand up, then do so; if the doctor is sitting down, maybe you should sit also. You may also ask the doctor to sit down with you. It may improve the way you communicate with the doctor.

Q29: Does the doctor respond to your questions with the attitude that you are out of place in questioning him because he has the medical degree and you do not? Did he react coolly to your questions or speak to you as if he were chastising you for questioning him?

It is your health, body, life, and future that are being discussed. Probably not his. You or someone is paying for the doctor to provide you with his expertise, and you should receive it through word or action as your case necessitates.

Q30: Does the doctor show signs of drug or alcohol use? Was there alcohol on his breath? Was he slurring his words? Did he seem level-headed?

Q31: On what merits have you based your decision to allow this particular doctor to perform surgery on you?

Was your decision based on the doctor's charisma, wit, or charm? Do you believe he is trustworthy? Does he treat you like he owns you? Is he rude, or perverse, or does he act like you are inferior to him? Does he treat you like one of his best buddies? Does he seem too eager to do the operation? Has the doctor spoken of the operation as if it is some kind of secret magical procedure? Has the doctor made inappropriate sexual comments or touched you in a sexual way?

Some doctors will give you a questionnaire that asks your opinion on the doctor, his staff, and their services. Do not fill it out. It might be used against you if, for some reason, you end up taking the doctor to court.

Q32: Did he listen to your side of the story? Has the doctor answered all your questions to your satisfaction? Are there still things that are not clear to you?

Get answers.

• OTHER PATIENTS

Q33: Can you see photos of the doctor's former patients who have received operations similar to the one you are looking into?

Q34: Can you meet people he has operated on?

Q35: Has the doctor ever had a patient who had the operation you are requesting who was disappointed? Why was the patient disappointed?

Q36: What kind of complications has the doctor seen with his other patients who have undergone the same procedure as you are considering?

Is there the possibility that you may experience the same type of complication?

What can be done to lower the risk that you will experience the same complication?

Q37: Has one of the doctor's patients ever died as a result of any operation the doctor has performed?

It is a bold question. Depending on what type of doctor he is, for instance, if he is a cancer specialist (oncologist), a history of patient deaths is to be expected. But if he is a doctor who practices a less involved type of medicine — a dentist, cosmetic surgeon, or dermatologist — a patient death is much less acceptable.

Even if the doctor did have a patient die while that patient was undergoing surgery, this still does not mean the doctor was negligent. There may have been an adverse reaction to anesthesia, an underlying health condition, or the patient may have withheld information about his health that led to the death. On the other hand, the doctor may simply have been purely negligent and created a situation that caused a patient to die.

If you do ask the question you may be surprised by the doctor's candid honesty, or appalled by his arrogance or distasteful reaction to your question.

• WEIGHING THE BENEFITS AND RISKS

Q38: Are there any pamphlets or other literature that the doctor suggests you should read before you make a decision to have the operation?

Q39: If you are having this surgery to repair damage, will the surgery itself cause more damage and health risks than the original injury?

Q40: If you are going in for some operation that will supposedly save your life, what are the statistics regarding the surgery's success rate? Do people who have had the operation actually live longer? What is their quality of life?

Q41: Will the operation interfere with your sex life, in what way, and for how long? Is there a risk of sexually responsive nerves being cut or damaged during the surgery?

Q42: Could being more conscientious about diet and exercise eliminate what is causing you to consider this surgery?

For example, are you dramatically overweight and experiencing knee problems for which you are planning to undergo surgery?

Q43: Are there other ways to treat your condition that could be tried before surgery? Why did you choose this operation instead of another operation, or a non-surgical treatment?

Q44: Will having this surgery create a situation in which you will be more dependent on doctors? For instance, will you need yearly checkups on the surgical site, or are you getting some type of implant that may cause future problems?

On June 26, 1996 the US Supreme Court ruled that injured consumers can sue the makers of medical devices even though the products have been screened for use by the federal Food and Drug Administration.

Q45: If you are getting some sort of man-made material put into your body, do you know the risks involved with that implant?

Does the implant arrive from the manufacturer in a sterilized condition, or does it have to be sterilized by someone on the surgical team in the operating room or sometime before it is inserted into your body? How is it sterilized? Is there special equipment involved? Does the sterilization process involve heat or liquids? Is the liquid something that you can have a reaction to?

Is the implant altered in any way by the doctor or his staff? Is there any glue or other substance involved with these alterations? What type of glue is it? Can your body have a reaction to the glue?

There have been cases where medical supply companies have sold implant devices to unknowing doctors who were told by the supplier that the devices were FDA approved when they had not been.

Do you have the information from the manufacturer of the implant that lists the risks involved with placing the material in the human body? Some implants come with information that is meant to be given to the patient.

Q46: If something does go wrong with this surgery, how will it affect your family, job, finances, and other areas of your life?

Q47: What kind of burden will your family experience because of your surgery?

• MENTAL WELL-BEING

Q48: How will the operation affect you emotionally?

When a person is experiencing health problems he is also likely to experience some form of emotional upset. This may force a patient to face a lot of issues he has ignored or procrastinated on. Illness may also create tension in personal relationships, and cause family members to experience raw emotions. Crisis can bring people closer together, or may expose situations that will cause a relationship to fall apart.

As has been pointed out in other areas of this book, state of mind can play a large part in a person's recovery from illness. Depending on the surgeon and nurses to take care of your emotional needs will probably not provide you with the therapy you require. To become healthier a person may benefit from consulting with a psychologist.

Children may be able to express their feelings about surgery through art. Providing an ill child with crayons, pencils, and paper may help the parents and doctor to understand the concerns of the child. Once the child's concerns are known, steps can be taken to help the child cope with his inhibitions and concerns about his illness.

Q49: If you are in psychological counseling, have you discussed your plans to have this surgery with your therapist?

• YOUR MOTIVES

Q50: What do you expect to gain from this surgery?

Are you undergoing the surgery to increase your life expectancy? Increase your physical capabilities? Cure a disease? Increase your comfort level?

Q51: Have you distorted the need for this surgery?

Q52: What happens if you do not undergo the surgery?

Q53: Will the surgery create a long-term problem that does not currently exist?

Q54: What is the chance that more than one surgery will be needed to correct any problem arising from the original surgery?

Q55: Has someone tried to talk you out of the surgery, or simply told you that you should not have it done? Have you considered their viewpoint?

Q56: Are you having surgery because you know someone else who had it and you like that person's results?

Just because a surgery had a satisfactory result on one patient does not mean you will experience the same result.

Q57: Do you feel responsible or guilty for your health condition? Is this a motivating factor in your choice of treatment?

Q58: Are you being pushed into the operation by someone else?

    The operation should be done only for the person getting it. He will be the one who will be living inside the body for the rest of his life.

Q59: Has your decision to undergo surgery been influenced by the doctor's advertising, his staff, or testimonials of former patients of the doctor?

Q60: Is the doctor or his staff trying to convince you to have more done than you originally intended? Has the doctor responded to you as if he knows what is best for you regardless of what your goals of the surgery are?

Q61: Do you feel the doctor may have convinced you to undergo surgery for a medical condition that is not serious enough for surgical treatment?

Q62: Are you overly confident?

    This is where the person has already decided, before entering the surgeon's office, and before doing any real research and considering the risks involved, that he knows everything necessary and will undergo the surgery as a personal goal. He may bristle with enthusiasm and an unrealistic abundance of self-esteem. Altogether, he may refuse to accept that his calculations are incorrect, and be unwilling to accept that the decision to undergo surgery is in his best interest. The latter can drive him to seek out a doctor who will agree with his views.

    This enthusiasm may be a form of anxiety and anxiousness brought on by a person who has overestimated the benefits of the surgery. It also may be related to hypochondriasis, or to bipolar disorder (manic depression) where he has grandiose visions and is experiencing overly self-assured feelings that he can accomplish anything. These feelings of confidence exist until the person flips back into a depression. Surgery is not a treatment for these states of mind.

    No one should be in a hurry to get onto a surgeon's table. Cautious steps should be followed to ensure that the patient understands the risks and is making a decision that he will be happy with for the rest of his life. This includes the possibility of deciding against the operation.

Q63: Are there any other awkward situations or life difficulties that are driving you to make irrational or desperate decisions or impairing your judgment?

    If you are desperate to undergo cosmetic surgery, you may be overlooking many things that may be important later. You may have unrealistic visions of how good you are going to look after recovering from the surgery. You may not have paid enough attention to the risks of the operation. You may be placing too much trust in the doctor and have, in your excitement, not done enough of your own research to realistically know what can and cannot be done. You may not have asked for a second and third opinion by two other unrelated doctors, and may not have done enough background checking into the qualifications of the doctor, his operating room staff, and the qualities of the operating room.

Q64: Did you plan to have this surgery in the past and then cancel? What was the reason you decided not to have the operation? Does that reason still stand?

• SECOND AND THIRD OPINIONS

Q65: Did the doctor become impatient when you mentioned that you were going to have a second opinion?

    Do not submit yourself to surgery based on one doctor's opinion. Your insurance company may cover the cost of the second opinion because it helps to avoid unnecessary surgery.

    Always get a second opinion by a financially unrelated doctor whenever you are told that you need to undergo elective surgery and when no emergency exists.

    Ask the second opinion doctor what optional forms of treatment may be available instead of surgery.

Q66: If you have a family doctor, did you discuss your plans to have this surgery and ask him about the doctor you are considering for the surgery?

- Ask your family doctor if he knows anything about the surgeon you have chosen. A doctor may have some insight on who the good doctors are in your city.
- Ask him if he has any advice on the testing that should be done before you have the surgery, preparations you should make, location where the surgery will take place, what safety precautions you should take, and any other advice he can give you.

• OUTPATIENT SURGERY

Q67: Does the doctor have hospital privileges to perform the operation you are thinking about having?

When the doctor performs the operation in a hospital and the nurse sees him do something wrong, the nurse is obligated to inform quality control at the hospital. The hospital will then be prepared to protect itself by taking actions against the doctor, and possibly prepare for a lawsuit. When the doctor performs the operation in his office suite, there is no one higher up than himself. Any actions that can be taken against him because of his negligence will be the result of a malpractice lawsuit, the rare action by the state medical authorities, or by the Drug Enforcement Administration.

Call the hospital the doctor is associated with and find out if the doctor has privileges at the hospital to perform the specific procedure you are seeking.

Q68: Is the outpatient surgery center licensed by the state? Is it accredited by the Accreditation Association of Ambulatory Healthcare and/or the American Association for Accreditation of Ambulatory Plastic Surgery Facilities?

Surgery centers that are accredited by these associations have met various standards. Doctors have to pay to have their facilities inspected. A doctor who has gone through the extra effort to have his facility accredited is looking out for the safety of his patients.

Q69: Does the doctor have an emergency transfer agreement with a local hospital?

If you are having the operation in the doctor's office, or at an outpatient surgery center, and an emergency arises during the operation that requires more attention than he can give you there, he will need to transfer you to the hospital. Therefore, your doctor needs to have an emergency transfer agreement with a local hospital.

Q70: Are the elevators, doorways, and hallways of the doctor's surgical suite big enough to accommodate a surgical table, should an emergency arise that requires you to be moved on it?

Q71: Is there an emergency power supply for the operating room?

If, for some reason, the power in the building goes off, there should be an emergency power supply that can be used while the doctor finishes the operation. Equipment and lights should be able to run off this power supply without delay. Computerized equipment should have surge protectors and equipment that will prevent dips in the power levels.

Q72: If you are having outpatient surgery and there is a complication making it necessary for you to be transferred to a hospital, will your insurance cover the expense?

• THE HOSPITAL

Types of hospitals:
- **Specialty hospital**. Usually concentrates on one type of health concern, such as cancer or rehabilitation.
- **Private hospital**. Owned by a corporation, religious group or private individuals. Hospitals owned by insurance companies (such as Kaiser) fall under this category.

There is a difference between a private hospital that is not owned by an HMO and a hospital that is. The hospital that is *not* owned by an HMO makes more money with each procedure that is performed on the patients there and looks at each patient as income. The hospital that is owned by an HMO may receive a set amount of money for each patient and look at patients as a cost. This kind of hospital will want to keep procedures to a minimum so that the profit ratio is high. The less they do, the more money they can keep.

Many people believe that not-for profit private hospitals give the best care. In particular they believe that religious-affiliated hospitals are the best. The ethics committees of the religious hospitals tend to have an influence on bringing higher standards to the hospital. It may have something to do with the religious influence on helping the sick and caring for the disabled. They also may have more staff, and this results in higher costs being reflected in the patient bills.

- **University hospital.** Often on the grounds of a university and is used to help teach medical students. University hospitals may also be off a college campus such as when a university has purchased a hospital in a nearby community, or has a contract with a hospital off campus. Many of the doctors in university hospitals are involved in research studies and in treating patients as part of a research agenda. Teaching hospitals often have more up-to-date medical equipment and perform more tests on each patient. It is usually more expensive to be treated in a teaching hospital because they must cover the cost of training medical students and of purchasing the most current equipment. A patient in a teaching hospital has the right to refuse to allow students, interns, and residents from treating him.
- **Private hospital associated with a medical school.** A privately owned hospital as described above that has an affiliation with a medical school that uses the hospital to help teach its medical students.
- **Public hospital.** Owned by either the federal government, the state, county, or city. Public hospitals are often associated with medical schools. Patient bills at public hospitals are often paid in whole or in part by government agencies.
- **Veterans or military hospitals.** For military personnel, their spouses and children. They also may be used by politicians, such as those around Washington, DC.

Some hospitals are choosing to make dramatic changes in the way patients are treated. These hospitals apply more of a holistic approach to wellness and provide information on holistic therapies, such as acupuncture and massage. Patients are allowed to look at their charts and are encouraged to ask questions and become involved in their treatment. Overnight visitors may spend the night on reclining chairs, and the rooms feature radios, VCRs, and places to hang family photos. Family members may be encouraged to participate in the care of the patient to prepare for recovery at home. Separate visiting rooms resemble living rooms, and some patients and their visitors are allowed to prepare their own food in small kitchens. Entertainment is sometimes provided, and the furnishings include plants and artwork. Patients are allowed access to libraries that contain medical information and computers.

This new way of running a hospital was started by an organization called Planetree that is located in San Francisco. Part of the Planetree philosophy is to empower the patient with knowledge about his own treatment and to build a comfortable environment where patients spend their time. A couple of dozen hospitals, or portions of them, in the US have adopted the Planetree approach.

Q73: If you have health insurance, what hospitals are affiliated with your insurance? The hospital will be able to tell you if they are under contract with your insurance company, or you can call the insurance company and ask them for the names of the hospitals in your area that accept your insurance.

Q74: Can you sign the admission papers early, such as the week before surgery? Women who are going to have their babies in hospitals often sign the admission forms weeks before the baby is due. Admission forms can also be signed early by patients who are planning to undergo elective procedures. This can give a patient time to read through the paperwork and see what the fine print actually says.

Q75: If you are to stay in a hospital after the operation, have you visited and checked out the hospital, its staff, and its resources?

Contact the hospital's public relations or administration office. Ask to see a copy of the hospital's admittance form and other printed material concerning your rights and responsibilities as a patient. The hospital may have a *Patient's Handbook* or a formal *Statement of Patient's Rights* or a *Patient's Bill of Rights* that you can see or obtain a copy of.

The American Hospital Association supplies its member hospitals with its *Patient's Bill of Rights*. To get a copy of this document, call the AHA at the phone number given in the *Research Resources* section of this book under the heading *Accrediting Healthcare Facilities and Setting Healthcare Standards*. Compare the document you receive from the AHA with the document you obtained from the hospital, and make note of any differences.

Q76: Is the hospital accredited by the American Osteopathic Association, Medicare, or the Joint Commission on Accreditation of Healthcare Organizations (or all three)?

Accreditation is a voluntary procedure the hospitals pay for to show that the facility has passed certain standards.

A hospital that is accredited through the JCAHO goes through an inspection at least every three years. If a hospital has "conditional accreditation" from the JCAHO, this means that the facility did not pass the inspection but has been given a set period of time to correct certain shortcomings. The JCAHO will tell you if a hospital is accredited, conditionally accredited, or not accredited. They will also tell you the date of the hospital's last survey and when it is up for renewal. As of October 1994, the JCAHO began making the detailed facility performance reports available to the public for a cost of $30.

A hospital that has been accredited by the JCAHO is automatically accepted by the federal government as qualified to participate in the Medicare program, and by most states as qualifying for state licensure.

The JCAHO is not a government agency and is financed and run by the medical industry. There have been JCAHO-accredited hospitals that have failed government inspections.

To find out if the hospital has gained or lost accreditation, look in the state register at your local library. The hospital or licensing heading of the register should contain this information.

(The phone number to the JCAHO is in the *Research Resources* section of this book under the heading of *Accrediting Healthcare Facilities and Setting Healthcare Standards*.)

Q77: Is the hospital a teaching hospital? This means that the hospital is associated with a local medical school and students take part in treating the patients.

A teaching hospital is more likely to have the latest equipment and a staff that is familiar with the latest developments in their field. The medical students and student nurses are supervised by doctors and hospital staff. The residents and interns often move (rotate) among the various units within the hospital so they get experience in various areas of medicine.

If you are being treated by an intern (a recent medical school graduate), be aware of the presence of the "attending" or "supervising physician." Any crucial medical decisions should be made by the attending physician, and not solely by the intern. Also, if there are any invasive procedures that are being performed, the attending physician should be closely supervising the procedure. Regardless, whenever you are being treated by an intern, the attending physician should be in the building and not "on call" at home, at church, or out playing golf.

Q78: Who will be attending you in the hospital?

If anyone comes into your hospital room you believe should not be there, call the hospital operator, state what room you are in and that you want the person out of your room immediately.

If a nurse, medical student, lab technician, or other person comes into your room and tells you he has orders from your doctor to give you a pill, a shot, a test, or other procedure and you believe he is mistaken, call your doctor and clear up any confusion. Do not be intimidated into taking a pill, having a shot, or undergoing a procedure that may not be in your best interest.

New interns and residents arrive in teaching hospitals at the beginning of July to begin a year of their postgraduate medical training. There they will gain experience through their work with the hospital patients. It is "hands-on training" in the purest form and it is part of the way medical students who become doctors learn their profession. Patients who stay in teaching hospitals should expect to see medical students in the patient rooms. Patients also have the right to ask medical students to leave the room, and should do so without hesitation.

Lab technicians who take patients to undergo tests, x-rays, or other procedures may show up in the room unannounced. They may wheel you away in your bed, transfer you to another bed, or help you into a wheelchair. You will be taken to the imaging or testing department, have the procedures done, and returned to your room. If you think they are being impersonal, or you do not know what they are there for, ask questions. Make sure it is you they want, and not the person in the next bed.

In addition to the doctors, nurses, interns, residents, lab technicians, housecleaning staff, and hospital administrators who may come into your room, there also may be representatives from pharmaceutical companies and medical device manufacturing companies. They may be there on a sales visit, or to check up on their companies' products as part of their research and development processes, and to see if the equipment is being used properly. There also may be others in the hospital who are involved in your care but you do not see. These include members of the hospital quality-assurance committee who review your records to keep track of the procedures done in the hospital. Pharmacists may review your hospital chart to see what medications have been prescribed. Pharmacists may also make their rounds of each patient room to check patient charts for medication errors. The pharmacist may accompany a doctor or nurse, or may work independently. Patients concerned about their medications may request to speak with the hospital pharmacist.

The nurses and others who tend to you in the hospital follow your doctor's orders that are detailed in your chart. This way they will know what drugs you are taking and when to give them to you, what tests to give you, and what physical activity and dietary needs you have. A specific nurse may be assigned to you and will coordinate your care as directed by your doctor. The nurse who is caring for you will also have several other patients to take care of. The nurse will be supervised by the head nurse of the hospital unit you are in. If you are having difficulty communicating with the nurse who is caring for you, the head nurse may be able to help settle your concerns.

Another nurse in the hospital who may be involved in your care is one who works in the utilization review department. She may review your chart on a daily basis and see to it that treatments, testing, and therapy are done on a timely basis to fit the needs of the hospital.

As in other industries, the medical industry is increasingly dependent on temporary workers. One reason for this is the increased pressure by HMOs to lower costs. Hospitals no longer have to keep a full staff of nurses and doctors on the payroll. They can use healthcare temp agencies to hire temporary nurses, doctors, therapists, and other staff as they are needed. These temporary workers may be used to fill in for vacationing hospital staff, or employed during the winter season when people tend to get sick more often.

If you are in a hospital that has a religious affiliation, there may be a nun, a priest, or other type of minister stopping by your room to say hello. If you are not associated with that church you should not feel obligated to spend time with this minister, unless you would enjoy the company. Otherwise, if you are trying to rest, kindly let the minister know that you would like to be left alone. You are there to receive medical treatment, not to be preached to. Additionally, the hospital may have a small chapel on the premises where you can go to pray or meditate if you are allowed to travel that far from your room.

Q79: How long should you expect to stay in the hospital?

Patients do not stay in the hospital as long as they did just a few years ago. This is due in part to the advances in surgery techniques and surgical instruments that inflict less trauma on the body.

Though it is probably in your best interest to remain in the hospital until the doctor says it is safe to go home, no one can stop you from leaving. If you do leave earlier than the doctor advises, you are then leaving "against medical advice." A patient wanting to leave a hospital earlier than the doctor advises could be unsatisfied with the treatment, or may have business or family matters that need his attention. Whatever the reason is, checking out of the hospital against medical advice may interfere with your medical insurance coverage. If negligent treatment was what motivated the patient to leave the hospital early, the patient may be wise to consult with another doctor or a lawyer to document the unsatisfactory treatment.

Unless you are a criminal detained in the jail ward of the county hospital or mentally unstable, you cannot be held in a hospital against your will. You have the right to walk out of the hospital without paying your bill, and without signing any paperwork. Some of the workers at the hospital may tell you that you "must" sign the release form. You do not have to sign anything unless you want to.

If you have been told by the nurses that it is time for you to leave the hospital and you feel too sick to leave, ask to speak to your doctor. There may be a complication that the nurses are unable to recognize that would require you to receive close medical attention, and a longer hospital stay.

Q80: If you are going to be traveling from out of town, does the hospital have an arrangement for discount rates at a local hotel?

This hotel arrangement may be helpful to your family if they are traveling with you. You also may not have to check into the hospital until the morning of the surgery and staying in the hotel the night before may be convenient. You may also need to stay in town some days after surgery.

Q81: Will you be on pain medication during your stay in the hospital?

Pain medication can distort your judgment. If there are any major decisions that you need to make during your time in the hospital, is there a relative, friend or lawyer who can help you with your decisions?

Pain medication may interfere with your balance. When you get out of your bed, you may need a cane, a walker, or a person to help you walk.

Q82: Does the hospital keep a doctor on staff who deals specifically with infections?

Q83: Are you allergic to any foods? Will the hospital accommodate any of your special dietary needs, such as vegetarianism? Can you speak to the hospital dietitian if you have any questions about dietary needs?

A patient should remember that nutrition is a very important part of healing — a concept that many hospital kitchens have yet to discover. A body that has been through major surgery uses more calories than usual and needs to be fed nutrients that it can use to repair itself.

There is no law that says you must eat the food served to you in a hospital. Many hospitals promote the idea of having patients order food from local restaurants that deliver or have friends or family supply meals. This can be particularly helpful if the patient is a vegetarian, or is sick of the stuff that hospitals refer to as "food."

Some hospitals will allow a long-term patient to bring in a small refrigerator. Some hospitals have small refrigerators available for rent.

If you have visitors while you are in the hospital, do not let them eat the food on your tray without letting the nurse know. The nurse may be keeping records of what you eat and drink. Similarly, if you are visiting someone in the hospital, do not give them food or drinks that you bring in without first asking the nurse. The food may interfere with medication, the patient may not be allowed any food, or the patient may be limited to certain types of food.

If the patient is not allowed to eat food, he will be taking nutrients through an intravenous drip that will also help replace fluids that are lost through breathing, urine, and the stool.

Q84: Will you be in a private room or will you have a roommate? Does the room have privacy curtains that surround the bed and are they in working order?

Private rooms usually cost extra. If you have an infectious disease you will be in a private room.

Your roommate may be quiet, or so drugged out that you may never have a conversation. Or you may have a roommate who talks so much and has so many visitors that it will interfere with your rest. If you have a roommate that you cannot tolerate, request that your room be changed.

Q85: Where are the emergency buttons located in the patient rooms? Are you going to be able to reach them from your bed?

Calling the nurse when you need help is just part of staying in a hospital. If you require too much of the nurses' attention, you may find yourself ignored, or your requests delayed. There is no rule that says one patient must be attended to first. Being liked or disliked by a nurse can play a part in your hospital stay. Remember that nurses are usually caring for several patients at one time. All patients must wait their turn.

Q86: Are there private bathrooms in each patient room? Does the shower or bathtub have safety bars so you can steady yourself while you are in the shower? Are there anti-slip surfaces on the bathtub or shower floor and on the bathroom floor? You are likely to be on pain medication and this may affect your balance.

Q87: Do the patient rooms or the bathrooms have mirrors?

Depending on what you are having done, it may be a good idea to avoid mirrors.

Q88: Are there security guards on the hospital grounds?

If you do not want someone to know you are in the hospital, tell the hospital admissions clerk that you need to be registered under a pseudonym. If the admissions clerk is unable to help you, ask to speak to a social worker at the hospital. Demand that no one be told that you are registered at the hospital unless you want them to know. The social worker can help ensure your safety and this can include arranging for a protective restraining order to help bar anyone who may try to harm you during your stay in the hospital.

Q89: If the surgery requires a child patient to stay overnight in the hospital, does the hospital have a security tracking system?

Some hospitals and nursing homes now have systems that can prevent patients who are wearing a wristwatch-type monitor from going through certain doorways. The monitor triggers a sensor that locks the door when the person wearing the monitor approaches the door. The monitor can both protect a child from wandering through the halls of the hospital and prevent the child from being kidnapped from the hospital.

Q90: How do you exit the hospital in case of an emergency?

Q91: Where do you park while you stay in the hospital? Is there a charge for parking?

Q92: What are the visiting hours at the hospital and where do your guests park?

Some hospitals have limits on what hours a patient may have visitors. Some limit children under a certain age from visiting — but rules can be challenged.

Q93: Do you feel as if you are being ignored during your time in the hospital? Call the hospital operator, state what room you are in and that you need help. If you still have a problem, contact the nurse manager, the hospital administrator's office, your doctor, or your insurance company. Patients who are extremely dissatisfied with their hospital care sometimes switch hospitals.

• NURSING STAFF

Q94: Are the staff nurses and other personnel who will be present during and after the surgery trained in emergency services, such as cardiopulmonary resuscitation?

This question may sound out of place, but there have been lawsuits based around patients not receiving the most basic forms of emergency treatment when it was needed while they were undergoing medical care.

Q95: What educational degree does the nurse carry?

The more help the doctor receives while he is operating on you, the more attention he can give you. A registered nurse has more training than a practical nurse.

The nurse should have gone to a legitimate school. You should not trust yourself with a surgery room nurse who received his degree from some third-rate career training center or correspondence school.

Q96: If the registered nurse (RN) is certified through the American Nurses Credentialing Center, what year was he certified?

A certification is valid for five years. After five years the nurse will have to be recertified to show he has continued to maintain an up-to-date knowledge of the profession.

Q97: Does your state have a Board of Nursing, and if not, what health authority regulates the nurses in your state?

Does this authority release information on disciplinary actions taken against specific nurses?

Q98: Is the nurse who is caring for you legally working in the country?

The Commission on Graduates of Foreign Nursing Schools administers an English language and nursing proficiency exam to nurses who received their education in a foreign country and who seek to practice as registered nurses in the US.

Q99: How long has the nurse worked at the hospital or with the doctor?

A temporary nurse who is filling in for the regular nurse may not be familiar with the layout of the hospital or where the emergency supplies are stored.

Be careful of what the nurse writes on the record. The doctor may base his decision on inaccurate information that was written on your record by other people.

• THE SURGICAL TEAM

Q100: Is the entire surgery performed by the surgeon you selected, or is part of it to be performed by a surgeon who is in training, or another person?

To have a less expensive operation, you can go to a medical school and have a student operate on you with a physician's supervision. If you want only the full-fledged doctor you hired to perform the operation, include this requirement in the consent form.

Q101: Will there be any students, medical equipment company representatives or other people present during the operation who are there simply to observe the procedure?

Q102: Will a registered, licensed, board certified anesthesiologist or a registered nurse certified anesthetist be present during the operation?

Again, the more well-educated help the doctor has in the operating room, the more attention he can give you. An anesthesiologist or nurse anesthetist can be very valuable if there is a complication during the operation.

You want the person administering the anesthesia to have a thorough knowledge of the complexity of anesthesia.

- If you choose a physician-anesthesiologist, find out if he is board certified by checking with the American Board of Anesthesiologists. The phone number is in the *Research Resources* section of this book under the heading Anesthesiology.
- If you choose a nurse-anesthetist, find out if he is a registered nurse and a member of the American Association of Nurse Anesthetists. The phone number is in the *Research Resources* section of this book under the heading *Nurses*, and the heading *Anesthesiology*.

• PRICE, PAYMENT AND INSURANCE

Q103: Is the price you are quoted all-inclusive, or are you going to have to pay separately for the doctor, the anesthesiologist, the operating room, and the post-surgical care?

Ask the doctor's office manager if you can get a discount on the price you are paying for the surgery. If you are paying for the surgery in cash, you may be able to get a discount.

Q104: What is the total cost of having the surgery? How will it affect your financial status?

This includes the doctor's fee, the operating room, the anesthesiologist, the medicines, any money spent because of the surgery, and the amount of money being lost by time spent off work.

Q105: Does the doctor accept your insurance? Is your insurance going to pay for any of this?

Some doctors have become rich by supplying false information to insurance companies. Some doctors will make their patients think they are doing them a favor by getting the insurance to cover part or all of an operation by supplying the insurance company with inaccurate information. Sometimes this act is legitimately sympathetic and helps the patient out of a struggle. Other times the doctor may be doing it out of greed. The doctor gets the money while the patient receives an operation he does not need, and is further inconvenienced by the recovery and possible complications. Where is the favor in that?

Q106: Do you need to supply the doctor's office with the insurance forms?

Q107: Will the surgery interfere with any future health insurance coverage?

Q108: If you are financing the operation on credit, how much will you need to pay per month? How much is it going to cost altogether with the interest charges added in? How many years will you be making payments?

Q109: Does the hospital have a patient services department that will help you sort through insurance forms and medical bills? Call the hospital billing department if you have any questions about your bill. (See the *Billing Problems* heading of the *Research Resources* section of this book for the phone number of companies that can help you figure out your medical bills and show you how to correct overcharges.)

• SIGNING THE CONSENT FORM

Q110: Can you get a copy of the consent form weeks or days ahead of time so that you can read it carefully and make sure it describes the operation you are to have?

Does the doctor have any apprehension about your making alterations to the consent form to make sure you get what you want?

One way to protect yourself is to cross out anything on the consent form that you do not agree to. Customize it to fit your needs so it is in your best interest. Make sure the doctor knows the changes you have made, and discuss the changes with the doctor.

Q111: Have you had the name of the doctor who is to perform the surgery written into the consent form?

Q112: Have you written into the consent form that an anesthesiologist or nurse anesthetist is to be present to administer the anesthesia and is to remain immediately physically available during the surgery, and physically present at the time the surgery is finished until you have recovered from the surgery?

Q113: Have you had it written into the consent form what side of the body the operation is to be performed on?

   If you are undergoing surgery that is to take place only on one side, be sure to have this noted in the consent form. Medical mistakes are known as "misadventures" in the medical community. A hospital in Florida that had admitted to mistakes where doctors amputated the wrong foot on one patient and operated on the wrong knee of another implemented the practice of writing "NO" in black felt pen on the side that is not to be operated on. Many patients are now writing instructions on their skin with a black marker to make sure there is no mistake during surgery, such as removal of the wrong organ or limb.

Q114: Is the doctor asking you to sign a waiver or release that aims to limit the legal action you can take in case the doctor or the medical team is negligent?

   Contact a malpractice lawyer and ask for advice before signing anything that seeks to limit your legal abilities.

• WILLS

Q115: Have you made out a will?

   You can find information about wills at the library, or your local bookstore. There are also lawyers who specialize in this area.

Q116: Do you have a living will and does the doctor know about it?

   See the *Living Wills* and *Final Relief* headings in the *Research Resources* section of this book.

Q117: Have you signed a "donor card" so your healthy organs can be given to someone else who needs them if you die?

   See the heading *Organ Donation and Transplants* in the *Research Resources* section of this book.

Q118: If you are nursing a baby, what is the waiting period for the anesthetic to clear your system before you can nurse again? Will any other medications interfere with your child's needs?

   Ask the obstetrician or pediatrician about these concerns.

• MEDICATIONS/PRESCRIPTIONS (Also see the *Prescriptions* heading in the *Research Resources* section of this book)

- Do not take medications that have been prescribed to another person.
- Do not assume taking three pills is better than taking two pills. Overdoses of medications can occur even with over-the-counter drugs. Risks with drugs vary from an upset stomach to a fatal reaction. When in doubt about prescriptions and over-the-counter drugs, ask your pharmacist.
- Do not mix medications without first asking your doctor and/or pharmacist if the two medications are safe to take at the same time. This includes over-the-counter medicines. One medication may intensify the effects of another. Some medications increase blood pressure. One interaction some people learn about in the most inconvenient way is that antibiotics interfere with contraceptive pills. Even some foods can amplify or cancel out the effects of certain medications.

- Do not expect your doctor to remember all the prescriptions he may have written for you. The average doctor writes thousands of prescriptions every year. If you are receiving prescriptions from more than one doctor, this increases your chances of taking a dangerous mix of medications.

    If you use the same pharmacist all the time, he may have your prescription history in his computer database and can warn you when you may be "crossing medications" in a way that would cause a harmful interaction.

- Dispose of medications at their expiration date. Some medications lose their potency as they age, and others may become toxic. Keep medications out of the reach of children and pets.

- Fetuses are vulnerable to both the effects and the side effects of drugs. Some drugs cause birth defects. If you are pregnant, do not take medications without first getting the approval of your doctor. This includes medications you have purchased over-the-counter. Your pharmacist may also be able to tell you what medications may be dangerous to the fetus.

- Do not give adult medications to children.

- Find out if you are supposed to take the medication with food or water or if the medication is supposed to be taken on an empty stomach. Ask your pharmacist.

- If you are on a medication that has to be injected, do not use the same needle twice, and never use a needle that has been used on another person. Dispose of needles immediately after use in a container that is not accessible to children.

- Keep your medications out of the reach of both children and pets.

- Keep your medications stored in a dry place. The bathroom is not a good place for medicines because the steam from the bath or shower can spoil them.

- Keep your medications away from heat.

- Some medications must be refrigerated. Read the label.

- Do not put more than one kind of pill in the same bottle.

- Turn the light on when you are taking your medications so you know you are taking the correct one and the correct amount.

- Generic drugs sometimes vary in quality. When a pharmacist asks you if you want to switch to a generic brand, find out what the differences are.

- Salesmanship and incentives to sell particular brands go on behind the drug counter just as they do at the car sales lot. When a pharmacist asks you to switch to a generic brand, remember that he may be acting in his own interests more than your own. The pharmacist may be making a bonus for increasing the sales of a generic drug.

- Your insurance company may reimburse you only for the price of the generic version of any drugs that you are prescribed. Check with your insurance handbook or call your insurance company to find out if there is such a requirement.

- If you have any concerns about the medication you are taking, ask your pharmacist and doctor.

    Pharmacists spend several years in school learning about medications. Doctors learn about medications in classes mixed in with their other training. In other words, the pharmacist is likely to know more about your medication than your doctor.

- If you are going to be staying in the hospital, ask about how you are supposed to handle your medication schedule. The nurses may not want you to be taking the medication on your own. Handing the prescriptions over to the nurses while you stay in the hospital may be best for you. The nurses can dispense the medications on schedule and this will reduce the risk of your taking the medications at the wrong time, or taking two medications that may result in an adverse reaction. They can mark the medication schedule and delivery on your chart. When your hospital stay ends, you can take whatever remaining drugs there are home with you. Some hospitals are now storing patient medications in the patient rooms. This reduces the chance that the nurse will mix your medications with those of another patient.

Q119: Do you have a history of addiction to alcohol or drugs? Have you undergone treatment for drug or alcohol addiction?

Do not be shy in letting the doctor know that you have been addicted to substances. He should then be careful with what type and amount of medication he prescribes. Be sure to inform the doctor that you are letting him know delicate information. If he writes about your drug or alcohol addictions in your medical record, this information may be made available to people whom you do not want informed of this.

Q120: Are there any foods or medications you should avoid in the weeks or days before and after the operation?

Q121: How often do you have to take the medications?

If you are prescribed a drug that is to be taken four times a day, taking four pills all at the same time in the morning is not an option, and may be dangerous. Find out if you are to take the medications on a timely basis. For instance, will you have to wake up in the middle of the night to take the medication?

Q122: Has the dosage been adjusted for your weight and height?

If you are five feet tall and 100 pounds, common sense only tells you that you should be taking a different dosage of medication than someone who is six-feet-five and 240 pounds. Medications should be personalized to your needs.

Q123: What are the side effects of the medications?

Have you been taking any medication in the last few months that will interfere with the medication? Inform the doctor of any over-the-counter or prescription medications you have taken within the past few months.

What happens if you do have side effects?

Be aware that some of the positive information you may find out about a medication may be that published by the manufacturer or another party who will make money if people choose to use the product. Information from those sources may be misleading. (A book titled *Worst Pills/Best Pills* is available through Public Citizen's Health Research Group. For ordering information see the *Prescriptions* heading in the *Research Resources* section of this book. It may also be available at your local library.)

If it is a new drug, all the side effects may not have been discovered.

If a drug carries possible serious side effects, a decision on whether to take it must be weighed against the benefits of taking the drug. The more serious the health problem that is being treated, the more the side effects of a drug can be justified.

Q124: How long will you have to continue to take the medication after the surgery?

Q125: What happens if you run out of medication and you need more? If the doctor is going out of town, and you will not be able to speak with him directly, does he have an arrangement with another doctor who will take care of your prescription needs?

Q126: Is the medication sold to be prescribed for your condition, or is the doctor prescribing a medication that is meant to treat some other condition?

Some drugs are being prescribed for conditions other than what the drug was tested and approved for. This is called prescribing a drug "off label."

• TESTS

Q127: Has the doctor performed all the necessary tests to confirm his diagnosis?

Do you know if the doctor has looked at the test results? Did you take the test results with you when you obtained your second opinion?

Q128: How much do the tests cost? The testing lab may require payment before a test is performed, or they may bill you or your insurance company directly.

Q129: Does the doctor own or is he a part owner of the testing equipment or facility where the tests are done?

Q130: Do they plan on taking x-rays of you? What does the doctor expect to find on the x-ray? Are there x-rays of the same body part that another doctor or medical facility has already taken of you that can be sent to the doctor so you can avoid repeat exposure to the radiation that x-rays emit?

Are the personnel who operate the x-ray equipment formally trained about radiation safety and hazards through an approved course that teaches how to correctly operate x-ray equipment? Have the personnel attended continuing education courses to keep updated on radiographic techniques and new developments?

Every time you are given an x-ray you are exposed to radiation. Some of this radiation remains in the tissues of your body. This can lead to future health problems. X-rays should be given only when they are essential.

Most states do not monitor the personnel who take x-rays, many states do not conduct radiation safety inspections of x-ray equipment, and many do not know if something is out of place unless a patient makes a complaint with the proper authorities.

When undergoing an x-ray make sure:
- The person operating the machinery is properly trained.
- You are wearing a protective apron.
- If you are undergoing x-rays of the teeth, make sure the technician is using a disposable/sterilization film holder to lower your risk of contracting hepatitis.
- The radiology technician who is giving you the x-ray is wearing a radiation monitoring film badge that records his exposure to radiation.

Q131: Does the test involve injection of a dye, such as iodine? Are you allergic to iodine, or to any of the substances contained in the injection?

Q132: Will experiments be done on any of the tissue that is removed from your body? What is the purpose of these experiments? Is your tissue being used by other people in a way that will bring them financial gain?

Get pathology reports on any tests done on tissue removed from your body.

Q133: How long does it take for the test results to come back?

Do not let the doctor forget to inform you of the test results. If you are not scheduled for an appointment when the test results are expected back, call to find out what the test results are. Get a copy of the results for your personal records.

• FOOD INTAKE

Q134: When is the last time you can eat before surgery?

Usually there will be a limit on food and liquid intake for several hours and as much as a day or two before the surgery. This will prevent some complications with anesthesia, and the possibility of vomiting during surgery. If the surgeon tells you not to eat, do not eat or you may create problems for yourself. If you vomit during surgery some of the vomit can be breathed (aspirated) into your lungs and this may cause pneumonia. The surgery may be canceled or delayed if you ate too close to the time of surgery.

During surgery the nurse may wet your mouth by putting a wet paper towel in it. This prevents you from getting too dry. When this is done during nasal, sinus, or oral surgery it can make it easier to swallow the blood that will be gathering in your throat. As the blood coagulates, it can irritate the throat and give the feeling of a sore and dry throat, and make you cough. Sometimes people who undergo nose jobs vomit up this blood during or after the operation.

Q135: When can you eat after the operation?

Facial surgery patients may be told to avoid foods that require chewing so the muscle movement does not interfere with healing. If the person has had any facial bone damage caused by the surgery and those bones have been set into place, the chewing motion may interfere with the healing of the bone.

There may be other limitations on what you can and cannot eat. Ask the doctor.

• THE SURGICAL PROCEDURES

Q136: What is the name of the procedure you are looking into?

Doctors do not all use the same terms when describing operations, and do not all use the same techniques.

Q137: What will you be wearing during the operation?

You may be in your street clothes during the operation, or you may have to change into a gown. Whatever you wear, it should be loose fitting and not anything that you will have to pull over your head. Avoid tight clothing, nylons, shoes that need to be tied, or any clothing that is difficult to remove. Children may be allowed to keep their underwear on, and if it needs to be removed, this can be done after they are under anesthesia.

Q138: What position will you be in during the operation? Will there be any restraints put on you during the surgery to keep your arms, legs, torso, or head immobile?

Some operations require that the patient be tied, or braced, down to prevent any type of movement that could interfere with the operation.

If you have a physical injury, such as a back problem that would require limitations on the position you are in during the surgery, arrangements can be made for your comfort and safety.

Q139: Are any of the procedures experimental, or considered to be in an experimental stage?

If it is a new technique, where did the doctor learn it? Who did the original research? Who came out with the technique? Where can you learn more about it?

Q140: Would it be safer to undergo the surgery in stages?

For instance, if you are to undergo eye surgery, would it be better to have one eye operated on and let it fully heal before undergoing surgery on the other eye?

Q141: How long does the operation take?

Q142: What are the steps of the operation from beginning to end?

Q143: Will there be needles or tubes placed in your arms or other areas (between the toes, in the thigh, in the neck, on the tops of the hands, or other areas)? Will you be fed intravenously? Will there be a portacath implanted (this device provides an opening where the nurse can easily draw blood and administer medication)? Will these be placed while you are awake? How long will they remain in place? What kind of pain is involved?

Q144: Do the intravenous pumps have free-flow safety clamps to safeguard against overdoses of medications and IV liquids?

Make it an absolute requirement that any IV used on you be equipped with a free-flow protection device. It can save your health and may save your life.

Q145: Will you have a breathing tube at any time during or after surgery?

When a patient has a tube that goes into the mouth and down the windpipe so a machine can breathe for the patient, it is called being "intubated" or "tubed." The other end of the pipe is connected to a respirator that pumps out oxygen. The tube is called an "ET," or endotracheal tube. The oxygen can also be pumped into the tube manually with a balloon-type device that a nurse squeezes.

The patient is not able to talk during the time the tube is in place. For this reason, you may need to have a pen and writing pad to be able to communicate with others.

Q146: Will any part of your body be shaved? Why, when, and by whom? Are you sensitive to razors, or do you easily develop skin rashes? Have you experienced sensitivity to shaving creams? Do you have coarse, curly, thick-stranded hair that twists back into the skin when it is shaved and that causes pimpling or infected hair follicles? These may cause or contribute to infection. The abrasions left over from the razor will also increase your risk of infection. Chemical hair removal has a lower risk of infection.

Q147: What are the side effects of the anesthesia being used?

Q148: How will the anesthetic be given?

Q149: Will there be music playing during the operation? If not, could you bring your own headset and listen to music of your choice?

A study by University of Buffalo behavioral researcher Karen Allen, published in the September 21, 1994, issue of the *Journal of the American Medical Association* reported that doctors' stress levels dropped when they played music during surgery.

One man who underwent surgery heard what was said between the doctor and the nurses during the surgery. The conversation was about another patient who had cancer and was expected to die. The man undergoing surgery could not move or open his eyes, and could not feel pain. But he could hear. In the confused state of mind that was the result of being drugged by the anesthesia, he thought the doctor was talking about him and that he was going die.

While music that is playing in the operating room may help the doctor relax, wearing your own headphones during surgery and listening to your choice of relaxing music can drown out any sounds you will hear during the operation, such as the conversations of the surgery team that may confuse or frighten you.

Q150: What kind of sterility procedures are taken in the operating room? Are the instruments heat-treated, or sterilized with liquids? Who prepares the instruments?

Post-operative infections are among the leading causes of post-operative death. Improperly cleaned instruments are among the leading causes of post-operative infections. Infections that are acquired in the medical facility where a patient received treatment are called "nosocomial infections."

There are more and more preventative measures being taken to help avoid contamination of a surgical wound. During some surgeries the surgical team wears what resemble space suits with filtered air tubes hanging off the back. Some instruments are sealed in a sterile package and disposed of after being used once.

Q151: Where and how will the incisions be made?

Are there different techniques to making the incisions for the operation you are getting? Will a laser or a scalpel be used to make the incisions? Will there be efforts taken to create the most minimal scar possible?

If the doctor says the scars will be invisible, you should question what he means by this. Scarring after any incision can be expected. Scars may not end up being very noticeable after a few years, and may fade a lot, but more than likely they will always be noticeable upon close inspection.

Many surgeries that once required making a large incision are now being done through very small incisions with the use of laparoscopic instruments. These laparoscopic techniques make use of video monitors that display the inside of the body where the tools are positioned. Saline solution or carbon dioxide gas is used to inflate the cavity where the surgery is being performed. Even complex surgeries, such as kidney removal, are being done this way. The kidney is removed by placing the organ in a bag within the body and then using an instrument to destroy the kidney within the bag and pulling this out through the small incision.

Patients who undergo laparoscopic procedures recover faster and experience less pain than those patients who undergo open surgery. The incisions may need to be protected only with a Band-Aid during the healing process. During some laparoscopic procedures a problem may arise requiring that the surgery be "converted" into an open surgery by making a larger incision (the old-fashioned way).

There are certain operations where the incision is made in an area not commonly seen (inside the nose for instance if a nose job is being performed). Other incisions can be made where there are naturally occurring folds in the skin (in the folds of the eyelids for instance if eyelid surgery is being performed). Some of the most noticeable scars created by surgery occur after surgery takes place on areas of the body where there are no natural folds, such as the torso. Some people arrange for a plastic surgeon to be on hand when it is time to close an incision.

Of course a patient should not be concerned about the vanity issue of scars if the operation is something that will overwhelmingly improve the health of the patient.

Q152: Does the operation entail the cutting of any muscles that will then no longer function?

Q153: Is there a chance the surgery will rupture or damage another organ, or nerves that control an organ or function of the body?

Q154: Will there be any flesh, muscle, cartilage, or bone removed during the operation?

Know what parts of you are going to be altered during the operation so there are no surprises later. One of the rudest surprises after surgery is when a patient finds the doctor did more and took away more than the patient ever expected. Later the patient finds out that the doctor's definition of a slight change was very different from his own. Once something is cut off the body, it cannot be put back.

Q155: What kind of bleeding occurs during the operation? Is there any chance that you will need to receive blood?

Q156: What kind of suture material is used? Are the stitches permanent, or dissolvable, or will you have to come in to have them removed? Will there be any staples used instead of sutures on any of the incisions?

There are various thicknesses of suture material (surgical thread). The closer to the number 100 the suture material is, the thinner it is.

Q157: Will there be any drains inserted at the site of the surgical wound? How long will the drains be left in place?

Sometimes drains are used that remain for a few days. This is done so that any excess blood can be eliminated, thus reducing the risk of hematomas and infection.

Sometimes large blood clots will form inside the body where it has been operated on. These clots may need to be surgically removed. Blood clots can also travel to other parts of the body. If they settle in the lungs they can halt breathing.

Q158: What kind of bandages are used?

Some bandages are made out of cotton, whereas others are a cotton-synthetic blend. Some people are allergic to synthetic materials. This may interfere with healing.

• SURGICAL WOUNDS

Q159: What kind of swelling, bruising, and bleeding should you expect to have?

When seeing your bruised and swollen body, or face, you may wonder what you did to yourself. It can sometimes look as if you have been in a horrible accident, which can incite or contribute to post-surgical depression.

Many patients are surprised by the amount of swelling and bruising that occurs in the days after their surgery. You want to be prepared for the vision of yourself being bruised and swollen. The doctor may have photos that he can show you of other patients at the peak of their swelling and bruising period after they have gone through a similar surgery.

Any uneven or excessive swelling or pain, or pain that comes on suddenly, may be a sign of complications. You should inform the doctor if these occur.

Q160: Are you supposed to apply ice packs to the wound to control swelling?

This may require that you purchase plenty of plastic zipper bags to put the ice in. Frozen peas, frozen corn, or small ice cubes may be better to use on facial wounds than large ice cubes because they are lighter. It may be wise to have a variety of 20 or 30 ice packs prepared and stored in your freezer. A thin cloth over the skin so the ice bag is not directly on it will prevent the skin from getting too cold and will also absorb any dripping water that should not get on the wound.

• POST-SURGICAL CARE

Q161: How will the bandages be applied? Are you supposed to change the bandages when they become dirty, or is the doctor or his staff supposed to do that?

If you are going to have to change your bandages, you will have to know what supplies you will need. Purchase everything days before you undergo the surgery so that you or someone caring for you will not have to run around buying them when you should be in bed recovering.

Q162: How are you to keep the area of the incisions clean?

You may need to clean the incision areas gently with a sterile cotton swab, or gauze dipped in hydrogen peroxide. Ask the doctor what he recommends and purchase these materials before the surgery.

You may be limited in the way you can shower, bathe, and wash your hair for days or weeks after surgery.

If you had surgery on your scalp, the use of hair sprays, gels, creams, and lotions will also be limited before and after surgery until the stitches have been removed. Ask your doctor when it will be safe for you to start using hair products.

Q163: Who is going to take care of you and be with you for the first one to ten days after the surgery?

Because you may be on medication that can distort your judgment, or you may be overwhelmed by the surgery, it is important to have someone around you who can make a responsible and safe decision as to what medical attention you need during this initial healing period.

If you are going to need a visiting nurse, physical therapist, or other person to come to your home to treat and assist you after the surgery, the discharge planner or social worker at the hospital, your insurance company, or your doctor may arrange for this or supply you with the phone number of an agency that offers the services you will need.

Q164: Will you need any special equipment (wheelchair, hospital bed, oxygen, crutches, cane, etc.) for your recovery at home?

Where can you get this equipment? Can it be rented, or do you have to purchase it? Do you need a backup power supply to run the equipment in case the electricity in your home or neighborhood fails?

Q165: Is the doctor available for you to call if you have questions during your recovery? Who will answer the phone when you call if there is an emergency after office hours? Does the doctor carry a pager? Is the doctor going to be in town during the first two weeks after your surgery?

If the doctor is going out of town within two weeks after your surgery you will want to know about it. In case there is a problem of some sort, you want to have access to a doctor who can give you the attention you need. The doctor may have an arrangement with one or more doctors who take over for him when he goes out of town. Other doctors may use a *locum tenens* doctor — who is hired from a temp agency that supplies medical professionals to fill in for workers who are sick, on vacation, or when there is a need for more personnel.

If you need to call the doctor after hours, his phone will likely be answered by an answering service telephone operator. The operator will probably ask if you are having a medical emergency. If so, you will be told to call an ambulance, or to get to the emergency room of your local hospital. If it is not a medical emergency and you need to talk to the doctor, the operator will page the doctor to call you. The answering service operators have no medical training. Do not depend on them for medical advice.

Q166: Will there be a day or more when you will be confined to your bed before or after the operation?

Q167: What kind of activities should be avoided in the days, weeks, and months following the operation?

Q168: If you are having a facial operation, will wearing glasses interfere with any of the healing processes?
    Some surgeries of the face and ears require that the person avoid wearing glasses during the healing process. There is an eyeglass cradle available that attaches to the forehead and keeps the glasses off the face. This is not helpful after ear-pinning surgery (otoplasty) because the glasses would still sit on the ears. Check with the doctor to see what the limitations will be if you wear eyeglasses.

Q169: Will the operation prevent you from being able to wear makeup for any period of time?
    You may be told to clean the surgery area well the night before the surgery, and again on the morning of the surgery. No creams, lotions, oils, perfumes, powders, or makeup should be applied to the area that will be operated on. Makeup will probably need to be avoided for a few days after the stitches are removed.
    If you perm, die, tint, or bleach your hair, it is a good idea to do this no later than a few days before surgery if the surgery is being performed on the face or head. Hair coloring and perms may also need to be avoided for several weeks after the surgery so they don't irritate the wound or tattoo the scar.

Q170: How many days will you need to remain off work? Everyone heals differently. One person getting the same operation as you may or may not have the same amount of swelling, bruising, soreness, and bleeding. Adequate rest and nutrition are important for healing.

Q171: What is the chance that you will experience post-surgical depression, or surgically induced posttraumatic stress disorder?
    Have former patients of the doctor gone through a depression after undergoing surgery similar to yours?
    Does the doctor recommend that you consult with a therapist before the surgery?
    People who are sick recover better if they are exposed to people who care about and pay attention to them. If you are undergoing breast cancer surgery, statistics show, and a study done at Stanford University Medical School found, that you will recover better if you attend a breast cancer support group. Patients undergoing many types of physical-health problems attend and benefit from group psychotherapy sessions. If you have a life-altering disease or other health problem, the doctor, his office, or the hospitals' patient relations office may be able to put you in contact with a support group that deals with your condition.
    Painkillers are "downers" and can contribute to post-surgical depression. Limit your use of painkillers to the amount that is necessary to relieve pain. The residue from the pain medication will remain in the body tissues and can contribute to lingering post-surgical depression.
    The same caution should be taken with sleeping pills. If you do not need them, do not take them. If you are staying overnight in the hospital, be cautious of a nurse who wants you to take a sleeping pill when you do not need one. The doctor may have prescribed sleeping pills for you if you need them, but this does not mean that you must

absolutely take them. The nurse may want everyone to be sedated on sleeping pills so he does not get bothered during his shift.

Be aware of your demands on the nurse who is caring for you. Nurses who work in hospitals are constantly on their feet, and this is very tiring. When they work in a large hospital, they can easily walk several miles during one day at work.

Q172: Does the doctor recommend that you undergo physical therapy after the operation?

Before you undergo the surgery, would it be helpful for you to check out physical therapists and the types of therapy that might be beneficial to your recovery?

What does this therapy cost, how long and how often will you need it, and will your insurance pay for it? Does the physical therapist come to your home, or do you have to go to a physical therapy center?

Q173: What will the schedule of follow-up visits be after the operation?

Q174: Who will drive you to your follow-up appointments if you cannot drive yourself?

Q175: If there is a problem with the surgery, or if you do not like the results, what will the arrangement be if a second operation is needed or requested?

If the doctor did something to you that you do not like, or that he is not satisfied with, he may offer you a free operation to correct it after you have gone through a healing period of what could be months or years. A safe waiting period before undergoing a second operation is usually six months to two years, during which the operation site can heal, revascularize, and relax. Your specific needs might dictate that you need surgery sooner. Having a second operation too soon on the same area may cause complications including vascularization problems (restricted blood supply) and increased risk of infection.

Letting a surgeon operate on you after he has botched one operation on you is probably not a wise thing to do. Get a second opinion from an unrelated doctor, and investigate your options.

• YOUR MEDICAL FILE

Q176: Have you obtained a copy of the doctor's file on you?

The patient medical records in a doctor's office belong to that doctor. Some doctors sell information from patient records to pharmaceutical companies and medical equipment manufacturers. Other times the records are sold for medical research purposes. Patient names and other identifying information may have been removed from the records before they were sold. Some doctors may have a paper that you sign explaining that his records on you will not be released to anyone other than you unless the doctor's office has your permission. This is good for you and a doctor who does this is saying that he understands your need for privacy.

It is your legal right to have a copy of your medical record. A doctor's office may request that you pay a small fee for copying your records. A small charge is understandable, but if they want a dollar or more per page, question them on this. They may be trying to discourage you from getting copies.

If you want copies of x-rays or medical tests, you should request a copy at the time these are done. If the doctor's office refuses to give you a copy of your record, contact one of the patients' rights groups listed in the *Research Resources* section of this book under the heading *Patients' and Consumers' Rights*.

11 • STRATEGIC PLANNING

Preparing Yourself for Surgery

If you decide to have any type of elective surgery, the chances of a successful result are greatly improved if you understand the procedures and the risks, get a second opinion, do background checks on the doctors, make sure the operating facilities are adequately equipped, and prepare yourself for a properly restful recovery period.

The following are suggested ways of preparing for surgery. Following the steps that apply to your situation can increase your confidence that the surgery will be successful, can reduce last-minute stress, and may speed your recovery.

A.   Write down the names of all the people you are dealing with at the doctor's office, and the names of the staff who are going to be in the operating room.

Know what each person's job is, and make sure the staff members are qualified to do their jobs. Remember that you are hiring them and they are making money from you. You have a right to know what you are paying for, and you have the right to refuse treatment from any health professional.

When you are in the hospital, keep a notebook of information on the names of all the people who are involved in your care. When people are aware that you know their name they may perform their job better.

B.   Try to schedule your surgery to take place early in the week.

You are more likely to receive better treatment if you undergo surgery in the first three days of the week. If you are in the hospital over the weekend, you may be cared for by a part-time, or temporary, nurse who may not be familiar with the hospital, the doctor, or the care you need. Hospitals also have reduced staffs on the weekend.

C.   In the days before the surgery you will have to give blood samples and possibly tissue and urine samples for lab testing. Get a copy of the lab results when they come back. Have the doctor explain the test results, and ask him if they were okay. Sometimes a doctor forgets to look at the test results.

If the lab report indicates a serious health concern, get a second doctor's opinion. If no emergency exists, assure that surgery is necessary by having another lab go over the test results, or order more test results from a separate test facility before undergoing invasive treatments.

D.   When you have your exam and your blood pressure is taken, find out what it is and keep a record of this for yourself. It will consist of two sets of numbers: a lower figure, the diastolic pressure that occurs between the heart beats, and a higher figure, the systolic pressure that occurs during the heart beats.

Depending on your health condition, you may want to purchase your own blood pressure cuff at a medical supply store.

Blood pressure should be measured in both arms, because some people consistently have higher blood pressure in one arm.

E. Request that you be given your own copy of any "before" photos that are taken. Also request copies of any photos, or videos, that are taken during the surgery.

Consider taking your own diary of photos before surgery, during the recovery period, and after healing has taken place.

F. Take care of as many things as possible days before the surgery both at work and at home so you will not be rushing around at the last moment. You do not want to be so rushed that you forget anything that could interfere with the outcome of your surgery. When you first decide to go through with the surgery, start making a list of the things you need to do. Prioritize the list and review it throughout the days before the surgery to make sure you are not overlooking anything.

If you are going to be staying in the hospital for a long period, remember to:

- Store valuables, such as jewelry, with a trustworthy relative or friend, or in a safety deposit box at your bank.
- Arrange for your paycheck to be mailed to you, or directly deposited into your bank account.
- Arrange for someone to take care of your pets, and have enough food for the pets to make it through your recovery.
- Make sure your plants, gardening, and other household needs such as collection of newspapers and mail are taken care of.

G. Get any prescriptions days ahead of the surgery. Bring the medications with you when you get the operation in case you need them.

Make sure the doctor knows what other prescriptions and over-the-counter medications you are taking. Make a list of them. This list should include every type of medication you are taking including eye drops, cold remedies, birth-control pills, and pain killers such as aspirin or Tylenol.

Read the information about the medication that is supplied by the manufacturer.

Know what you cannot eat with the medications, when you are supposed to take them, and what the side effects are for each medication.

Know what the pills look like, what they are supposed to accomplish, how much to take, and when you are supposed to take them.

Avoid taking medication in the dark. One of the most common mistakes made in hospitals has to do with patients being given the wrong medication or an improper amount of the right medication. If someone else is giving you the pills, make sure they are giving you the right ones.

It may be helpful to create a checklist calendar for taking medications according to the proper time intervals so you know you have taken them and do not take double doses. This is especially true if you are taking a medication that can distort your judgment, or if you are in and out of sleep.

Make note of any changes in your mood, mental capabilities, vision, and any physical changes you experience after taking a medication. Physical changes may include a rash on the skin, nausea, breathing difficulties, dizziness, or rapid heartbeat. Tell your doctor if you experience these types of side effects.

Some people experience side effects with antibiotics. If you experience nausea or other sickness from the antibiotics or other drugs, do not just stop taking the medications. Notify your doctor of the problem. There may be different types of medication you can take, there may be ways to avoid the side effects, or you may no longer need the medication.

H.   Get a thermometer and take your temperature two or three times a day while you are recovering (normal body temperature stays around 98.6° Fahrenheit). Keep a chart and note any changes. Contact the doctor if there is any unexpected change.

A fever is not necessarily a bad thing, as it is part of the body's defense mechanism against bacteria and viruses. White blood cell and antibody production increases during a fever, and these help fight infection. You should still let the doctor know if you have a fever. Fever can be a sign of an infection and underlying problems. A fever above 106° can result in death. Trying to lower a fever by placing the person in ice water is not recommended. A person with a fever should drink fluids to prevent dehydration. Children with a fever should **NOT** be given aspirin.

Fever can impair judgment and cause confusion in people of any age. Therefore, it is a good safety measure to have someone with you, or who can easily be contacted to help you in case you have any emergency during your recovery from surgery.

Other changes and symptoms to be concerned about that you should report to your doctor:
- If you have injured the surgical wound, especially if it starts to bleed, or if you have damaged the sutures.
- If your incision burns, especially if pus is present on the wound, or the area around the incision turns red.
- Skin rash.
- Prolonged rapid heartbeat.
- Chills and cold sweat.
- Heavy sweating, trembling, dizziness, nausea, or breathing difficulties.
- You fainted.
- Inability to eat food, and especially if this is accompanied by forceful vomiting.
- Diarrhea.
- Sensitivity to sound or to light.
- A continuous headache.
- Unmanageable pain, and especially pain that comes on suddenly.
- The arm or leg where your surgery was performed becomes numb or turns blue.

- Pain when urinating or defecating, or inability to urinate or defecate. Be careful not to use too much force during these times, because the pressure may break open sutures and cause incisions to bleed. Ask about the possibility of using stool softeners to relieve constipation.
- Bloody stool or bloody urine.
- Unexpected swelling or bruising beyond what the doctor told you to expect.
- Inability to focus your eyes, or blurred or double vision.
- Loss of function, such as speech, or inability to move a limb.
- If your condition does not improve the way the doctor said it would even though you have done everything he has told you to do.

   Complications, such as infection, or bleeding, can lead to serious threats to your health. They should be given prompt attention.
   Many lawsuits have been brought against doctors who did not respond to situations where patients' health was at risk, and many patients have died after complications were ignored. If you are experiencing complications and are concerned that the doctor dismisses your concerns too quickly, does not seem to know how to manage your pain, or may not be giving you the attention you need (he seems to be overwhelmed with his workload or for some other reason), it may be time to find the medical attention you need by contacting another doctor, or by checking into the local emergency room.

I.   Have a few clean hats handy that you can wear if you are having a surgery that prevents you from washing your hair. Baseball caps partially hide the face and provide some protection to anyone with a facial operation. If the surgery is going to make the upper head swell, the hats will need to be larger to accommodate any swelling. Do not wear a hat that rubs against an incision or surgical wound. Scarves and bandannas may also be helpful.

J.   Pay attention to your nutrition. Your body is going to need nutrients so it can heal itself. Check with your local library or healthfood store for the latest books on nutrition.

K.   Spend some time days before the surgery making meals and freezing them in individual meal-size containers that can be reheated. If you are having a surgery requiring that you do not chew for a certain number of days or weeks, you may be restricted to soups and liquid foods. Some surgeries may require you to avoid hot foods. Get a juicer or blender to make fresh vegetable or fruit juice. Fresh juices are also full of the nutrients your body can use to heal itself.
   You may be restricted to bland foods for the first twenty-four hours after surgery. This is likely to be because you will feel nauseated by the anesthesia. Bland foods include plain rice, soft bread, and clear soups. From there you may want to try plain steamed vegetables, plain crackers, or milk. In one to three days you may be ready to begin eating your normal food.
   Do not plan to eat a large meal after surgery in some kind of victory celebration. Your body will need nourishment, but several small meals will be better than one large one.

L.   If you are going to stay in the hospital, prepare a bag containing what you will need during your stay. Take only inexpensive items.

Items you may want to bring to the hospital:
- A list of phone numbers you may need during your stay.
- An inexpensive watch.
- An inexpensive pillow that you will not miss if lost or damaged. This will avoid the possibility of having to settle for hospital pillows that may be uncomfortable.
- Toiletries, such as your own soap, shampoo, toothpaste, toothbrush, stick deodorant, brush, comb, small mirror, razor, skin lotion, and other items you may need. The hospital may supply these things, but they may not be your choice — and they will charge you premium prices for every item you use.
- Do bring your glasses or contacts, dentures, and hearing aids if you use any of these. You will be asked to remove them before surgery, but may need them once you recover from the anesthesia.
- Pajamas. Depending on what you are having done, you may not be able to wear anything other than the hospital gown, but you may be able to wear your own pajamas and slippers. Some people bring a robe with them to the hospital and wear this over the hospital gown, or over their own pajamas.
- An inexpensive book to occupy your time. Do not bring library books or expensive books, as they may be lost or damaged during your hospital stay.
- Magazines. The hospital store may carry a variety of newspapers and magazines.
- A cheap hand radio with headphones so you can listen to it at any time without disturbing other patients.

    You may want to use a tape player or CD player instead of a radio. This way you can choose what you want to listen to during surgery, such as soft relaxing music, sounds of nature, or suggestion tapes. Listening to the radio may not be a good idea during surgery because a song may come on that you do not like, or a breaking news story may cause stress. A tape player may run out of tape before the surgery is over. A CD player can be adjusted to replay the CD over and over again until you turn the player off. (Make sure the batteries are new so they do not fade during the surgery.)
- A sketch pad and drawing pencils. This may be especially important for children who may be able to express their concerns about their illness and surgery through art.
- Playing cards.
- Something to write with and something to write on.
- Children (and some adults) may want to have a stuffed animal, or a familiar blanket.
- A copy of this book.

M. Do not bring jewelry with you when you go to be operated on. You are going to be unconscious in a room full of strangers — and this is not the time to try and look attractive. Leave jewelry at home, or in a safety deposit box at your bank. Using a safety deposit box may be the best choice. There will easily by more than a dozen people involved in your care during your hospital stay.

There may also be neighbors and others who will know that your home may be empty and vulnerable to robbery.

N. Stock up on books, videos, stationery, postage stamps, hobbies, puzzles, and pillows, and put your phone next to your bed. Get access to a tape player or CD player so you can listen to soothing music while you rest.

There are now many good books available on cassette tape that can be listened to. These can be particularly useful to a person who has had eye surgery. Headphones can be used so that other people will not be disturbed if they are sleeping.

A company called Radio Memories sells cassette tapes of old radio plays including dramas, comedies, and serials. Each cassette is sixty minutes and they are very reasonably priced. (Radio Memories, 1600 Wewoka St., N. Little Rock, AR 72116; (501)835-0465; Fax (501)835-0118; Net: http://www.old-time.com/davenpor.html)

O. Remember that one of the key complications that can arise after surgery is infection. Infection is caused by impurities getting into your system. To limit your exposure to germs, thoroughly clean all the rooms in your home where you will be spending your recovery time. Use hot water (unless otherwise indicated by the manufacturer of the product) to wash bed linen, towels, and any clothing you will be using during your recovery. If you are spending a lot of time in bed during your recovery, you may want to change your bed linens — or have someone change them for you — every day.

P. Prepare your bathroom and other rooms in your house so things are easily reached in case your movements are limited after the surgery.

Remove anything on the floor that can cause you to trip or slip, such as a rug or electrical wires. Install a night light in the bathroom. Find out whether you will need to place a stool or chair in the bathtub in case you cannot bend over, sit, or stand (a plastic chair or stool that will not float in the tub may be useful; you may be able to rent one from a medical equipment and supplies store). Apply slip guards to your bathtub or shower (these can be bought at most hardware stores). Washcloths can come in handy if you have an operation that prevents you from taking a full bath or shower.

If you cannot get into your bed, you may need to rent a bed from a medical supply company, or from the hospital, for your recovery.

Q. Ice packs can relieve some of the bruising and swelling. (Check with the doctor to see if you will benefit from applying ice packs). If you are to use ice packs on the area of the operation, make sure you have enough ice or a source for it that will last for as many days as you need it, at all hours of the day. Make individual ice packs using plastic zipper bags. Some people who undergo facial surgery use frozen peas or frozen corn instead of ice. Adding a little water to the ice bags at the time you use them will help them conform to the shape of the body part you are laying it on. Wrapping the bag in a thin cloth, as in a handkerchief or bandanna, will absorb any water drops, and will prevent the area from becoming too cold. Binder-paper clamps are helpful for clipping the bag in place. You will also need someone with you to replace the ice for you so you do not have to keep getting up.

R. A daily massage during your recovery on areas that have not been operated on, even if it is limited to the hands, feet, or scalp can keep you from getting too uncomfortable when spending a lot of time in bed, can help prevent stiffness, can aid body circulation, can relieve tension, and can help prevent bed sores.

S. Let the doctor's office know how and where you can be contacted the day and night before surgery. The doctor, the anesthesiologist, or the doctor's staff may need to contact you.

T. With a relative or friend present, have one last conversation with the doctor before the operation to clear up any concerns you have. You can always delay or back out of an operation and leave.

If the anesthesiologist, or anesthetist, fails to show up, refuse to have the operation.

U. When you arrive for the surgery, be prepared to have your paperwork reviewed, and to have a nurse give you a short physical exam. The nurse will make sure the information on your chart is correct. She will also check your vital signs including your pulse, respiration, temperature, and blood pressure.

You will be asked about when you last ate food and drank liquid. If you are having surgery on your intestines or digestive tract, you will have already cleared your system with oral laxatives, and may have been given an enema. Be sure to tell the truth about whether you have eaten or drunk anything because if you have, it may cause very serious complications with the surgery. It is better to tell the truth and have the surgery delayed, or canceled, than to risk the complications that may arise.

Before or after this exam, you will be asked to change from your clothes to a medical gown. You may then have time to relax before the surgery takes place, or there may be more testing or medical imaging procedures to be done before the surgery is performed.

You may be transferred to the operating room in a wheelchair or on a gurney unless you are able to walk.

V. You may feel more secure, and also feel comforted, if you have arranged for someone you trust to be in the waiting room while you undergo surgery. Let the doctor know your friend or relative is waiting.

If you are having outpatient surgery (where you go home right after the surgery), you will need someone to drive you home, and to stay with you for at least twenty-four hours.

You should not drive after surgery because you will have narcotics in your bloodstream. It is dangerous to drive after surgery, and you can be arrested. Your surgery may be canceled if you arrive at the outpatient surgery center without someone to take you home after the surgery.

W. Do not enter the operating room, and do not let the anesthesiologist or anyone else stick needles into your arm until you are sure everything is clearly understood by you and the doctor. Do not be sweet-talked into the surgery room before all your questions are answered.

There should be no discussion of changes to the planned alterations of your body once you are in the operating room. If the doctor starts talking about doing things differently, or doing more things to you than you had already agreed to, that is your cue to leave.

Once the anesthesia makes its way through the needle and into your arm, it is too late to change your mind, and the outcome of the surgery is something you will have to live with for the rest of your life. Any freedom you give the doctor to do what he wants can be an invitation for a big surprise when the bandages are removed. You do not want to find out after the operation that there was a misunderstanding. Having botched surgery is not a pleasant experience.

X.   Get a copy of the operation report. It may be referred to as the "doctor's operative summary" or "op report." This is the typed version of what was done to you during the surgery. Also, get a copy of the pathologist's report (if there is one) that would show the results of any tests performed on tissues removed from your body. Keep copies of them for your own records.

A doctor who writes false information on insurance forms may also write false information on the operation report. This may affect your future insurance eligibility.

Y.   Depending on your operation, some activity may help you recover faster, and some walking and light exercise may help circulation and prevent blood clots, pneumonia, and constipation. Spending too much time in bed will lead to loss in muscle strength. Getting up and walking several times a day, and doing other activities, may be beneficial to the condition of your body, as well as your mind. Ask the doctor what activities would be appropriate during your recovery.

Z.   The period of recovery after surgery is a good time to learn more about health. Learn what areas of behavior may have contributed to your illness. If you have not been eating healthfully, learn more about nutrition. If you have not been exercising properly, learn more about ways to exercise. If there are other areas of your life that need to change, work on changing them. Make plans. Set goals. Heal your life.

12 • RESEARCH RESOURCES

Educating Yourself

A person experiencing a health problem can feel a loss of control. Taking steps to understand the health problem and the therapies that are offered can restore a sense of control. Being well informed can also play a part in recovery, as studies show that well-informed patients recover faster.

If you are considering any elective surgery procedure, doing your own research can answer a lot of questions. Any good doctor would not feel attacked by a patient who has made the effort to become informed by doing research.

The medical professional you are communicating with may not be aware of all the options out there for treating your condition because that person may not have read all the information available on your condition. Many procedures and forms of treatment have been developed after a patient inflicted with a condition was relentless in finding a way to improve his health. You might end up being one of those patients who is paramount in the development of a new form of treatment or operational technique.

Some doctors think that the patient should know only so much, beyond that, the patient should put his trust in the doctor. That is one way to open the door to future disappointment. If, after surgery, you discover that the operation was not what you expected, or that the procedure was an outdated technique, then it is too late to do library research, ask questions, get second and third opinions, assure that you understood every word of the informed consent form, and receive detailed explanations from the doctor of his intentions for you.

When you consider that many patients spend thousands of dollars on operations to repair what other doctors have done to them, that other patients are stuck with bad results from surgery that they cannot afford to have fixed, or is beyond repair, and that people have been injured, maimed, and killed during surgery, you should see clearly that doing your own research before having any elective surgery is a wise thing to do.

Do not be surprised if during your research you find out something that the doctor does not know. The human body is a very complex mechanism and no one person knows everything about it. There are also new procedures being developed and new discoveries about the body being found every day by the many people around the world who are dedicated to the study of the human body.

If you are planning to undergo elective surgery, you should take responsibility to protect yourself from bad medicine by first considering alternatives to surgery, and by investigating the doctor's training and experience, what the operation entails, what the risks are, what kind of injury it can cause, the details about the healing process, what the outcome can be, and what can be done to fix the problems that can arise if the operation does not turn out right.

Doing your own research and studying medical books found in any good library or bookstore can prepare you to deal with the world of medicine. No matter what your health concern is, there is information somewhere that can help you understand it and find the best help.

Library research

A librarian can help you locate reference books that can guide you to specific information. Most libraries have a variety of directories, indexes, and encyclopedias that cover many health topics.

Some doctors, medical schools, and hospitals may let you use their private libraries for your medical research. The National Network of Libraries may be able to help you locate a library that contains the information you need (800)338-7657. Or try contacting the Health Sciences Libraries Consortium (University City Science Center, 3600 Market St., Ste. 550, Philadelphia, PA 19104-2646).

- **Directories that include information on associations**

  There are thousands of support and specialty information groups that exist to help people who have specific health needs. Associations provide a valuable network of resources through publications and services, such as newsletters, conferences, seminars, and professional journals. Many of their publications contain the most recent developments in medicine. The majority of US health groups are listed in this book.

- **Computers for research**

  Some libraries have computers that you can use to find information about specific health subjects. Check your local library and see what computer systems are available for your use.

  There are also computer programs used by doctors to help find medical information. Names of these programs include Apache, QMR, and Help. Your doctor or hospital may give you access to the computers they use for researching on these programs.

- **Online services**

  One way to obtain current medical information is by using a home computer, or a computer at your library, that is hooked into the Internet. There is a tremendous amount of health-related information available on the Internet, and more becomes accessible every day.

  By accessing the Internet, you can talk to other people in a discussion group that is focused on a specific health topic, and search for information on online services such as America Online, Prodigy, or CompuServe, which charge by the hour.

  Some Internet sites called "bulletin boards" allow you to communicate with health professionals and medical organizations by posting a question and receiving an answer. Other areas called "chat rooms" allow you to communicate with other people who have, or are concerned with, specific health problems. Newsgroups allow you to subscribe to a type of interactive newsletter.

  Some libraries, medical schools, and facilities are connected to a database called *Medline*. *Medline* can also be accessed through America Online.

  A person who is dealing with a serious health problem may also want to search the database of the National Library of Medicine, (800) 638-8480, which has been hooked up to the Internet. This database includes information from many medical journals from around the world.

  One of the largest and fastest growing Internet-oriented companies, Netscape, has started an online service called *Healthscape*, which will be providing medical information to anyone hooked up to the Internet.

  Many of the organizations listed in this book have their own Internet address that you can call up on a computer to access their databases and communicate with their staff. For more information about the Internet, see the *Online Health Information Resources* heading.

- **Books**

Many guidebooks, textbooks, and manuals on health are published annually. To find the names of books not in your local library check *Books in Print* , a directory of books currently available from publishers.

Medical information in books can become quickly outdated as advances in some areas of medicine are taking place rapidly.

- **Magazine, professional journals and newspaper articles**

Magazines, medical journals, and newspapers provide information that is often more current than that found in books and textbooks. There are a number of indexes available in libraries that can help you find specific articles in periodicals.

You may not be able to understand all the technical terms used in medical books. Medical language is filled with phrases, such as "in vitro fertilization," which simply means "in glass" — the term for test-tube babies. Using complicated terms is one way the medical community keeps itself ambiguous. Meanwhile, to find definitions of medical terms, look in a medical dictionary — or ask your doctor or nurse.

Do not judge the simplicity of an operation on the clean line drawings that are often used in medical texts to show how an operation is performed. A textbook understanding of a surgical procedure and actually performing the surgery are two very different things. Also, remember that medical books often use photographs of the worst case scenarios. So if you are diagnosed with a condition and are looking into a medical book and find photos of people who have experienced severe reactions to the same condition you have, do not assume that you will one day appear the same way.

Medical and Health Organizations, Information Resources, and Personal Support

I tried to include groups that deal with everything that is mentioned in the book. Some of the organizations listed here are nonprofit and support themselves solely by donations; therefore, they may welcome any kind of financial help you can give them (check with them before sending a donation). Some will require that when you request information, you send them a self-addressed, stamped envelope.

This section contains some of the organizations of surgeons and other physicians in the US. Membership in some of these groups does not guarantee quality of education, or of surgical and healing skills. Some are simply trade associations that work to represent the financial and political interests of the members.

Some organizations publish newsletters that you can subscribe to. When reading a newsletter, try to be aware of how the newsletter is funded, and from where the information in the newsletter originated. Some newsletters are financed strictly with the money coming in from subscriptions. Other newsletters may have a lower subscription rate and accept advertising to help pay for production costs. Some newsletters are funded by grants from private individuals, or through government agencies. Newsletters that are sent out by some organizations are paid for by drug companies — and this is where a conflict of interest may exist.

A drug company that is financing a newsletter is likely to have a financial interest in the disease that is discussed in the newsletter. For instance, the newsletter may be filled with articles that say you must take drug "A" if you are going to manage your disease successfully. This push to prescribe drug "A" may be expressed while the newsletter fails to inform readers of other treatment options, such as other drug or non-drug therapies, or dietary or lifestyle changes. The newsletter may discuss other treatment options, but always arrives at the same conclusion, that the best therapy is that with the drug manufactured by the funding drug company. The writers who are writing the articles appearing in the newsletters may be employed by the drug company, or otherwise may be receiving some form of compensation from them, even if the writer is a doctor. In this way the newsletter stands only as a clever advertisement for the drug company.

While it is true that some health newsletters would not exist, especially in some cases of rare disorders, if drug companies did not provide funding for the newsletters, there are guidelines that should be followed to ensure that the newsletter is not biased toward one health theory, and that funding sources are disclosed.

Health newsletters should include disclosure information telling how the newsletter is funded. The newsletters should feature a variety of articles written by people who do not hold a corporate interest in the treatment options that are discussed. When a conflict of interest does exist, it should be clearly stated where it exists, by including a paragraph stating for whom the writer works, or from where studies received financing. It would also be helpful if the newsletter contains legitimate letters to the editor so that a variety of opinions are expressed and responded to. Other related news, such as legislation and developments in the health area being discussed, are helpful, as are book reviews. And allopathic therapies of drugs and scalpels should not be the only ones explored within the pages of any health newsletter — otherwise the newsletter would be incomplete.

Medical scams cost consumers billions of dollars every year. People are always out to make money, and fraudulent persons can be very clever. Before giving your money to anyone, or signing any contracts or agreements, find out if you are dealing with a legitimate person and organization.

Always ask questions when doubtful of any services you are considering, and of any person who may provide you with medical treatment.
— The author

Phone numbers

Because phone numbers are subject to change, if any of the following phone numbers are inoperative, simply call information by dialing the area code followed by 555-1212, and ask for the new number.

To obtain information from a group that does not have a phone number listed, write a letter requesting the information you need.

Be aware that many organizations request that you send a self-addressed, stamped envelope when requesting information from them, and may also require a small donation.

Books

There are many books available on most health subjects. The books listed are some of those the author has read part or all of, and can generally be found in bookstores or libraries. More technically detailed books are available in medical libraries.

Organizations

Those organizations listed in this book are not necessarily completely legitimate. Consumers should take steps to protect themselves and check up on the credibility and safety of any service, business, association, or professional mentioned in this research section.

• ABBREVIATIONS USED IN MEDICAL RECORDS

a: before
aa: each
A and D: admissions and discharge
ABG: arterial blood gasses
ac: ante cibum (before meals)
ACLS: advanced cardiac life support
ad: to, up to

AD: auris dextra (right ear)
ad effect: until it is effective
ADL: activities of daily living
ad lib: as needed, as desired by patient
AF: auricular fibrillation
agit: shake, stir
AI: aortic insufficiency

AK: above the knee amputation
ama: against medical advice
amb: ambulatory
AML: acute myelogenous leukemia
amt: amount
Ap: appendicitis
AP: ante partum (before childbirth)
APC: aspirin, phenacetin, caffeine
APE: acute pulmonary edema
approx: approximately
aq: (aqua) water
ARC: AIDS-related complex
ARD: acute respiratory disease
AS: auris sinstra (left ear)
ASHD: arteriosclerotic heart disease
AU: auris unitas (both ears)
av: average
AV: arteriovenous, audiovisual
awa: as well as
B: black (African)
BE: barium enema
bid or **bis in die**: twice a day
BKA: below knee amputation
Bl. time: bleeding time
BM: bowel movement
BMR: basal metabolism rate
BP: blood pressure
BPD: bronchopulmonary dysplasia
BRP: bathroom privileges
Bx: biopsy
C.: centigrade
Ca: cancer or carcinoma
CABG: coronary artery bypass graft
CAD: coronary artery disease
cap(s): capsule(s)
CBC: complete blood count
CBD: common bile duct
CC: chief complaint
cc: cubic centimeter
CCU: coronary care unit
CHD: congenital heart disease; or coronary heart disease
CHF: congestive heart failure
Chol: cholesterol
Cl. time: clotting time
clin: clinical
CML: chronic myelogenous leukemia
CNS: central nervous system
comp: compound
cont rem: continue the medicine
COPD: chronic obstructive pulmonary disease
CP: chest pain
CPR: cardiopulmonary resuscitation
CSF: cerebrospinal fluid
CV: cardiovascular
CVA: cerebrovascular accident
CVP: central venous pressure

CXR: chest x ray
d: give
D and D: Diarrhea and dehydration
dbl: double
D&C: dilation and curettage
dd in d: from day to day
dec: pour off
dexter: the right
dil: dilute
disp: dispense
div: divide
DM: diabetes mellitus
DOA: dead on arrival
dos: dose
DT: delirium tremens (severe tremors)
dur dolor: while pain lasts
D/W: dextrose in water
Dx: diagnosis
ea: each
EEG: electroencephalogram
EENT: ear, eye, nose, and throat
EKG or ECG: electrocardiogram
EST: electroshock therapy
EM: electron microscope
EMG: electromyogram
emp: as directed
ENT: ear, nose, and throat
ER: emergency room
et al.: and others
F: female
F.: Fahrenheit
FBS: fasting blood sugar
febris: fever
FH: family history
Fx: fracture
GA: general anesthesia
garg: gargle
GB: gallbladder
GC: gonorrhea
GI: gastrointestinal
GL: glaucoma
GP: general practitioner
gm: grams
gr: grains
grad: by degrees
gravida: pregnancies
GSW: gunshot wound
gtt: drops
GTT: glucose tolerance test
GU: genitourinary
gutta or **gt**: drop
Gyn: gynecology
h: hour, or height
H: Hispanic
HASHD: hypertensive arteriosclerotic heart disease
Hb or Hgb: hemoglobin
Hct: hematocrit

HG: hemoglobin
HHD: hypertensive heart disease
HIP: headache, insomnia, and depression
HOP: head of bed
hora somni or **hs**: at bedtime
HPI: history of present illness
HPN: hypertension
HPV: human papilloma virus
HR: heart rate
hs or **hora somni**: at bedtime, before
retiring
HVL: half value layer
Hx: history
ICU: intensive care unit
I&D or I and D: incision and drainage
id: idem (the same), or in diem (during
the day)
IEP: immonoelectrophoresis
Ig: immunoglobulin
IJ: internal jugular
IM: intramuscular, or internal medicine
I.M.: infectious mononucleosis
ind: daily
I&O: intake and output of fluids
IOP: intraocular pressure
IPPD: intermittent positive pressure
breathing
IQ: intelligence quotient
IST: insulin shock therapy
IUD: intrauterine device
IV: intravenous
IVDA: intravenous drug abuse
IVP: intravenous pyelogram
IVU: intravenous urogram
k: constant
KUB: kidney, ureter, bladder
KVO: keep vein open
L: left
LD: lethal dose
LE: lupus erythematosis
liq: liquid
LKS: liver, kidney, spleen
LLE: left lower extremity
LLQ: left lower quadrant
LMD: local medical doctor
LMP: last menstrual period
loc cit: in the place cited
LOL: laughing out loud, or little old lady
LP: lumbar puncture (spinal tap), low
power, or latent period
LPN: licensed practical nurse
LUE: left upper extremity
LUQ: left upper quadrant
M: mix, or male
MA: mental age
MAP: mean arterial pressure
mb: mix well

MD: muscular dystrophy, or medical
doctor
MDR: minimum daily requirement
MED: minimum effective dose
m et n: morning and night
MF: main fluid
MFT: muscle function test
MFV: main fluid vein
mg: milligrams
MI: myocardial infarcation (heart attack),
or mitral insufficiency
MICU: Medical Intensive Care Unit
ml: milliliters
mm Hg: millimeters of mercury (as in
measuring blood pressure)
mor. dict.: in the manner directed
MS: morphine sulfate, or multiple
sclerosis
N: normal
NA: not applicable
neg: negative
N-G: nasogastric
NICU: Neonatal Intensive Care Unit
no.: number
non rep; nr: do not repeat
npo: non per os (nothing per mouth, or
nothing by mouth)
NS: normal saline
NSA: no significant abnormality
NSR: normal heart rate
N&V: nausea and vomiting
O2: oxygen
o: none
OBS: organic brain syndrome
OD or **oculus dexter**: right eye, or
overdose
od: once a day
O.L.: left eye
OOB: out of bed
OPD: outpatient department
OR: operating room
OS or **oculus sinister**: left eye
OT: occupational therapy
OU or **oculus uterque**: both eyes
P: probability
p: pulse
Pap: Papanicolaou
Para: number of births
Path.: pathology
PBI: protein-bound iodine
pc or **post cibum**: after meals
pCO2: carbon dioxide pressure, tension
PE: physical examination; or pulmonary
embolus
PFT: pulmonary function test
PI: present illness
PICU: Pulmonary Intensive Care Unit
PID: pelvic inflammatory disease

pil: pill
PM: post mortem (after death)
PMHx: past medical history
p.o. or **per os**: by mouth
pO2: oxygen tension, pressure
Post.: posterior
post-op: postoperative, after the operation
PPD: pelvic inflammatory disease
PPD: purified protein derivative (used as a skin test for TB)
PPD: packs per day — as in cigarettes
PR: pulse rate; or rectally
prn or **pro re nata**: as needed, as circumstances dictate, or as often as necessary
Prog.: prognosis
pt: patient
PT: physical therapy
PTA: prior to admission
PVC: premature ventricular contractions
PVD: peripheral vascular disease
Px: prognosis
q: every
qd or **quaque die**: every day
qh or **quaque hora**: every hour
q3h or **puaque 3 hora**: every 3 hours
q.4h: every four hours,
qid or **quarter in die**: four times per day
qn: every night
qod: every other day
qq or **quaque**: each, every
qs: proper amount, quantity sufficient
qv or **quantum vis**: as much as desired
R: right, or respiration
rbc: red blood cell
RBC: red blood cell count
rep: repeat
RES: reticuloendothelial system
RHD: rheumatic heart disease
RLQ: right lower quadrant
RN: registered nurse
RNA: ribonucleic acid
ROM: range of motion
RR: respiratory rate; or recovery room
RT: radiation therapy
rub: red
RUQ: right upper quadrant
RX: recipe (prescription, therapy, or treatment)
S: subject
S&A: sugar and acetone (a diabetic urine test)
SC: subcutaneous
Scop.: scopolamine
SDU: step down unit
sed: sedimentation
seq: sequela(e) (that which follows)

SH: social history
SI: Systeme Internationale (metric units)
SICU: surgical intensive care unit
sig: signa (label)
SIEP: serum immunoelectrophoresis
sing: of each
SOB: short of breath
sol: solution
solv: dissolve
SOP: standard operating procedure
S-O-R: stimulus-ordanims-response
SOS: can repeat in emergency
S-R: stimulus-response
ss: half
Ss: subjects
S&S: signs and symptoms
SSE: soapsuds enema
stat: statim (right away, immediately)
STD: sexually transmitted disease
STP: standard temperature and pressure
sub Q: subcutaneous
sum: let it be taken
suppos: suppository
SX: symptoms
t: time
T: temperature
T&A: tonsillectomy and adenoidectomy
tab: tablet
TAH: total abdominal hysterectomy
TAT: tetanus antitoxin
TB: tuberculosis
tere: rub
TFT: thyroid function tests
TIA: transient ischemic attacks
tid or **ter in die**: three times a day
tinct or **tinc**: tincture
TLC: tender loving care
TPR: temperature, pulse, and respiration
trach: tracheostomy
TURP: transurethral prostatectomy
Tx: treatment
TX: transfusion
U: unit
UCS: unconditioned stimulus
UGI: upper gastrointestinal
ung: ointment
UO: of undetermined origin
URI: upper respiratory infection or illness
ut dict: ut dictum (as directed)
UTI: urinary tract infection
UV: ultra violet
UVR: ultra violet radiation
V: volume
VD: venereal disease
vid: vide (see)
viz: videlicet (namely)
V/O: verbal order
VPC: volume packed cells

VS: vital signs
v/v: percent volume in volume
w: weight
w/: with
W: Caucasian
WBC: white blood cell

WC: wheelchair
WDWN: well developed, well nourished
wk: week
W/V: weight per volume
YO: year old

• ABUSE

Books :
- *Come Here: One Man Overcomes the Tragic Aftermath of Childhood Sexual Abuse*, by Richard Berendzen with Laura Palmer; Villard Books, 1993
- *Confronting Abuse*, by Anne L. Horton, B. Kent Harrison and Barry L. Johnson; Deseret Book Company 1993
- *The Courage to Heal: A Guide for Women Survivors of Child Sexual Abuse*, by Ellen Bass and Laura Davis; Harper Collins, 1993
- *Domestic Violence in America*, by Michael McKenzie; Brunswick Publishing Corporation, 1995
- *Family Violence*, by Mildred Daley Pagelow; Praeger, 1984
- *Hero or Victim*, by Meredith B. Mitchell, PhD; 1995
- *One Door Closes, Another Door Opens: Turning Your Setbacks into Comebacks*, by Arthur Pine with Julie Houston; Dell, 1995
- *The Right to Innocence*, by Beverly Engle, MFCC.; St. Martin's Press, 1989
- *The Sexually Abused Male*, by M. Hunter; Macmillan, NY, 1990
- *Silent Sons*, by Robert J. Ackerman; Simon & Schuster, 1993
- *Trauma and Recovery*, by J.L. Herman; Basic Books/Harper Collins, 1992
- *Verbal Abuse: Survivors Speak Out on Relationship and Recovery*, by Patricia Evans, 1994
- *The Verbally Abusive Relationship: How to Recognize It and How to Respond*, by Patricia Evans; Bob Adams, Inc., 1992
- *Victims No Longer: Men Recovering from Incest and Other Sexual Child Abuse*, by Mike Lew; Harper Collins, 1990
- *Wednesday's Children: Adult Survivors of Abuse Speak Out*, by Suzanne Somers; Putnam, 1992
- *Woman-Battering: Victims and Their Experiences*, by Mildred Daley Pagelow; Sage Publishers, 1981
- *You Can't Say That to Me!: Stopping the Pain of Verbal Abuse*, by Suzette Haden Elgin; John Wiley & Sons, 1995

Many people undergo surgery to repair physical damage that was the result of domestic violence. In 1990 the *Journal of the American Medical Association* reported that 22% to 35% of women who visit emergency rooms are there for treatment of injuries related to domestic abuse. According to the National Coalition Against Domestic Violence, injuries inflicted by husbands and boyfriends are the leading causes of injury to women — more common than automobile accidents, muggings, and rape combined. Children are the second most likely to need medical care for injuries sustained at the hands of parents, brothers, sisters, other family, or non-family members. Elderly individuals and men are the third and fourth most likely to seek medical care for injuries suffered from domestic violence.

People who have not been physically battered, but have been the subject of other forms of abuse, might also seek a physical transformation through cosmetic surgery to change the part of their physical structure that was the target of abusive criticism or cruel comments.

Health problems may be the result of stress in a person's life that was caused by mistreatment. Physical-health problems may bring a person to expose issues he has not dealt with from his past. Self-inflicted injuries, such as suicide attempts and substance abuse, may be signs that a person who has been abused in some way is trying to reach out for help.

Abuse and assault are about power and control. They can be manifested in several ways including sexual, verbal, psychological, physical, spiritual, social, ritual, and financial. The physical and emotional damage caused by domestic abuse makes it one of the most horrible violations a person can experience.

Simply leaving an abusive relationship does not cure a person from it. He takes a suitcase of memories that affect his thought patterns, dreams, actions, body language, and the way he relates to and treats other people.

Often a person who has regularly been mistreated in his own home does not recognize how serious the problem is and does not know the psychological damage that has been done to him. Many times he lacks healthy communication skills and proceeds to mistreat others, or allows others to mistreat him. He may have become so accustomed to unhealthy relationships that it becomes normal to him and is his familiar way of life.

In any instances of unhealthy relationships, becoming physically healthy can be aided by becoming mentally healthy so that the whole person feels better.

People involved in abuse should seek outside help through counseling and/or support groups.

The best understanding of abuse may come from people who have had to cope with severe abuse. There are many books about the different kinds of abuse. Reading those books written by people who have been through severe abuse may be very helpful to those currently experiencing it, or who need to work through their feelings about what happened to them in the past.

AMEND, 777 Grant St., Ste. 600, Denver, CO 80203; (303)832-6363

Association for the Treatment of Sexual Abusers, 10700 SW Beaverton Hillsdale Hwy., Ste. 26, Beaverton, OR 97005-3035; (503)643-1023.

Center for the Prevention of Sexual and Domestic Violence, 936 N. 34th St., Ste. 200, Seattle, WA 98103; (206)634-1903

Child Help USA, 6463 Independence Ave., Woodland Hills, CA 91367; (800)422-4453

Child Welfare League of America, 440 — 1st St., NW, Ste. 310, Washington, DC 20001; (202)638-2952

Coalition of Free Men (provides information about violence by women against men), PO Box 43954, Austin, TX 78745-5675

Daughters and Sons United, c/o Institute for Community as Extended Family, 232 E. Gish Rd., San Jose, CA 95112; (408)453-7616

Domestic Abuse Hotline, (800)288-3854

Family Violence Information Clearinghouse, PO Box 1182, Washington, DC 20013; (703)385-7565

Family Violence & Sexual Assault Bulletin, 1310 Clinic Dr., Tyler, TX 75701; (903)595-6600

For Crying Out Loud, 46 Pleasant St., Cambridge, MA 02139

Healing Hearts, 1515 Webster St., Oakland, CA 94612

Incest Survivors Anonymous, PO Box 17245, Long Beach, CA 90807-7245

Incest Survivors Resource Network, PO Box 7375, Las Cruces, NM 88006-7375; (505)521-4260

Life Skills International (for men who batter), (800)799-SAFE

Many Voices, PO Box 2639, Cincinnati, OH 45201-2639

National Association for Child Abuse and Neglect, (800)4-A-CHILD

National Center for Elder Abuse, 810 First St., Ste. 500, Washington, DC 20002; (202)682-2470

National Clearinghouse for Defense of Battered Women, 125 S. 9th St., Ste. 302, Philadelphia, PA 19107; (215)351-0010

National Coalition Against Domestic Violence, PO Box 18749, Denver, CO 80218-0749; (303)839-1852

National Council on Child Abuse and Family Violence, 1155 Connecticut Ave., NW, Ste. 400, Washington, DC 20036; (202)429-6695 or (800)222-2000

National Gay and Lesbian Domestic Violence Victim's Network, 3506 S. Ouray Circle, Aurora, CO 80013; (303)266-3477

National Organization for Victim Assistance, 1757 Park Rd., NW, Washington DC 20010; (202)232-6682

National Victim Center, 2111 Wilson Blvd., Ste. 300, Arlington, VA 22201; (703)276-2880 or (800)FYI-CALL

On Our Own/Hear Our Cry, (312)435-1007

Parents Anonymous (helping parents overcome abuse and neglect issues), 675 W. Foothill Blvd., Ste. 220, Claremont, CA 91711

Rape Abuse & Incest National Network, (800)656-HOPE

The Survivor's Healing Center, PO Box 5296, Santa Cruz, CA 95063-5296

Survivorship: A Newsletter for Ritual Abuse Survivors, 3181 Mission St., Ste. 139, San Francisco, CA 94110

Survivors of Incest Anonymous, PO Box 21817, Baltimore, MD 21222-6817; (410)282-3400

Victims of Incest Can Emerge Survivors (VOICES) in Action provides information on assisting victims of incest and childhood sexual abuse to become survivors. They publish a newsletter called *The Chorus.*
VOICES in Action, PO Box 148309, Chicago, IL 60614; (312)327-1500

Women in Transition is a domestic violence and substance abuse prevention and intervention agency. They are not a mental health center or treatment clinic. They have a 24-hour hotline, support groups, individual counseling, and family counseling. They publish a quarterly newsletter called *Transitions.*
Women in Transition, 21 S. 12th St., 6th Flr., Philadelphia, PA 19107-3606; (215)564-5301 ext. 130; Fax (215)564-5723

• ACCREDITING HEALTHCARE FACILITIES AND SETTING HEALTHCARE STANDARDS

Accreditation Association for Ambulatory Health Care, 9933 Lawler Ave., Skokie, IL 60077-3708; (708)676-9601

Accreditation Council for Continuing Medical Education, PO Box 245, Lake Bluff, IL 60044; (708)295-1490

Accreditation Council for Graduate Medical Education, 515 N. State St., Ste. 2000, Chicago, IL 60610; (312)464-4920

Accreditation Review Committee on Education for Physician Assistants, 515 N. State St., Chicago, IL 60610; (312)464-4623

Accreditation Review Committee on Education in Surgical Technology, 7108-C S. Alton Way, Englewood, CO 80112; (303)694-9262

Accrediting Bureau of Health Education Schools, Oak Manor Office, 29089 US 20 W., Elkhart, Indiana 46514; (219)293-0124

Accrediting Commission on Education for Health Services Administration, 1911 N. Fort Myer Dr., Ste. 503, Arlington, VA 22209; (703)524-0511

American Academy of Medical Administrators, 30555 Southfield Rd., Ste. 150, Southfield, MI 48076; (810)540-4310

American Association for Accreditation of Ambulatory Plastic Surgery Facilities, 1202 Allanson Rd., Mundelein, IL 60060; (708)949-6058

American College of Health Care Administrators, 325 S. Patrick St., Alexandria, VA 22314; (703)549-5822

American College of Healthcare Executives, 840 N. Lake Shore Dr., Ste. 1103 W., Chicago, IL 60611; (312)943-0544

American College of Medical Quality, 9005 Congressional Crt., Potamic, MD 20854; (301)365-3570

For a free brochure that emphasizes the importance of seeking answers from your physician, and from hospitals, and for a copy of the *Patients Bill of Rights of the American Hospital Association*, send a letter requesting these items along with a self-addressed, stamped business-sized envelope to the
American Hospital Association, Order Processing Dept., 840 N. Lake Shore Dr., Chicago, IL 60611; (312)280-6000

American Managed Care and Review Association, 1227 — 25th St., NW, Ste. 610, Washington, DC 20037; (202)728-0506

American Medical Peer Review Association, 810 First St., NE, Ste. 410, Washington, DC 20002; (202)371-5610

American Osteopathic Hospital Association, 1454 Duke St., Alexandria, VA 22314; (703)684-7700

Association for Ambulatory Healthcare, 9933 Lawler Ave., Skokie, IL 60077-3702; (708)676-9610

The *Consumer's Guide to Hospital's* is published by the Center for the Study of Services and contains information compiled by the Health Care Financing Administration which collects data on hospital mortality rates. The book is available for $12 through the
Center for the Study of Services, 733 — 15th St., Ste. 820, Washington, DC 20005; (800)475-7283

Commission on Accreditation of Rehabilitation Facilities, 2500 Pantzano Rd., Tucson, AZ 85715; (602)748-1212

Foundation for Healthcare Evaluation, 2901 Metro Dr., Ste. 400, Bloomington, MN 55425

Healthcare Financing Administration, Health Standards and Quality Bureau, 2-D-2 Meadows E. Bldg., 6325 Security Blvd., Baltimore, MD 21207; (410)966-1133

The Joint Commission on Accreditation of Healthcare Organizations (JCAHO) was formed in 1951 with representatives from five groups — the American College of Physicians (ACP), the American Hospital Association (AHA), the American Medical Association (AMA), the American College of Surgeon (ACS), and the Canadian Medical Association (CMA). The CMA withdrew from the JCAHO to form its own accrediting organization. The JCAHO is currently sponsored by the AMA, AHA, ACP, ACS, and the American Dental Association.

The JCAHO originally evaluated hospitals and operating rooms. The accrediting program has been extended to include laboratories, home care, ambulatory care, mental health care, and long-term care facilities. In 1994 the JCAHO began an accrediting program to assess the ethical, medical, and business practices of healthcare networks.

The JCAHO offers educational programs for people in the healthcare industry, and inspects medical facilities to see if they are in compliance with national standards. The survey consists of more than 2,000 quality standards, including safety of the buildings, infection control, patient services and records, staff training, use of pharmaceuticals, and administrative procedures. The survey does not cover specific medical procedures and their outcomes. About 80% of US hospitals are accredited.

The JCAHO will tell you whether a particular hospital is accredited. In October 1994, the commission agreed to begin to make once-secret report cards issued to 11,000 US hospitals, nursing homes, and other health facilities available to the public. This action drew complaints from hospitals about the fairness of the reports and claims of

inconsistencies in the inspections conducted by the commission. The detailed performance reports, which are prepared every three years with participating facilities, were previously confidential. The cost of obtaining a report is $30.
Joint Commission on Accreditation of Healthcare Organizations, 1 Renaissance Blvd., Oakbrook Terrace, IL 60181; (708)916-5800 or 5600 or (312)642-6061

The National Committee for Quality-assurance accredits Health Maintenance Organizations. The Committee keeps report cards on HMOs. The report cards are based on an evaluation system called the HEDIS Indicators. HEDIS (Health Plan Employer Data and Information Set) was developed in 1989 by major corporations to compare health plans. These report cards may be available directly from the HMOs and can be helpful in evaluating the services a person may receive under a particular HMO plan. The NCQA has four levels of quality assurance. These include: Full Accreditation, lasts for three years; Accreditation with Recommendations, when there needs to be improvement before Full Accreditation is given; One-Year Accreditation, granted when an organization is in significant compliance with the standards but is not in full compliance standards; Provisional Accreditation, awarded for 15 months and the organization is surveyed again within 12 months to determine if deficiencies have been corrected.
National Committee for Quality-assurance, 1350 New York Ave., NW, Ste. 700, Washington, DC 20005; (202)955-3500

To find out whether a hospital has been certified by Medicare, contact your local Medicare office (a Social Security office can supply you with the phone number). Your state health department can tell you if a hospital has been suspended from participating in Medicare, or is on probation.

The United States Government Printing Office prints a yearly *Medicare Information Report*. It is available in some libraries, or can be purchased through the
United States Government Printing Office, Superintendent of Documents, PO Box 371954, Pittsburgh, PA 15250-7954; (202)512-1800; Fax (202)512-2250

• ADDISON'S DISEASE

National Adrenal Diseases Foundation, 505 Northern Blvd., Ste. 200, Great Neck, NY 11021; (516)487-4992; Net: http://medhlp.netusa.net/www/nadf.htm

• AIDS

Books:
- *The Gravest Show on Earth: America in the Age of AIDS,* by Elinor Burkett; Houghton, 1995
- *The Invisible Epidemic: The Story of Women and AIDS,* by Gena Corea; Harper Collins, 1992
- *National Directory of Bereavement Support Groups and Services,* by Mary M. Wong; ADM Publishing (PO Box 751155, Forest Hills, NY 11375-8755; [718]657-1277; E-mail: adm pub@internetmci.com)
- *Sometimes My Heart Goes Numb: Love and Caring in the Time of AIDS,* by Charles Garfield; Jossey-Bass, 1995
- *Start the Conversation: The Book About Death You Were Hoping to Find,* by Ganga Stone; Warner Books, 1996

AIDS/HIV Information Service, Net: http://www.ircam.fr/solidarites/sida/index-e/html

AIDS Information, Net: http://nearnet.gnn.com/wic/health.03.html

AIDS Online Databases, Net: http://www.nlm.nik.gov/top_level.dir/nln_online _info.html

AIDS Patients Project, Net: http://patients.cnidr.org.welcome.html

AIDS-Related World Wide Web Pages, Net: http://www.seanet.com/Users/jbrian /aids.html

AIDS Resource Fund for Children, St. Clare's Home for Children, 182 Roseville Ave., Newark, NJ 07107; (201)483-4250

Americans for a Sound AIDS Policy, PO Box 17433, Washington, DC 20041; (703)471-7350

Bastyr University Center for Alternative Medicine Research in HIV/AIDS, (800)475-0135

Being Alive : People With HIV/AIDS Action Coalition, Net: http://www.mbay.net/~bngalive/index.html

Center for AIDS Prevention Studies, Net: http://www.caps.ucsf.edu/capsweb

Centers for Disease Control and Prevention, National AIDS Hot Line (800)342-AIDS; Spanish (800)344-7432; TTY (800)243-7889

Gay Men's Health Crisis, 129 W. Twentieth St., New York, NY 10011; (212)807-6664

HIV/AIDS Information, Net: http://vector.casti.com/QRD/html/AIDS.html

National AIDS Information Centers for Disease Control and Prevention Clearinghouse, PO Box 6003, Rockville, MD 20849-6003; (800)458-5231

National HIV and AIDS Information Service, American Social Health Association, PO Box 13827, Research Triangle Park, NC 27709; (800)342-AIDS

National Minority AIDS Council, 300 — 1st St., NE, Ste. 400, Washington, DC 20002; (202)544-1076

For a free booklet titled *Every Question You Need to Ask Before Selling Your Life Insurance Policy,* contact the
National Viator Representatives' Thinking Positive Newsletter, 56 W. 57th St., Flr. 4, New York, NY 10019; (800)932-0050; Net: http://www.nvrnvr.com

Pediatric AIDS Foundation, 1311 Colorado Ave., Santa Monica, CA 90404; (310)395-5149

• ALLERGY AND ASTHMA

Books:
- *An Alternative Approach to Allergies,* by Theron G. Randolph and R.W. Moss; Bantam Books, 1987
- *Catching My Breath: An Asthmatic Explores His Illness,* by Tim Brookes; Vintage, 1995
- *The Complete Guide to Food Allergy and Intolerance: Prevention, Identification, and Treatment of Common Illnesses and Allergies Caused by Food,* by Dr. Jonathon Brostoff and Linda Gamlin; Crown Publishers, 1989
- *Sinus Survival: The Holistic Medical Treatment for Allergies, Asthma, Bronchitis, Colds, and Sinusitis,* by Robert S. Ivker, DO; Putnam Books, 1995

Action Against Allergy, 24-26 High St., Hampton Hill, Middlesex, Greater London, England TW12 1PD

Allergy, Net: alt.med.allergy

Allergy Alert Newsletter (published quarterly), Allergy Foundation of Canada, PO Box 1904, Saskatoon, SK, Canada 57K 3S5; (306)652-1608

Allergy and Asthma Network, 3554 Chain Bridge Rd., Ste. 200, Fairfax, VA 22030-2709; (703)385-4403 or (800)878-4403

Allergy Control Products, 96 Danbury Rd., Ridgefield, CT 06887; (800)422-DUST

Allergy Foundation of America, 801 Second Ave., New York, NY 10017; (212)684-7875

Allergy Immunology Medical College of Georgia, Net: gopher://lab.allergy.mcg.edu:70/1

Allergy Research Group, 400 Preda St., San Leonardo, CA 94577-0489; (510)569-9064 or (800)545-9960

American Academy of Allergy, Asthma, and Immunology, 611 E. Wells St., Milwaukee, WI 53202; (414)272-6071 or (800)822-2762

American Association of Certified Allergists, 800 E. Northwest Hwy., Ste. 1080, Palatine, IL 60067; (708)359-3919

American College of Allergy and Immunology, 85 W. Algonquin, Ste. 550, Arlington Heights, IL 60005; (708)427-1200 or (800)842-7777

American Osteopathic College of Allergy and Immunology, 3030 N. Hayden, Ste. 26, Scottsdale, AZ 85251; (602)949-8898

Asthma and Allergy Foundation of America, 1125 — 15th St., NW, Ste. 502, Washington, DC 20005; (202)265-0265 or (800)7-Asthma

Asthma Information Center, PO Box 790, Springhouse, PA 19477-0790; (800)727-5400

Canadian Society of Allergy and Clinical Immunology, Victoria General Hospital, PO Box 5375, 800 Commissioner's Rd. E., London, Ontario, N6A 4G5 Canada; (519)685-8167

The Food Allergy Network, 4744 Holly Ave., Fairfax, VA 22030

Gluten Intolerance Group of North America, PO Box 23053, Seattle, WA 98102-03543; (206)325-6980

International Foundation for Homeopathy, 2366 Eastlake Ave. E., Ste. 301, Seattle, WA 98102; (206)324-8230

National Institute of Allergy and Infectious Diseases, 9000 Rockville Pike, Bldg. 31, Rm. 7A-50, Bethesda, MD 20892; (301)496-5717

National Jewish Center for Immunology and Respiratory Medicine, 1400 Jackson St., Denver, CO 80206; (800)222-5864

Santa Fe Center for Allergy and Environmental Medicine, 141 Paseo Peralta, Ste. A, Santa Fe, NM 87501; (505)983-8890

ZAND Herbal Formulas, PO Box 5312, Santa Monica, CA 90409; (310)822-0500

• ALLOPATHIC EDUCATION ORGANIZATIONS

Accrediting Bureau of Health Education Schools, 29089 US 20, W., Elkhart, IN 46514; (219)293-0124

The Association of American Medical Colleges administers the *Medical College Admissions Test.* The test evaluates the qualifications of those who wish to attend allopathic medical schools in the US.

Association of American Medical Colleges, 2450 N St., NW, Washington, DC 20037-1126; (202)828-0400 or (202)828-0600

Educational Commission for Foreign Medical Graduates, 3624 Market St., Philadelphia, PA 19104; (215)386-5900

Society of University Surgeons, PO Box 7069, New Haven, CT 06519; (203)932-0541

University of Texas System, Medical and Dental Application Center, 702 Colorado, Ste. 620, Austin, TX 78701

Ontario Universities' Application Centre, P.O. Box 1328, 650 Woodlawn Rd. W., Guelph, Ontario, N1H 7P4 Canada

• ALTERNATIVE, AYURVEDIC, HOMEOPATHIC, NATUROPATHIC, AND OTHER HOLISTIC HEALTHCARE

(Also see *Aromatherapy; Chiropractic; Herbal and Plant-based Medicines/Therapies; Manipulative Therapies: Massage, Rolfing, Reflexology & Yoga;* and *Oriental Medicine*)

Books:
• *A Consumer's Guide to Alternative Healthcare,* by Craig Clayton and Virginia McCullough; Adams Publishing, 1995
• *Alternative Health & Medicine Encyclopedia,* by James Marti, Visible Ink Press, 1995

- *Alternative Medicine: The Definitive Guide*, compiled by the Burton Goldberg Group; Future Medicine Publishing, 1994
- *Alternative Medicine Yellow Pages: The Comprehensive Guide to the New World of Health*; Future Medicine Publishing (98 Main St., Ste. 209, Tiburne, CA 94920)
- *The Assault on Medical Freedom*, by Joseph Lisa; Hampton Roads Publishing ([800]766-8009), 1994
- *Ayurveda: A Way of Life*, by Vinod Verma; Samuel Weiser, Inc., 1995
- *The Book of Ayurveda: A Holistic Approach to Health and Longevity*, by Judith H. Morrison; Fireside Books, 1995
- *The Consumer's Guide to Homeopathy: The Definitive Resource for Understanding Homeopathic Medicine and Making it Work for You*, by Dana Ullman; Tarcher/Putnam, 1996
- *Encyclopedia of Natural Medicine*, by Michael Murray, ND, & Joseph Pizzorno, ND; Pima Publishing, 1991
- *The Family Guide to Homeopathy — Symptoms and Natural Solutions*, by Andrew Lockie; Fireside/Simon & Schuster, 1993
- *The Heretics Feast*, by Colin Spencer; University Press of New England, 1995
- *Living Beyond Limits: A Scientific Mind and Body Approach to Facing Life-Threatening Illness*, by Dr. David Spiegel; Random House, 1993
- *The Medical Mafia: How to Get Out of it Alive and Take Back Our Health & Wealth*, by Guylaine Lnctot, MD; Here's the Key, 1995
- *Natural Alternatives to Over-the-counter and Prescription Drugs*, by Michael T. Murray; Morrow, 1994
- *Natural Health, Natural Medicine: A Comprehensive Manual for Wellness and Self Care*, by Andrew Weil MD; Houghton Mifflen, 1995
- *Natural Prescriptions: Dr. Giller's Natural Treatments & Vitamin Therapies for over 100 Common Ailments*, by Robert M. Giller MD, and Kathy Matthews; Crown, 1994
- *The Practical Encyclopedia of Natural Healing: Hundreds of Natural Remedies for Common Health Problems*, by Mark Bricklin; Fine Communications, 1992
- *Racketeering in Medicine: The Suppression of Alternatives*, by James P. Carter, MD; Hampton Roads Publishing ([800]766-8009), 1993
- *Spontaneous Healing: Enhance Your Body's Natural Ability to Maintain and Heal Itself*, by Andrew Weil MD; Alfred A Knopf Publishing, 1995
- *Why I Left Orthodox Medicine: Healing for the 21st Century*, by Derrick Lonsdale; Hampton Roads Publishing ([800]766-8009), 1994

Academy for Guided Imagery, PO Box 2070, Mill Valley, CA 94942; (415)389-9324 or (800)726-2070

Academy of Natural Healing, 1443 S. St. Francis Dr., Santa Fe, NM 87501; (505)982-8398

Actual Natural Resource, Net: http://floralsnw.ark.com/health.html

Alexandra Health Center, Net: http://www.aescon.com/alexandra/index.html

   The Alternative Health Group specializes in finding insurance coverage for holistic treatments.

Alliance for Alternatives in Healthcare/The Alternative Health Plan, PO Box 6279, Thousand Oaks, CA 91359-6279; (805)494-7818 x 14; Alternative Health Insurance Services, (800)966-8467

Alternative and Complimentary Therapies, Mary Leibert, Inc., 2 Madison Ave., Larchmont, NY 10538; (914)834-3100

Alternative Care, Net: http://www.servint.com/altcare/whatsnew.html

Alternative Health and Medicine, Net: http://werple.mira.net.au/sumeria/health.html

Alternative Medicine Association, 7909 SE Stark St., Portland, OR 97215; (503)253-4031

Future Medicine Publishing markets several books on alternative medicine and publishes the monthly *Alternative Medicine Digest*. Subscriptions to the digest are $30. *Alternative Medicine Digest,* Future Medicine Publishing, Inc., 1640 Tiburon Blvd., Ste. 2, Tiburon, CA 94920; (415)435-0992 or (800)320-0512; Net: http://www. alternativemedicine.com

The Alternative Medicine Homepage from Falk Library of the Health Sciences at the University of Pittsburgh, Net: http://www.pitt.edu/~cbw/altm.html

Alternative Medicine Upcoming Events, Net: http://www.teleport.com/~amrta /events.html

Alternative Therapies in Health and Medicine, 101 Columbia, Alizo Viejo, CA 92656; (800)345-8112 or (800)899-1712

American Association of Ayurvedic Medicine, PO Box 344, 679 George Hill Rd., Lancaster, MA 01523; (508)365-4549

American Association of Naturopathic Physicians, 2366 Eastlake Ave., Ste. 322, Seattle, WA 98102; (206)323-7610; Net: http://infinity.dorsai.org/Naturopathic .Physician/AANPWeb.htm/

American College for Advancement in Medicine, 23121 Verdugo Dr., Ste. 204, Laguna Hills, CA 92653; (800)532-3688

American Holistic Medical Association, 4101 Lake Boone Trail, Ste. 201, Raleigh, NC 27607; (919)787-5181 or 5146

American Holistic Nurses Association, 4101 Lake Boone Trail, Ste. 201, Raleigh, NC 27607; (919)787-5146 or (800)878-3373

American Institute of Homeopathy, 1585 Glenco St., Ste. 44, Denver, CO 80220-1338; (303)898-5477 or 312-4105

American Preventive Medical Association, PO Box 211, Takoma, WA 98401-2111; (800)230-APMA

American School of Ayurvedic Sciences, 10025 NE 4th St., Bellevue, WA 98004; (206)453-8022

Ayurvedic Institute, PO Box 23445, Albuquerque, NM 87192; (505)291-9698

Bastyr University was founded in 1978. It offers a four-year program in naturopathic medicine, bachelor's degrees in the natural health sciences, and master's degree programs in nutrition, botanical medicine, and acupuncture. Midwifery is also taught. Bastyr Publications publishes and distributes the internationally-recognized *Textbook of Natural Medicine,* a two-volume, over 1,000-page reference work with regular updates. Bastyr also publishes the *Encyclopedia of Natural Medicine,* a 632-page consumer reference discussing natural treatments for common health problems. The Bastyr Bookstore offers mail order service of titles on natural health therapies. **Bastyr University,** 144 NE 54th St., Seattle, WA 98105; (206)523-9585; Net: http:// www.bastyr.edu

Biofeedback Certification Institute of America, 10200 W. 44th Ave., Ste. 304, Wheat Ridge, CO 80033; (303)420-2902

Boericke & Tafel (homeopathic medicine products), 2381 Circadian Way, Santa Rosa, CA 95407; (800)876-9505

Canadian Association of Ayurvedic Medicine, PO Box 749, Ottawa, Ontario K1P 5P8, Canada; (613)837-5737

Canadian College of Naturopathic Medicine, 60 Berl Ave., Etobicoke, Ontario M8Y 3C7, Canada; (416)251-5261

Canadian Holistic Medical Association, 491 Eglinton Ave. W., Ste. 407, Toronto, Ontario M5N 1A8 Canada; (416)485-3071

Canadian Naturopathic Association, PO Box 4520, Calgary, Alberta T2T 5N3, Canada; (403)244-4487

Center for Integrative Medicine, PO Box 40006, Tucson, AZ 85717; (520)626-5077

Center for Mind Body Medicine, 1110 Camino del Mar, Ste. G, Del Mar, CA 92014; (619)794-2425

Center for Mind-Body Medicine, 5225 Connecticut Ave., NW, Ste. 414, Washington, DC 20015; (202)966-7338

Citizens for Health works to protect consumers' rights to maintain access to a wide range of healthcare products and services relating to wellness and preventive healthcare. Citizens for Health publishes a newsletter ($25 a year), a Vitamin E Factbook ($3.50), and a handbook for grassroots activists that lists key government telephone numbers and addresses ($8.25). They publish a bi-monthly newsletter titled *The Digest of Drugless Therapies.*

Citizens for Health, PO Box 1195, Tacoma, WA 98401; (206)922-2457 or (800)357-2211

College of Synotic Optometry (light therapy), 1200 Robertson St., Fall River, MA 02720-5508; (508)673-1251

In 1994, the Columbia University College of Physicians and Surgeons, the oldest medical school in the United States, became the first university allopathic medical school to open a school of alternative medicine.

Columbia University College of Physicians and Surgeons School of Alternative Medicine, 630 W. 168th St., New York, NY 10032; (212)544-1306

Complimentary Medicine Homepage, Net: http://galen.med.virginia.edu/~pjb3s /ComplimentaryHomePage

Complimentary Medicine International/Alternative Medicine Journal, 470 Boston Post Rd., Westin, MA 02193-1569; (617)899-2702; E-mail: DeVitoR@aol.com — or — E-mail: 76150,1602@compuserve.com — or — Net: radjr@netcom.com

Cranial Academy, 8606 Allisonville Rd., Ste. 130, Indianapolis, IN 46250; (317)594-0411

Dr. Bower's Complimentary Medicine Homepage, Net: http://galen.med.virginia .edu/~pjb3s/ComplimentaryHomePage.html

Foundation for Homeopathic Education and Research, 2124 Kittredge St., Berkeley, CA 94704

General Complimentary Medicine, Net: http://www.forthrt.com/~chronicl /archiv.htm#5

Good Medicine Online, Net: http://none.coolware.com/health/good_med /NovIssue.html

Hahnemann Medical Clinic and Pharmacy (homeopathic), 828 San Pablo Ave., Albany, CA 94706; (510)524-3117

Health and Longevity, Net: http://www.sims.net/organizations/naturopath/ naturopath.html

Health Awareness Resource Center is a non-profit information service for those who want to learn more about holistic medicine. They publish a newsletter called *Awareness Update.*

Health Awareness Resource Center, 18 Old Padonia Rd., Cockeysville, MD 21030; (410)560-6864; Compuserve: 74464.145@compuserve.com

Health Information Network International, 4213 Montgomery Dr., Santa Rosa, CA 95405; (707)539-3967 or (800)743-6996

Holistic Dental Association, PO Box 5007, Durango, CO 81301; (303)259-1091

Homeopathic Academy of Naturopathic Physicians, PO Box 69565, Portland, OR 97201

Homeopathic Educational Services runs a store in Berkeley and publishes a catalog of homeopathic medicines, books, tapes, and other products. A directory of US and Canadian homeopathic professionals is $5.

Homeopathic Educational Services, 2124 Kittredge St., Berkeley, CA 94704; (510)649-0294; Net: http://www.homeopathic.com

Homeopathic Internet Resources List, Net: http://www.dungeon.com/home/cam/interlst.html

Homeopathy Homepage, Net: http://www.dungeon.com/home/cam/homeo

International College of Applied Kinesiology, PO Box 905, Lawrence, KS 66044-0905; (913)542-1801

International Foundation for Homeopathy, PO Box 7, Edmunds, WA 98020; (206)776-4147

Institute for Natural Medicine, 66 1/2 N. State St., Concord, NH 03301-4330; (603)225-8844

The Journal of Alternative and Complimentary Medicine: Research and Paradigm, Practice, and Policy, Mary Leibert, Inc., 2 Madison Ave., Larchmont, NY 10538; (914)834-3100

Life Extension Foundation, Net: http://aeiveos.wa.com/lef/

Maharishi Ayur-Veda Medical Center, PO Box 282, Fairfield, IA 52556

The National Center for Homeopathy provides an information package that is available for $6 which includes a directory to homeopathic practitioners, pharmacies, bookstores, and study groups throughout the US and Canada. They publish a magazine titled *Homeopathy Today* which comes out 11 times per year. Subscription is part of a $40.00 yearly membership. They also sell a number of books covering various areas of homeopathy.
National Center for Homeopathy, 801 N. Fairfax St., Ste. 306, Alexandria, VA 22314; (703)548-7790

National College of Naturopathic Medicine, 11231 SE Market St., Portland, OR 976216; (503)255-4860

Natural Health Magazine, PO Box 57320, Boulder, CO 80322-7320

Natural Medicine, Complimentary Healthcare and Alternative Therapies, Net: http://wwwteleport.com80/~amrta

The Natural Way Magazine, 566 Westchester Ave., Rye Brook, NY 10573; (914)939-2111

Nature's Medicine, Net: http://www.halcyon.com/jerryga/welcome.html

Naturopathic Physicians, Net: http://www.infinite.org/Naturopathic.Physician

New Age Publishing is the publisher of the *Holistic Health Directory* and *New Age Journal Magazine.*
New Age Publishing, 42 Pleasant St., Watertown, MA 02172; (617)926-0200 or (800)782-7006; E-mail: editor@newage.com — or — Net: http://www.spdcc.com/home/newage/index.html

New Center for Holistic Health, Education, and Research, 6801 Jericho Trnpk., Syosset, NY 11791-4413; (516)364-0808

New England Journal of Homeopathy, 115 Elm St., Ste. 210, Enfield, CT 06082; (203)253-5040 or (800)NESH-440

New Health News is a newsletter put out by the publishers of *Delicious,* and *Natural Foods Merchandiser* magazines. It reports on developments in alternative healthcare, natural products, remedies, and preventative medicine.
New Health News, 1301 Spruce St., Boulder, CO 80302; (303)939-8440 or (800)933-8440

Newton Homeopathic Medicine, 612 Upland Trail, Conyers, GA 30207; (800)448-7256

Office for the Study of Unconventional Medical Practices, National Institutes of Health, Bldg. 31, Rm. 2B25, Bethesda, MD 20892; (301)496-7498

Office of Alternative Medicine, National Institutes of Health, 6120 Executive Blvd., EPS Ste. 450, Rockville, MD 20892; (301)402-2466

The People's Place, Net: http://peopleplace.com

Physicians Committee for Responsible Medicine, 5100 Wisconsin Ave., NW, Ste. 404, Washington, DC 20016; (202)686-2210

Sharp Institute for Human Potential and Mind-Body Medicine, 1110 Camino Del Mar, Del Mar, CA 92014; (800)82-SHARP

Smart Health (discount homeopaths and vitamins), (800)371-0027

Southwest College of Naturopathic Medicine, 6535 E. Osborn Rd., Scottsdale, AZ 85251; (602)990-7424

Standard Homeopathic Company, 210 W. 131st St., Los Angeles, CA 90061; (213)321-4284 or (800)624-9659

The Trager Institute, 33 Millwood, Mill Valley, CA 94941; (415)388-2688

Vital Communications Natural Medicine Update, 15401 SE 54th Court, Bellevue, WA 98006; (800)488-0753

Wellness Plan (holistic medicine health insurance), 1950 Elkhorn Crt., San Mateo, CA 94403-1308; (800)925-5323

World Natural Medicine Foundation, 9904 — 106 St., Edmonton, Alberta, Canada T5K 1C4; (403)424-2231

World Wide Wellness, Net: http://www.doubleclickd.com/wwwellness.html

• ALZHEIMER'S DISEASE

Books:
• *Defense Against Alzheimer's Disease: A Rational Blueprint for Prevention,* by H.J. Roberts; Sunshine Sentinal Press (PO Box 8697, West Palm Beach, FL 33407), 1995
• *Therapeutic Caregiving: A Practical Guide for Caregivers of Persons with Alzheimer's and Other Dementia Causing Diseases,* by Barbara J. Bridges, RN (E-mail: FGXK82A@prodigy.com; BJB Publishing ([800]799-3414), 1996
• *The 36-Hour Day: A Family Guide to Caring for Persons with Alzheimer's Disease, Related Dementing Illnesses, and Memory Loss in Later Life,* by Nancy L. Mace and Peter V. Rabins; Johns Hopkins University Press, 1991

Alzheimer's Association, 919 N. Michigan Ave., Ste. 100, Chicago, IL 60611-1676; (312)335-8700 or (800)621-0379 or (800)272-3900 or in Illinois call (800)572-6037; Net: http://www.alz.org/

Alzheimer's Disease International, 919 N. Michigan Ave., Ste. 1000, Chicago, IL 60611; (312)335-5777

• AMPUTATION

AFTER Rehabilitation and Training Center for Limb Birth Deficiencies and Amputations, 2559 Fairway Island Dr., W. Palm Beach, FL 33414; (407)790-3589

American Amputee Foundation, Box 250218 Hillcrest St., Little Rock, Arkansas 72225; (501)666-2523

Amputee Shoe and Glove Exchange, PO Box 27067, Houston, TX 77227

Amputees in Motion, PO Box 2703, Escondido, CA 92033; (619)454-9300

National Amputation Foundation, 73 Church St., Malverne, NY 11565; (516)887-3600; Fax (516)887-3667

• ANESTHESIOLOGY

Upon request, the American Association of Nurse Anesthetists will send you pamphlets that will familiarize you with anesthesia, and the process of preparing for the administration of and recovery from anesthesia. The name of the pamphlets are: *Anesthesia: Certified Registered Nurse Anesthetists Answer Your Questions; Before Anesthesia: Your Active Role Makes a Difference;* and *After Anesthesia: Your Active Role Assists Your Recovery.*

Prior to entering the Master's Degree nurse anesthesia educational program, these advanced practice specialty nurses must have at least one year's acute care experience. Additional continuing education is required for recertification every two years.
American Association of Nurse Anesthetists, 222 S. Prospect Ave., Park Ridge, IL 60068-4001; (847)692-7050 or (800)543-AANA

American Board of Anesthesiology, 100 Constitution Plaza, Hartford, CT 06103; (203)522-9857

American Dental Society of Anesthesiology, 211 E. Chicago Ave., Ste. 948, Chicago, IL 60611; (312)664-8270

American Osteopathic Board of Anesthesiology, 17201 E. Hwy. 40, Ste. 204, Independence, MO 64055; (816)373-4700

American Society of Anesthesiologists, 520 Northwest Hwy., Park Ridge, IL 60068-2573; (708)825-5586

American Society of Post Anesthesia Nurses, 11512 Allecingie Pkwy., Ste. C, Richmond, VA 23235; (804)379-5516

American Society of Regional Anesthesia, 1910 Byrd Ave., PO Box 11086, Ste. 100, Richmond, VA 23230-1086; (804)282-0010

Anesthesiology, Net: gopher://eja/anes.hscsyr.edu:70/1

Anesthesiology, Net: http://www.med.nyu.edu/ruskin/ruskinintro.html

Anesthesiology Medicine Biosciences, Net: http://gasnet.med.nyu.edu/index .html

Canadian Anesthetists' Society, 1 Eglinton Ave. E., #209, Toronto, Ontario M4P 3A1 Canada; (416)480-0602

Society of Cardiovascular Anesthesiologists, PO Box 11086, Richmond, VA 23230-1086; (804)282-0084

• ANIMAL CONCERNS

Books:
* *Animal Factories: The mass production of animals for food and how it affects the lives of consumers, farmers, and the animals themselves,* by Jim Mason and Peter Singer; Crown Publishers, 1980
* *Animal Liberation,* by Peter Singer; Random House, 1990
* *Beyond Beef: The Rise and the Fall of the Cattle Culture,* by Jeremy Rifkin; Plume, 1992
* *Old MacDonald's Factory Farm,* by C. David Coats; Crossroads Publishing ([212]532-3650)

Animals' Agenda, PO Box 6809, Syracuse, NY 13217

Biodiversity Legal Foundation, PO Box 18327, Boulder, CO 80308-1327

Colorado Wolf Tracks, Sinapu, PO Box 3243, Boulder, CO 80307; (303)447-8655

Earth First, PO Box 1415, Eugene, OR 97440; (503)741-9191; Fax (503)741-9192; E-mail: Earthfirst@igc.apc.org

Farm Animal Reform Movement, PO Box 30654, Bethesda, MD 20824; (301)530-1737

Farm Sanctuary, PO Box 150, Watkins Glen, NY 14891-0150; (607)583-2225

Friends of the Amazon Forest, PO Box 625, Cambridge, MA 02140

The Fund for Animals, National Campaign Office, 850 Sligo Ave., Ste. 300, Silver Spring, MD 20910; (301)585-2591 — or — The Fund for Animals, National Headquarters, 200 W. 57th St., New York, NY 10019; (212)246-2096

Fund for Wild Nature, PO Box 1657, 254 SW Madison Ave., Corvallis, OR 97339; (541)757-1780

Greenhouse Crisis Foundation, 1130 — 17th St., NW, Ste. 630, Washington, DC 20036; (202)466-2823

Greenpeace, 847 West Jackson Blvd., Chicago, IL 60607; (312)563-6060; Fax (312)563-6099

Humane Farming Association, PO Box 3577, San Rafael, CA 94912 — or — 1550 California St., San Francisco, CA 94109; (415)771-CALF

To read the Pulitzer Prize winning "Boss Hog" report on the damage done by big business hog farming that appeared in the News & Observer newspaper, you can sign on to

News & Observer Boss Hog series, Net: http://www.nando.net/sproject/hogs/hoghome.html

People for the Ethical Treatment of Animals, PO Box 42516, Washington, DC 20015; (202)726-0156

United Poultry Concerns, PO Box 59367, Potomac, MD 20859; (301)948-2406

Wildlife Damage Review, PO Box 85218, Tucson, AZ 85754; (520)884-0883; E-mail: PREDheads@aol.com

• AROMATHERAPY

Books:
- *Aromatherapy and the Mind: An Exploration Into the Psychological and Emotional Effects of Essential Oils,* by Julia Lawless; Harper Collins, 1994
- *Aromatherapy Scent and Psyche: Using Essential Oils for Physical and Emotional Well-Being,* by Peter and Kate Damian; Inner Traditions, 1995
- *The Complete Book of Essential Oils and Aromatherapy,* by Valerie Ann Worwood; New World Library, 1991
- *Essential Aromatherapy,* by Susan Worwood; New World Library, 1995
- *The Illustrated Encyclopedia of Essential Oils: Complete Guide to the Use of Oils in Aromatherapy and Herbalism,* by Julia Lawless; Element Books, 1995

While aromatherapy may not play a major role in bringing a person to better health, it may help establish a good feeling in an ailing person. The sense of smell is very powerful and may stimulate both physical and psychological responses. A pleasing scent may help calm the nerves, establish comfort, and influence emotions and dreams. In this way aromatherapy has a place in holistic health. Scents used in aromatherapy come from extracts of flowers, plants, and trees. They can be heated in a special holder to spread the aroma through a room, used in bath water, or during massage.

Some companies are now using the definition of aromatherapy loosely and putting out products that contain chemical aromas. This is to jump on the bandwagon to make money in this area by increasing sales to people seeking aromatherapy products. The companies listed below should be fairly reliable in providing aromatherapy products that are made from natural ingredients (plants, flowers, and trees).

American Society for Phytotherapy and Aromatherapy, Box 3679, South Pasadena, CA 91031; (818)457-1742

Aroma Land, Inc., Rte. 20, Box 29, Santa Fe, NM 87501; (800)933-5269

Aromatherapy International, 3 Seal Harbor Rd., Ste. 735, Winthrop, MA 02152; (800)722-4377

The Aromatherapy Quarterly (publication), PO Box 421, Inverness, CA 94937-0421; (415)663-9519

Aromatic Thymes Magazine, 75 Lakeview Pkwy., Barrington, IL 60010; (847)526-0456; E-mail: aromatic@interaccess.com

Aroma Vera, 5901 Rodeo Rd., Los Angeles, CA 90016-4312; (310)280-0407 or (800)669-9514

Earth Essentials, PO Box 35284, Sarasota, FL 34242; (941)346-3220 or (800)370-3220

Flower Essence Society, (800)548-0075; E-mail: fes@nccn.net

Hands On Aromatherapy, 1558 Nantahalla Ct., NE, Atlanta, GA 30329; (800)331-6457

National Association for Holistic Aromatherapy, PO Box 17622, Boulder, CO 80308-7622; (800)566-6735

Natural Oils Research Association, BGB Plaza, Ste. H, 894 Rte. 52, Beacon, NY 12508; (914)838-4340; E-mail: norassoc@aol.com

North American Flower Essences, PO Box 1769, Nevada City, CA 95959; (916)265-0258 or (800)548-0075; E-mail: FES@nccn.net

Original Sunrise Aromatics, Box 606, San Rafael, CA 94915

Rosa, Olfaction, Scent & Aromatherapy, 219 Carl St., San Francisco, CA 94117; (415)564-6787 or fax (415)564-6799

True Essence Aromatherapy, 2203 Westmount Rd., NW, Calgary, Alberta, Canada T2N 3N5; (800)563-8938

The Very Essence, PO Box 22929, San Diego, CA 92192-2929; (800)237-7362

• ARTHRITIS

Aids for Arthritis (catalog of products), 3 Little Knoll Court, Medford, NJ 08055; (609)654-6918

American College of Rheumatology, 17 Executive Park Dr., NE, Ste. 480, Atlanta, GA 30329

American Juvenile Arthritis Organization, 1314 Spring St., NW, Atlanta, GA 30309; (404)872-7100

Arthritis Consulting Services, 4620 N. State Rd. 7, Ste. 206, Ft. Lauderdale, FL 33319; (305)739-3202 or (800)327-3027; E-mail: HBT@GATE.NET.

The Arthritis Fund, 5106 Old Harding Rd., Franklin, TN 37064-9400; (615)646-1030; Net: Mall-net.com/arth

Arthritis Foundation, PO Box 7669, Atlanta, GA 30357-0669; (404)872-7100 or (800)283-7800; Net: http://www.arthritis.org

Arthritis Newsgroup, Net: alt.med.arthritis

Arthritis Society, 250 Bloor St. E., Ste. 401, Toronto, Ontario, M4W 3P2 Canada; (416)967-1414

National Arthritis and Muscoloskeletal and Skin Diseases, Information Clearinghouse, 1 AMS Circle, Bethesda, MD 20892-3675; (301)495-4484

Spondylitis Association of America, PO Box 5872, Sherman Oaks, CA 91413; (800)777-8189

• BACK AND SPINE

Books:
• *The Back Almanac;* Celestial Arts (PO Box 7123, Berkeley, CA 94707), 1992
• *Back Care Basics: A Doctor's Gentle Yoga Program for Back and Neck Pain Relief,* by Mary Pullig Schatz; Rodmell Press (E-mail: RodmellPrs@aol.com), 1992
• *Freedom from Back Pain,* by Edward Abraham; Rodale Press, 1986
• *Relax & Renew,* by Judith Lasater; Rodmell Press (E-mail: RodmellPrs@aol.com), 1995

Next to the common cold, back problems are the leading reasons that people see doctors. Pain can occur anywhere on the spine, but the lower back is the most common area of back pain and is the region that carries the most weight and supports muscle activity. Certain types of back pain can be a sign of kidney problems (they are located on the sides of the back inside the lower rib cage), heart disease, or other internal health problems. The most common back pains are caused by emotional tension, physical strain, lazy posture and seating habits, bad sleeping positions, lack of exercise, being overweight, and having weak abdominal muscles. More serious causes of back pain are compressed or injured disks, arthritis, bone deformities, osteoporosis, fractures, tumors, infections, and nerve problems. When a slipped disk presses against the nerves in the spinal cord, the person can experience pain in the rear and down the leg.

Preventive measures that can be utilized to maintain a healthy back include massage and exercise. Massage can help relieve stress that may contribute to back strains. Taking 10 to 20 minutes every day to perform back-strengthening exercises is better and safer than doing a lot of exercise once in awhile. Exercises that may help the back are swimming, abdominal exercises, and leg-lift and tummy-scrunch exercises performed while hanging from a chin-up bar. Mild yoga-type stretching is also helpful.

Visiting with a well-trained physical therapist or chiropractor who can teach you how to strengthen your back with an exercise program can be very beneficial. The right exercise and treatments done the wrong way, the wrong combination of movements, or doing too much too soon, may do more damage than good. Some back injuries may become irritated by certain exercise positions or movements, so learning the best form of exercise for your type of injury is important.

The US Public Health Service's Publication Clearinghouse will send you a free copy of a pamphlet titled *Understanding Acute Low Back Problems*.
Agency for Health Care Policy and Research, US Dept. of Health and Human Services, PO Box 8547, Silver Spring, MD 20907-8547; (800)358-9295

American Association of Spinal Cord Injury Nurses, 75-20 Astoria Blvd., Flushing, NY 11370-1177; (718)803-3782

American Association of Spinal Cord Injury Psychologists and Social Workers, 75-20 Astoria Blvd., Flushing, NY 11370-1177

Because it is low-impact and creates the least amount of stress on the back of any exercise, swimming is a good form of exercise for people with back problems. For $16.95, plus $6 shipping, the American Lap Swimmers' Association will send you their publication called *A Swimmer's Guide* that lists over 1,200 exercise pools, including locations and hours of operation.
American Lap Swimmers' Association, 5755 Powerline Rd., Ft. Lauderdale, FL 33309; (800)431-9111

American Paralysis Association, 500 Morris Ave., Springfield, NJ 07081; (800)225-0292; Net: http://www.apa.uci.edu/paralysis

American Spinal Injury Association, 250 E. Superior, Rm. 619, Chicago, IL 60611; (312)908-3425

American Syringomyelia Alliance Project, PO Box 1586, Longview, TX 75606-1586; (903)236-7079

Back Pain Hotline, (800)247-BACK

Citizens Against Pedical Plates & Screws, PO Box 842, Carson, WA 98610

Families of Spinal Muscular Atrophy, PO Box 1465, Highland Park, IL 60035-7465; (708)432-5551

Feldenkrais Guild (movement therapy), PO Box 489, Albany, OR 97321; (503)926-0981

Gravity Plus (catalog of products to help treat and prevent back problems), PO Box 2182, La Jolla, CA 92038; (619)454-1626 or (800)383-8056; E-mail: gravity@sd.znet.com

Mensendieck Enterprises produces and distributes video programs which demonstrate back exercises and teach back pain therapies that do not rely on drugs or medical procedures.
Mensendieck Enterprises, PO Box 9450, Stanford, CA 94305-9450

Miami Project to Cure Paralysis, Spinal Injury Research Center, (305)243-6001

National Scoliosis Foundation, 72 Mt. Auburn St., Watertown, MA 02172; (617)926-0397

National Spinal Cord Injury Association, 545 Concord Ave., Ste. 29, Cambridge, MA 02138; (617)441-8500 or (800)962-9629; Fax (617)441-3449

North American Society of Teachers of the Alexander Technique, PO Box 3992, Champaign, IL 61826; (217)359-3529

Rehabilitation Learning Center, Net: http://weber.u.washington.edu/~rlc/

Relax the Back Stores are retail stores specializing in products for the relief and prevention of back pain. They sell hundreds of products including special pillows, supports for the car, ergonomically designed office furniture, massage products, braces, and back exercise videos. To find a store near you, contact the headquarters at **Relax the Back Store Franchising Co.,** 3355 Bee Cave Rd., Bldg. 7, Ste. 705, Austin, TX 78746; (800)290-2225

Scoliosis Association, PO Box 811705, Boca Raton, FL 33481-1705; (407)994-4435 or (800)800-0669

Scoliosis Research Society, 6300 N. River Rd., Ste. 717, Rosemont, IL 60018

Spina Bifida Association of America, 4590 MacArthur Blvd., NW, Ste. 250, Washington, DC 20007; (202)944-3285 or (800)621-3141

Spina Bifida Association of British Columbia, 9460 140th St., Surrey, British Columbia, V3V 5Z4 Canada; (604)584-1361

Spinal Cord Society, RR 5 Box 22A, Fergus Falls, MN 56537-9805

Texas Back Institute, Dallas, TX; (800)247-2225

• BILLING PROBLEMS

Book:
* *Getting the Most for Your Medical Dollar,* by Charles Inlander and Karla Morales; People's Medical Society (462 Walnut St., Allentown, PA 18102; [610] 770-1670)

Although some overcharges might be honest mistakes, most hospital bills contain errors and these are usually not in the patients' favor. Often these charges are false and some charges are of tests and procedures that were ordered and never carried out because they were overlooked or were canceled. When services are not coded correctly it can cause interference with insurance coverage.

When you cannot get clear definitions of the codes and abbreviations on your hospital bill, you may want to contact the hospital billing department, the doctor, or the claims representative of your insurance carrier to find out what it is you are being charged for. Keep a record of who you spoke with, the date, and what was said. If all else fails you might want to contact your state's insurance commissioner.

If you send your medical records to one of the private auditing services, be sure to request that your records be returned to you, unless you posses your own copy. Whenever possible, keep the originals for your own files and send copies to the auditing service.

Make the hospital aware of any errors in the bills they have sent to you. If they are requesting payment from you, pay the part of the bill that you are not disputing and hold off on the unresolved charges until they are explained to you and, if in error, removed from your bill.

Bills Project, Ocean Park Blvd., Santa Monica, CA 90405; (310)475-0883; E-mail: network @primenet.com. — or — Net: http://www.primenet.com/~network

CostReview Services is a company with three medical price review departments. CostReview works with insurance companies, MedResolve works with doctors, and MedReview works with patients.

MedReview will review bills from hospitals, doctors, clinics, and laboratories. A person using MedReviews' service sends the company copies of medical records, itemized billing statements, and any records relating to each bill. A nurse-auditor will make a report of the discrepancies and work with the patient to straighten out the bill. If a claim for adjustment or reimbursement is appropriate, MedReview will act as your advocate in filing an appeal. The fee for the audit of hospital bills is based on the amount billed by the hospital. All fees, for both hospital and physician reviews, are subject to 8% sales tax.

According to the US General Accounting Office, there are discrepancies on 98% of hospital bills that are sent to patients.

MedReview, 3724 Executive Center Dr., Ste. 101, Austin, TX 78731; (512)338-9196 or (800)397-5359

Trusting Your Health Insurance company Too Much

Insurance companies count on the fact that we, the public, trust them implicitly when it comes to our medical benefits. They count on us not to fight. We are far too passive when it comes to dealing with insurance companies. We take their word when they don't reimburse us enough, leaving us with heavy out-of-pocket expenses. We even trust that they will follow up on our requests without having to remind them. We forget that insurance companies are in the business of making money. We must learn to question them when they deny our benefits. And never to accept their 'No' as a final answer.

Unfortunately, statistics prove that insurance companies are correct: Most of us do blindly accept their decisions, without protest. Only a small percentage of people ever question their insurance companies, and consequently, most people do not get the money that is rightfully theirs.

There are five steps to what I call my "battle plan," and it is important to follow all these steps in order to maximize your insurance reimbursements.

1. Know what your benefits are, and are not, before you need them. What you don't know can hurt you. It can also help the insurance company save money.

2. Keep meticulous records of conversations with both insurance company personnel and medical providers. Document everything that happens to avoid claim problems and possible denials down the road.

3. Track all your medical expenses, and follow up with your insurance carriers in a timely manner to assure that they pay all your claims. Too many claims fall through the cracks and into the garbage can because of faulty follow-up.

4. Be persistent and assertive. Don't give up your benefits. Fight back and never take the first "NO" you receive as your final answer.

5. Never pay a bill until you know that you really owe the money. Remember, once you have paid the money — even if you have paid it in error — you will have to fight to get it back.

— by Gail Glink, medical claims advocate and the owner of ProMediClaim

ProMediClaim is not associated with an insurance agency. The company founder describes the company as "a medical claims management and advocacy company that helps patients and their families minimize the confusion and frustration surrounding the filing and collection of health insurance benefits."

ProMediClaim, 113 McHenry Rd., Ste. 274, Buffalo Grove, IL 60089; (708)634-6212

• BIRTH-CONTROL

Association for Voluntary Surgical Contraception, 79 Madison Ave., New York, NY 10016; (212)561-8000

Office of Population Affairs Clearinghouse, PO Box 30686, Bethesda, MD 20824-0686; (301)654-6190

Ovulation Method Teachers Association, PO Box 101780, Anchorage, AK 99510-1760

• BLOOD

American Association of Blood Banks, 8101 Glenbrook Rd., Bethesda, MD 20814; (301)907-6977

American Blood Commission, American Hospital Association, 840 N. Lakeshore Dr., Chicago, IL 60611; (312)280-6000

American Blood Resource Association, PO Box 669, Annapolis, MD 21404-0669; (410)263-8296

American Society of Hematology, 1200 — 19th St., NW, Ste. 300, Washington, DC 20036-2401; (202)857-1118

Aplastic Anemia Foundation, PO Box 22689, Baltimore, MD 21203; (800)747-2820

Children's Blood Foundation, 333 E. 38th St., Ste. 210, New York, NY 10016; (212)297-4336

Council of Community Blood Centers, 725 — 15th St., NW, Ste. 700, Washington, DC 20005-2109; (202)393-5725

Dept. of Health and Human Services, Public Health Service, Food and Drug Administration, Office of Public Affairs, 5600 Fishers Lane, Rockville, MD 20857

Foundation for Blood Irradiation, 1315 Apple Ave., Silver Spring, MD 20910; (301)587-8686

Foundation for Blood Research, Scarborough, ME; (207)883-4131

Fanconi Anemia Research Fund, 1902 Jefferson St., Ste. 2, Eugene, OR 97405; (541)687-4658 or (800)828-4891; Fax (541)687-0548; E-mail: fafund@rio.com

Hemochromatosis Foundation, PO Box 8569, Albany, NY 12208; (518)489-0972

Hepatitis B Foundation, PO Box 464, New Hope, PA 18938

Members of the Jehovah's Witness Church are opposed to blood transfusions. The Jehovah's Witness-run Hospital Information Services Dept. can supply information on ways of limiting blood loss during surgery.
Hospital Information Services Dept., Watchtower Bible and Tract Society of New York, 25 Columbus Heights, Brooklyn, NY 11201

Hypoglycemia Association, 18008 new Hampshire Ave., Ashton, MD 20861-0165

International Society of Hematology, 920 Hilton, 200 — 1st St., SW, Rochester, MN 55905; (507)284-3937

Leukemia Society of America, 600 Third Ave., New York, NY 10016; (800)955-4LSA

National Blood Resource Education Program, Information Center, 4733 Bethesda Ave., Ste. 530, Bethesda, MD 20814

National Hemophilia Foundation, 1101 — 17th St. NW, Washington, DC 20036; (202)833-0085 — or — 110 Green St., Ste. 303, New York, NY 10012; (212)219-8180

National Hypoglycemia Association, PO Box 120, Ridgewood, NJ 07451; (201)670-1189

A phlebotomist obtains patients' blood specimens and may collect other clinical laboratory specimens. They are employed by hospitals, health and medical clinics, group practices, HMO's, and public health facilities. The position does not require a degree. The National Phlebotomy Association educates and certifies phlebotomists, and offers continuing education programs for them. The certified membership is about 20,000. According to NPA literature, there are over 200,000 persons working as phlebotomists who have not been certified. The lack of certified workers in this field is particularly troubling since AIDS has become an epidemic and is a risk factor for those working in the field of phlebotomy. There have been dozens of healthcare workers who have been infected with HIV by needlestick injuries. The newsletter of the NPA is called the *Tourniquet.*
National Phlebotomy Association, 5616 Landover Rd., Hyattsville, MD 20784; (301)699-3846; Fax (301)699-5766

National Rare Blood Club, 99 Madison Ave., New York, NY 10016; (212)889-4455 or (800)722-8668

The Red Cross, (800)974-2113

Sickle Cell Disease Association of America, 200 Corporate Point, Ste. 495, Culver City, CA 90230-7633; (310)216-6363 or (800)421-8453; Fax (310)215-3722

• BONES AND ORTHOPEDICS

American Board of Orthopedic Surgery, 737 N. Michigan Ave., Ste. 1150, Chicago, IL 60611; (312)664-9444

American Bone Fracture Association, 2416 E. Washington St., Ste. D-3, Bloomington, IL 61704; (309)663-6272

American Academy of Orthopaedic Surgeons, 6300 N. River Rd., Rosemont, IL 60018; (800)824-BONE (2663)

American Association of Orthopedic Medicine, 5147 Lewiston Rd., Lewiston, NY 14092

American Orthopaedic Society for Sports Medicine, 6300 N. River Rd., Ste. 200, Rosemont, IL 60018; (708)292-4900

American Society for Bone and Mineral Research, 1101 Connecticut Ave., NW, Washington, DC 20036; (202)857-1161

Association of Bone and Joint Surgeons, 6300 N. River Rd., Ste. 727, Rosemont, IL 60018-4226; (708)698-1636

Paget Foundation for Paget's Disease of Bone and Related Disorders, 200 Varick St., Ste. 1004, New York, NY 10014-4810; (212)229-1582 or (800)23-PAGET; E-mail: paget fdn@aol.com

• BOOKSTORES, MAIL ORDER, AND ONLINE

This book and many of the books listed in this book can be purchased with a credit card over the phone through the following bookstores:

Harry W. Schwartz Bookshops, 409 East Silver Spring Dr., Milwaukee, WI 53217; (414)274-6400

Healing Pages Bookstore, 600 W. McGraw St., #2, Seattle, WA 98119; (206)283-7621

Malaprop's Bookstore, 61 Haywood St., Asheville, NC 28801; (704) 254-6734

Madea Books, Santa Cruz, California, (408)425-0913

Midnight Special Bookstore, 1318 — 3rd St. Promenade, Santa Monica, CA 90401; (310)393-2923; E-mail: books@msbooks.com — or — Net: http://msbooks.com/msbooks

Parents Choice Book Center, 57 Stevens St., Stoneham, MA 02180; (617)438-8791 or (800)722-2939

Powell's Bookstore, 1005 W. Burnside, Portland, OR 97209; (503) 228-4651

Red Wing Books sells a large variety of books on acupuncture, aromatherapy, Chinese herbal medicine, energetic arts (aikido, t'ai chi, taoist, and yogic), holistic health, homeopathy, macrobiotics, manual therapies, nutrition, naturopathy, natural medicine, Oriental healing arts, and Western herbal medicine. They also sell natural food cookbooks.

Red Wing Books, 44 Linden St., Brookline, MA 02146; (617)738-4664 or (800)873-3946; Fax (617)738-4620; Net: redwing@oa.net

Tattered Cover Bookstore , 1536 Wyncoop, Denver, CO 80202; (303) 322-7727 or (800)833-9327

Bookstores on the Internet:
- **Alternative Books Superstore,** E-mail: altbooks@aol.com — or — Net: http://web-star.com/alternative/books.html
- **Amazon,** E-mail: content-dept@amazon.com —or — Net, http://www.amazon.com/
- **Barnes & Noble on Compuserve,** Net: go BN
- **Basement Full of Books:** E-mail: bfob@greyware.com
- **Bestbooks Online,** E-mail: mike@speaking.com — or — Net: http://www.bestbooks.com
- **Book Reviews Digest on Compuserve,** Net: go BOOKREVIEW $$

- **Bookserve**, E-mail: Bookserve@nashville.net — or — Net: http://www.bookserve .com
- **Books In Print on Compuserve**, Net: go BOOKS $$
- **BookSite**, Rob@booksite.com — or — Net: http://www.booksite.com
- **Book Stacks Unlimited**, E-mail: afinet@books.com — or — Net: http://www .books.com/
- **Bookstores at Intertain**, E-mail: bookstore@intertain.com — or — Net: http:// www.intertain.com/store
- **Book Zone**, E-mail: bookzone@bookzone@com — or — Net: http://bookzone.com
- **The Electric Bookstore**, Net: http://www.cadvision.com/bookstore/electric.html
- **Info Cafe Online Bookstore**, E-mail: fandre@infocafe.com
- **The Online Bookstore on America Online**, Net: key-word BOOKSTORE
- **Oxford Books Online**, E-mail: webmaster@oxfordbooks.com — or — Net: http:// www.oxfordbooks.com

• BRAIN

Books:
- *From the Ashes: A Head Injury Self-Advocacy Guide*, by Constance Miller & Kay Campbell; The Phoenix Project (206)329-1371
- *Living With Head Injury: A Guide for Families*, by Richard C. Senelick and Cathy Ryan; Demos Publications ([212] 683-0072), 1995

American Brain Tumor Association, 2720 River Rd., Des Plains, IL 60018; (708)827-9910 or (800)886-2282

Aneurysm Information Project of Columbia University, Net: http://www.columbia .edu/~mdt1/

Brain Injury Association, 1776 Massachusetts Ave., NW, Ste. 100, Washington, DC 20036; (202)296-6443 or (800)444-6443

Brain Injury Hotline, 212 Pioneer Building, Seattle, WA 98104; (206)621-8558; Net: http://www.headinjury.com

Brain-Pituitary Foundation of America, 281 E. Moody Ave., Fresno, CA 93720-1524

Family Caregiver Alliance operates within Northern California and assists families of adults stricken with chronic or progressive brain disorders. FCA resource specialists can help locate services for caregivers in other parts of the country.
Family Caregiver Alliance, 425 Bush St., Ste. 500, San Francisco, CA 94108; (415)434-3388

Harvard's Whole Brain Atlas, http://www.med.harvard.edu:80/AANLIB.home .html

Illinois Head Injury Association, 1127 S. Manheim Rd., Ste. 213, Westchester, IL 60154; (708)344-4646

Memory and Disorders Clinic, c/o Dr. Arnold Starr, 154 MedSearch, University of California at Irvine, Irvine, CA 92717; (714)824-8650

National Brain Tumor Foundation, 785 Market St., Ste. 1600, San Francisco, CA 94103; (415)284-0208 or (800)934-2873

National Hydrocephalus Foundation, 1670 Green Oak Circle, Lawrenceville, GA 30243; (404)995-8982 or (800)431-8093; E-mail: AnnLiakos@aol.com

Pituitary Tumor Network Association, 16350 Ventura Blvd., Ste. 231, Encino, CA 91436

• BREAST CANCER

Books:
- *The Breast Book: The Essential Guide to Breast Care & Breast Health for Women of All Ages*, by Miriam Stoppard; DK Publishing, 1996

- *Breast Cancer: What You Should Know (But May Not Be Told) About Prevention, Diagnosis and Treatment*, by Steve Austin and Cathy Hitchcock; Prima Publishing (PO Box 1260, Rocklin, CA 95677), 1994
- *Breast Cancer, The Complete Guide*, by Yashar Hirshaut and Peter I. Pressman; Bantam Books, 1993
- *Breast Cancer? Let Me Check My Schedule!: Ten women meet the challenge of fitting breast cancer into their busy lives*; Innovative Medical Education Consortium, Inc.
- *The Breast Connection: A Laywoman's Guide to the Treatment of Breast Disease by Chinese Medicine*, by Honora Lee Wolfe; Blue Poppy Press ([800]487-9296; E-mail: 102151.1614 @compuserve.com), 1996
- *Celebrating Life: African American Women Speak Out about Breast Cancer*, by Sylvia Dunnavant; USFI, 1995
- *I Can Cope*, by Judi Johnson and Linda Klein; DCI Publishing, 1988
- *Keep Your Breasts!: Preventing Breast Cancer the Natural Way*, by Susan Moss; Source Publications, 1994
- *Long-Term Tamoxifen Treatment for Breast Cancer*, by V. Craig Jordan, MD; The University of Wisconsin Press (Madison, WI 53715), 1995
- *Dr. Susan Love's Breast Book*, by Susan M. Love; Addison-Wesley, 1991, revised 1995
- *Preventing Breast Cancer*, by John W. Gofman; San Francisco Committee for Nuclear Responsibility (PO Box 421993, San Francisco, CA 94142), 1995
- *Save Yourself From Breast Cancer*, Robert M. Kradjian, MD; Berkeley Publishing Group
- *Spinning Straw Into Gold: Your Emotional Recovery From Breast Cancer*, Ronnie Kaye; Lamp Post Press, 1991
- *Surviving Cancer*, by Danette G. Kaufman; Acropolis Books, 1989

According to the American Cancer Society, breast cancer is the most common form of cancer in America. (Women are more likely to develop, and die of, heart disease.) It is estimated that breast cancer now afflicts 182,000 American women a year and causes 46,000 deaths. Women who get breast cancer when they are young are more likely to die from it. One in nine American women who live to their full life expectancy are expected to develop some form of breast cancer. Whereas three-fourths of all breast cancer cases occur in women over 50, the incidence of breast cancer has risen steadily among women in every age group. About 70% of women who get breast cancer have no risk factors.

Because of medical advances, most women who do get breast cancer will not die of it. Additionally, women with breast cancer who attend support groups have a better chance of surviving the disease than women who do not attend support groups.

While doing research for this book, I compiled the following list of items, obtained from various sources, which may play a part in determining whether a woman does or does not develop breast cancer:
- Taking the pill (though some studies show that the pill reduces the incidence of ovarian and uterine cancers).

A study by scientists at the National Cancer Institute that was published in the June 7, 1995 issue of the *Journal of the National Cancer Institute* found that women under the age of 35 who use oral contraceptives have a slightly greater chance of getting breast cancer.
- Having a family history of breast cancer.

In September 1994, it was announced that researchers at the University of Utah identified a gene, now called BRCA1, that may play a part in the development of breast cancer.

Researchers Mark Skolnick, Lisa Cannon-Albright, and David Goldgar were aided by genealogy records kept by Mormon families in Utah who are known for keeping detailed family history charts that go back for centuries. Using records from Mormon families, the Utah Genealogical Data Base was specifically set up to be used for genetic research.

Some question whether making a widely available test that screens for BRCAI would result in emotional stress for the women who have it, and a false sense of security for those who test negative for the gene, when only a small percentage of women with breast cancer have a family history of it.

A second gene that is believed to play a part in inherited breast cancer was identified in December 1995. It has been named BRCA2.

- Having an induced abortion (may increase risks).

A limited study done by the Fred Hutchison Cancer Center in Seattle, printed in the *Journal of the National Cancer Institute*, found that among 1,815 women studied, women who had an abortion were 50% more likely to develop breast cancer. If the abortion was before age 18, the women were 150% more likely to develop breast cancer. The risks were higher if the pregnancy had proceeded beyond eight weeks.

The risk may be related to the proliferation of breast cells in the first half of the pregnancy and how the cells differentiate later in pregnancy to allow for milk production. The cells are not allowed to differentiate when the woman experiences a miscarriage, or has an abortion.

Some criticize the studies on breast cancer and abortions because they rely on women to admit having had an abortion, and for mixing statistics from women who had induced abortions with those who had spontaneous miscarriages. Additionally, other studies, such as one conducted by the Slone Epidemiology Unit at Boston University School of Medicine, have concluded that there is no relation between abortion and breast cancer.

The Y-Me National Breast Cancer Organization has said that "there is no evidence of a direct relationship between breast cancer and either induced or spontaneous abortions" (Y-Me Newsletter, March 1996).

- Having children early in adulthood (lowers risks).
- Breast feeding (may lower risks).
- Regular exercise (lowers risks).

A 1986 study done by Rose E. Frisch of the Harvard School of Public Health and Center for Population Studies came to the conclusion that long-term athletic training establishes a lifestyle that somehow lowers the risk of breast cancer, and cancers of the reproductive system.

A study done by Leslie Bernstein at the University of Southern California's Norris Comprehensive Cancer Center, published in the September 1995 issue of the *Journal of the National Cancer Institute*, concluded that exercising at least four hours a week significantly reduces breast cancer risks. Working out lowers the levels of estradiol (a form of estrogen) and progesterone, both of which can play a part in breast tumor formation, and subsequently diminishes the breast's exposure to hormones.

- Having estrogen replacement therapy (ERT) after hysterectomy (increases risks).

The most common estrogen product is Premarin, made by Wyeth-Ayers Laboratories. It is horse estrogen and is derived from the urine of pregnant horses. Estrogen may be beneficial in preventing heart disease and osteoporosis, but also may promote breast cancer (*New England Journal of Medicine*, June 15, 1995; also in the *Journal of the American Medical Association*, July 12, 1995). Women who take estrogen supplements have a 30% to 80% greater risk of breast cancer.

ERT is often prescribed to prevent bone loss and heart disease. A woman can help prevent bone loss and heart disease by not smoking, eating a low-fat vegetarian diet, avoiding coffee, cutting the salt in her diet, losing excess weight, and exercising every day.

A hormone called progesterone, derived from soybeans and yams, can increase bone density. Progesterone is available without prescription from Klabin Marketing , (800) 933-94400, or Women's International Pharmacy, (800) 279-5708).

For updated information on the subject of hormone replacement therapy, contact *A Friend Indeed* Publications, Inc., Box 1710, Champlain, NY 12919-1710; [514] 843-5730, Fax (514)843-5681. Ten issues a year are $30.

- A low-fat vegetarian diet that is free from all flesh foods and dairy products including milk and eggs (greatly lowers risks).

Numerous studies have concluded that the consumption of animal foods increases the risks of breast cancer as well as all major forms of cancer. Those

countries that consume the most amount of animal foods also have the highest rates of cancers of the breasts, colon, and other cancers. Many people believe animal foods are the number-one cancer risk factor women can eliminate from their lives by becoming strict vegetarians.
- Consumption of soy protein (lowers risks).
  The phytochemicals in soy products have been found to have anti-cancer properties (*Journal of the National Cancer Institute*, November 16, 1994).
- Having a diet that is low in nutrition, and especially low in fresh fruits and vegetables (increases risks).
  Women who eat a mostly vegetarian diet have lower levels of the kind of estrogens associated with breast cancer. According to the University of California at Los Angeles, a diet high in plant content helps prevent breast cancer because plant fiber slows down the reabsorption of hormones associated with increased risk of breast cancer.
- Having a diet that is high in fat (increases risks).
  A study of women in Greece that was done by epidemiologists at Harvard School of Public Health, and that was published in the *Journal of the National Cancer Institute*, reported that women who had consumed olive oil in their daily diets had a 25% lower risk of breast cancer compared to women who consumed olive oil less frequently. The study authors cautioned that they do not yet know what substances in olive oil may help prevent breast cancer. Olive oil does contain vitamins and is a monounsaturated fat, and these are known to protect against cancer.
- Eating foods that contain growth hormones, and other chemicals fed to farm animals (increases risks).
- Exposure to pesticides used on farms, in homes, and in businesses, and sprayed over cities (increases risks).
  The incidence of breast cancer has been on the rise since the 1940s and this is in proportion to the increase in chemical pesticides and fertilizers being used to grow food.
  Researchers at the Strang Cancer Prevention Center at Cornell University Medical School found that pesticides appear to raise levels of a harmful form of estrogen. The study was done with the expectation that it would show pesticides had no effect on estrogen.
  For more information on this subject, contact The Humane Farming Association at (415) 771-CALF, the Pure Food Campaign at (202) 775-1132, or *Food & Water Journal* (802) 563-3300.
- Consuming alcoholic drinks (increases risks)(April 1987 issue of the *Journal of the National Cancer Institute*).
  More women suffer from heart disease than breast cancer. Many studies have shown that there may be cardiovascular benefits in drinking moderately, especially red wine. But alcohol is known to cause many other serious physical and mental health problems, and these may outweigh the cardiovascular benefits for the large majority of people. Women who are pregnant should not drink alcohol because it may contribute to many birth abnormalities including acute myeloid leukemia (*Journal of the National Cancer Institute*, January 3, 1996).

The National Cancer Institute recommends that all women do monthly breast self-examinations (BSE) to feel for lumps or thickenings, swelling, puckering, skin irritation, and pain or tenderness of a nipple (over 80% of breast lumps are not cancerous, but should be checked by a doctor). For women who menstruate, the best time to examine the breasts is the week after the menstrual period ends, when the breasts are least likely to be tender or swollen. Women who no longer menstruate should examine their breasts at the same time each month. (As about 1,500 American men are diagnosed with breast cancer each year, and an estimated 300 men die each year from breast cancer (1996 figure), men too should regularly examine their breasts.) The breast exam should cover the entire chest area from underarm to underarm, and from the collarbones to the underside base of the breasts.

The NCI also recommends that starting in their teens, women should have breast exams performed by a doctor once every three years. The breast exam should include the area behind the areola, where many lumps are overlooked.

One way of finding a lump in the breast is through mammography. A mammogram is a special x-ray picture of the breast done with minimal amounts of radiation (.3 rad per film exposure, compared to as many as 35 rads in mammograms performed 30 years ago). Mammography is designed to find cancer in its earliest stages — even years before a person can feel a lump or have any other symptoms and sometimes when a lump is still the size of a pinhead.

Women who decide to have mammograms should have the procedure performed at facilities certified by the FDA (Food and Drug Administration). A facility that is certified by the FDA should have the certificate prominently displayed.

Most mammograms range from $70 to $150 for a routine screening mammogram, to $250 for a diagnostic mammogram for women with symptoms. Health insurance plans often cover the cost of a mammogram. Some insurance plans are required by law to cover the procedure. Self-insured corporations are exempt from these laws.

For those who cannot afford the procedure, the American Cancer Society may help locate healthcare facilities that offer low-cost or free mammography programs. The number is 1-800-ACS-2345. A Breast and Cervical Cancer Early Detection Program may also be located through the Department of Health in each state.

Quality standards for mammography were required by a law passed by Congress in 1992, and the deadline for certification was October 1, 1994. Facilities lacking such certification are operating illegally. To find an FDA-certified, accredited facility, call the Cancer Information Service at 1-800-4-CANCER.

A woman who is going in for a mammogram should not wear talcum powder, deodorant, or lotion near the breasts that day. If the woman has x-rays from previous mammograms, she should bring these with her to the appointment (and make sure they are returned to her afterward).

During the mammography procedure, the breast is placed between a compression paddle and an x-ray plate, and pressure is applied to flatten the breast in order to get a clear x-ray picture. Some women may feel a little discomfort while others may experience pain. The exam takes only a few minutes. During the same visit at which the mammogram is performed, a physical exam of the breast should be performed by the radiologist (not by the technician).

It has long been the advice of specialists in the area of breast cancer for a woman to have a first mammogram at about thirty-five years of age, then every other year during the forties and annually after age fifty. Other experts believe that the additional exposure to the radiation used during mammography can lead to breast cancer. Many people believe that there were major flaws in the Canadian study that was used to determine the age when mammography is most beneficial.

Some women refrain from ever undergoing mammograms because they expose the body to radiation that may cause cancer. The Illinois-based Cancer Prevention Coalition says that some studies show a link between exposure to premenopausal mammography and breast-cancer mortality.

Some women who were denied mammography through their insurance because they were too young later found that mammography would have detected the breast cancer that was later discovered.

The Food and Drug Administration encourages women with breast implants who are in an age group for which routine mammograms are recommended to be sure to have these examinations at the suggested intervals. Implants can easily rupture during mammography (no breast implants are safe). Women with implants should always inform the radiologist and technician about the implants beforehand. (Mammograms can rupture implants. Xeromammography and MRI are believed to be safer for women with breast implants.)

The best way for the doctor to read the mammogram film is for her or him to be able to see the films from your last mammogram. If you are going to a new facility, if at all possible, bring your prior films with you.
— From the National Alliance of Breast Cancer Organizations

- Breast tissue and cancerous tumors can have the same density.
- Mammography is more accurate in older women who have gone through menopause because their breasts are less dense and have more fatty tissue. While many promote the use of mammography as a way of finding breast abnormalities, some people recommend against exposing the breast to any level of radiation.
- When a lump is found, the use of high-resolution digital ultrasound can help distinguish between cancerous and non-cancerous lumps.
- Digital mammography that uses computers to sharpen mammographic images can make it easier to detect tumors of the breast.
- Magnetic resonance imaging (MRI), a high-powered imaging device, is helpful in detecting abnormalities within the body, and especially in screening for brain and spinal cancer. It is being used more regularly in detecting abnormalities within the breasts and around breast implants.

  At a cost of $1,000, MRI is more expensive than mammography, but has been shown to be more accurate in the diagnosis of a lump. MRI is more beneficial than mammography in detecting breast cancer in younger women because their breast tissue is more dense than that of older women. MRI can also help determine if breast cancer has spread to lymph nodes and bone marrow.

  Dr. Steven Harms of Baylor University Medical Center designed an MRI technique specifically designed to detect breast cancer, and which has detected cancer that did not show up in mammography. Unlike mammograms, MRI does not use radiation, which some people believe to be a major risk factor in breast cancer.

- In April 1996 the FDA approved the use of HDI (high-definition imaging) digital ultrasound for the evaluation of solid breast masses. HDI takes about 15-minutes and can help determine if a breast lump is malignant or benign. HDI relies on sound waves and does not use radiation.

The key to surviving breast cancer is early detection. The sooner a problem is found, the greater the chance of successful treatment. And, in many cases, less extensive surgery can be used to treat the disease, often saving the breast. When breast cancer has spread beyond the breasts and the lymph nodes, it usually settles in three places — the lungs, the liver, and the bones. The further it has spread, the lower the chances are of survival.

If a lump is found in your breast, ask if needle biopsy techniques (fine needle aspiration or core biopsy) are used in the doctor's office. Needle biopsies are less invasive than surgery. They have been common in Europe and are becoming more popular in America.

A procedure called stereotactic large core needle biopsy can be used instead of surgical biopsy to help diagnose abnormal breast tissue that is not palpable. A woman undergoing this procedure lies on an exam table. Her breast is positioned in an opening in the table and is placed between two Plexiglas paddles. X-rays are taken and the image is digitized onto a computer monitor. The abnormality within the breast is located. A grid helps determine the angle necessary for placement of the needle to remove samples of the tissue. This is done through a small incision made after a medication is used to numb the breast.

One of the following breast cancer information organizations may help you find a doctor in your area who is experienced in performing needle biopsies.

Some people believe the needle biopsies will trigger the cancer to spread.

Learn as much as you can about the procedure before making a decision.

Contact one or more of the breast cancer support groups for more information.

For a free copy of a booklet titled *Things to Know About Quality Mammograms*, call the US Government's
Agency for Health Care Policy and Research, (800)358-9295

Alta Bates Comprehensive Cancer Center, Cancer Risk Counseling Service, Berkeley, CA; (510)204-4286

The American College of Radiology is the certifying organization for radiologists and conducts a five-step accreditation process for mammography clinics.
American College of Radiology, Mammography Accreditation Program, 1891 Preston White Dr., Reston, VA 22091; (703)648-8900

Avon's Breast Cancer Awareness Crusade, Net: http:www.pmedio.com/Avon /avon.html

B&B Company (sells prostheses for mastectomy survivors), 2417 Bank Dr., PO Box 5731, Boise, ID 83705; (800)262-2789

Bosom Buddy sells breast forms that can be worn beneath clothing in place of what cancer has taken away. The prostheses are all-fabric, glass-bead weighted, and adjustable.
Bosom Buddy, PO Box 5731, 2417 Bank Dr., Ste. 201, Boise, ID 83705-0731; (208)343-9696 or (800)262-2789

Breast Cancer Advisory Center, PO Box 224, Kensington, MD 20895; (301)949-1132

Breast Cancer Discussion List Web Page, Net: http://nysernet.org/bcic/

Breast Cancer Fund, 1280 Columbus Ave., Ste. 201, San Francisco, CA 94133; (800)487-0492

Breast Cancer Information Clearinghouse of the New York State Education and Research Network, Net: http://nysernet.org/bcic/

Breast Cancer Research Foundation, Box 9236, GPO, New York, NY 10087-9236

Breast Lump & Cervical Cancer Information Hotline, (800)4-CANCER; In Alaska (800)638-6070

Dana-Farber Cancer Institute, Boston, MA; (617)632-2178

The Feminine Image (catalog of post-mastectomy clothing and products) 312 Crosstown Dr., Ste. 168, Peachtree City, GA 30269; (800)730-1123

International Breast Cancer Research Foundation, PO Box 5127, Madison, WI 53705-0127

Kingston Breast Cancer Committee, Kingston, Ontario, Canada; (613)549-1118

Rose Kushner Breast Cancer Advisory Center, PO Box 224, Kensington, MD 20895; (301)897-3445

Lombardi Cancer Research Center, Comprehensive Breast Center, Georgetown University, Washington, DC 20007; (202)687-2104 or 687-2113

Mammatech sells an educational kit that teaches how to properly do breast self-examination. The kit includes a video, and a silicone model of a breast.
Mammatech, PO Box 15748, Gainsville, FL 32604; (800)626-2273

Massachusetts Breast Cancer Coalition, 85 Merrimac St., Ste. 508, Boston, MA 02114; (617)624-0180 or (800)649-6222; Fax (617)624-0176

My Image After Breast Cancer, 6000 Stevenson Ave., Ste. 203, Alexandria, VA 22304; (703)461-9616

National Alliance of Breast Cancer Organizations, 9 E. 37th St., 10th Flr., New York, NY 10016; (212)719-0154; E-mail: NABCOinfo@aol.com — or — Net: http://www .nabco.org

National Breast Cancer Coalition, 1707 Market St., Ste. 1060, Washington, DC 20036; (202)296-7477

To obtain information about accredited facilities where mammograms are performed, call the National Cancer Institute. The Institute also provides information on comprehensive cancer centers.

National Cancer Institute, (800)4-CANCER

Susan G. Komen Foundation (breast cancer information), 5005 LBJ Freeway, Ste. 370, Dallas, TX 75244; (800)462-9273

SHARE/Self-Help for Women With Breast or Ovarian Cancer, 1501 Broadway, Ste. 720, New York, NY 10036; (212)382-2111

Sisters Network/African-American Breast Cancer Survivors Support Group, 8787 Woodway Dr., Ste. 4207, Houston, TX 77063; (713)781-0255

Terri's Post-Surgical Boutique Catalogue, 2570 N. McCarn Rd., Palm Springs, CA 92262-2240; (619)325-2612 or (800)925-3676

United Center for Breast Care, 333 N. Smith Ave., St. Paul, MN 55102; (612)220-8300; Fax (612) 220-7203

UCLA Breast Center, (800) UCLA-MD-1

A technique that involves injecting a blue dye into a breast tumor to determine if cancer has spread into the lymph glands was developed by surgeons at the John Wayne Cancer Institute. Often the lymph glands, part of the body's immune system, near the breast that is being removed are removed at the same time as the breast.

John Wayne Cancer Institute, 1328 — 22nd St., Santa Monica, CA 90404; (310)315-6125

Y-ME National Organization for Breast Cancer Information and Support, 212 W. Van Buren St., Chicago, IL 60607-3908; (708)799-8220 or (312)986-8228 or (800)221-2141; Spanish-speaking individuals can call (312)986-9505 or (800)986-9505; E-mail: Ymeone@aol.com — or — Net: http://www.y-me.org

• BREAST IMPLANTS AND SILICONE POISONING

Books:
- *Plastic Surgery Hopscotch: A Resource Guide for Those Considering Cosmetic Surgery,* by John McCabe; Carmania Books (PO Box 1272, Santa Monica, CA 90406-1272), 1995
- *The Silicone Breast Implant Controversy: What Women Need to Know Now,* by Frank B. Vasey and Josh Feldstein; Crossing Press

American Silicone Implant Survivors (AS-IS), 1288 Cork Elm Dr., Kirkwood, MO 63122; (314)821-0115

Breast Implant Litigation Group of the American Trial Lawyer's Association, 1050 — 31st St., NW, Washington, DC 20007-4499; (800)424-2725 or 2727

Coalition of Silicone Survivors, PO Box 129, Broomfield, CO 80038-0129; (303)469-8242

Food and Drug Administration Breast Implant Information Service, Office of Consumer Affairs (HFE — 88), 5600 Fishers Lane, Rockville, MD 20857; (303)443-5006; FDA Breast Implant Information Line (800)532-4440; To report problems with your breast implants, phone (800) FDA-1088

• BURNS

Advance Tissue Sciences has developed the technology to grow skin by using cells from the foreskins of circumcised infants.

Advanced Tissue Sciences, 10933 N. Torrey Pines Rd., La Jolla, CA 92037; (619)450-5730

American Burn Association, c/o Andrew M. Munster, MD, Baltimore Regional Burn Center, Francis Scott Key Hospital, 4940 Eastern Ave., Baltimore, MD 21224; (800)548-2876

Burns United Support Groups, 441 Colonial Court, Grosse Pointe Farms, MI 48236; (313)881-5577

Cinema Secrets sells cosmetics and wigs for burn survivors. The company is owned by movie makeup artist Maurice Stein. He has developed foundation makeup specifically for burn scars.
Cinema Secrets, 4400 Riverside Dr., Burbank, CA 91505; (818)846-0579

A company named Genzyme Tissue Repair can grow small pieces of skin for use on patients who have experienced severe burns. The company uses cells from a small piece of the patient's skin.
Genzyme Tissue Repair, 64 Sidney St., Cambridge, MA 02139; (617)494-8484; Fax (617)252-0650

International Society for Burn Injuries, 2005 Franklin St., Ste. 660, Denver, CO 80205; (303)839-1694

National Burn Victim Foundation, 32-34 Scotland Rd., Orange, NJ 07050

National Institute for Burn Medicine, 909 E. Ann St., Ann Arbor, MI 48104; (313)769-9000

Phoenix Society for Burn Survivors, 11 Rust Hill Rd., Levittown, PA 19056; (215)946-2876; burn survivors only may call (800)888-BURN

• CANCER

Books:
- *Bone Marrow Transplants: A Book of Basics for Patients,* by Susan K. Stewart; BMT Newsletter ([708]831-1913), 1995
- *Cancer & Natural Medicine: A Textbook of Basic Science and Clinical Research,* by John Boik (E-mail: johnboik@aol.com), Oregon Medical Press ([800]610-0768), 1996
- *Everyone's Guide to Cancer Therapy: How Cancer is Diagnosed, Treated, and Managed Day to Day,* by Malin Dollinger, MD, Ernest H. Rosenbaum, MD, and Greg Cable; Somerville House, 1995
- *Recalled by Life: The Story of My Recovery from Cancer,* by Anthony Sattilaro, MD; Houghton Mifflin, 1992
- *Rhythmic Walking: Exercises for People Living with Cancer,* by Maryl Winningham and Elaine Glass; for a free copy write to: Ohio State University Comprehensive Cancer Center, 300 W. 10th Ave., Ste. 1132, Columbus, OH 43210
- *The Wellness Community Guide to Fighting for Recovery from Cancer,* by Harold H. Benjamin, PhD; G.P. Putnam's Sons
- *World Oncology Directory and Source Book,* Oncology Directory (19 Raeburn Ave., Rochester, NY 14619), 1995
- *You Don't Have to Suffer: A Complete Guide to Relieving Cancer Pain for Patients and Their Families,* by Susan S. Lang and Richard B. Patt; Oxford University Press ([800]451-7556), 1995

A life free of smoking and other substance addictions, and that includes regular exercise and a nutritious, lowfat, high-fiber diet with whole grains, fresh fruits, and vegetables that are free from chemical processes improves overall health and lowers all cancer risks.

About cancer:
- There are more than 100 types of cancer.
- Cancer is an abnormal growth of cells.
- Benign tumors do not spread to other parts of the body and are not life threatening.
- Malignant tumors are cancerous. They invade and damage other tissues.
- Invasive tumors have invaded surrounding tissues.
- In-situ tumors are confined to the place where they originated.
- A metastasized tumor is one that has invaded other areas of the body.
- Cancers are also classified in the type of organ or cell where they started. These include
  - Carcinoma: cancer that originates in the skin or layers of cells covering the lining of the glands and organs.

- Melanoma: cancer that originates in the pigment cells of the skin.
- Sarcoma: cancer that originates in the supporting tissues, such as the muscles, bones, and blood vessels.
- Leukemia: cancer that originates in the blood forming tissues, such as the spleen, bone marrow, and the lymph nodes.
- Lymphoma: cancer that originates in the lymph system.
- Cancer often spreads by way of the lymph system. This is why some lymph nodes are often removed during cancer surgery. The lymph nodes are then examined to see if they contain cancer.
- The sooner a tumor is found, the better the possibilities are for successful treatment.
- Treatment depends on the type of tumor, its size, shape, location, whether it has spread to other areas, and the age and health of the person with the tumor. The desires of the patient should play the biggest role in how cancer is treated.
- A biopsy is a procedure in which some of the tissue believed to be cancerous is removed and examined by a specialist doctor called a pathologist.
- The pathologist documents the findings of the biopsy in a pathology report.
- A pathology report may include a description of the tissue and a diagnosis that tells what the pathologist believes the tissue contains.
- The pathology report may also include information on whether the tumor is of a low grade or aggressive, and in what stage of existence it is.
- Cancer patients undergoing allopathic care often are given what is called radiation therapy. This is done by using high energy radiation, such as x-rays, gamma rays, and electron beams. Radiation hampers the ability of cells to grow and divide. This form of treatment is delivered by an allopathic medical specialist called a radiation therapist. It is sometimes done before surgery is performed in an attempt to shrink a tumor. Most often it is done after surgery.

  Allopathic doctors also treat cancer patients with chemotherapy. This is done by using toxic chemical drugs. The drugs may be taken by mouth or injection. A patient who is receiving chemotherapy may need to stay in the hospital for a few days. The treatments are often continued at home. A period of chemotherapy treatment is called a cycle. (Chemotherapy drugs are so toxic that when they are eliminated from the body they often kill off the bacteria needed in home septic tanks to decompose waste.)

  Patients undergoing radiation and chemotherapy treatments often become tired, have skin reactions, and experience hair loss, nausea, and vomiting. Loss of appetite and painful swallowing may also occur.

  Chemotherapy reduces the level of blood platelets, making the patient anemic. This can cause bruising, internal bleeding, brain hemorrhages, strokes, and sometimes death. The chronic bleeding experienced by chemotherapy patients often forces doctors to slow or stop chemotherapy treatments. Patients may then be given blood transfusions, which can cost $1,000 per treatment and carry the risk of viral infections.

- The radiation and chemotherapy treatments and surgery also damage healthy cells. Because radiation and chemical drugs are known to cause cancer and other health problems, and surgery is always accompanied by risks, some people refuse radiation, chemotherapy, and surgery because they believe the radiation, chemotherapy, and surgery may do more damage than they can do good.

  Instead, they often seek holistic approaches to rid themselves of cancer.

  Holistic therapies for cancer focus strongly on eating, exercise, and state of mind to clean the body and strengthen the immune system. Holistic therapies eliminate animal products, saturated fat, refined sugar, stimulants (such as caffeine), and food additives from the diet. They concentrate on foods made from plants (vegetables, fruits, grains, and legumes), and on using nutritional supplements including amino acids and natural plant chemicals, such as isoflavones (such as genistein, genestin, and daidzin), phase 2 enzymes from cruciferous vegetables, and modified citrus pectin (MCP). Holistic cancer treatments may include hyperthermia, and the use of tumor energy deprivation therapies, such as hydrazine sulfate blocks, and the use of substances with anti-angiogenesis (blood vessel growth that feeds tumors) factors.

A person wanting to know about holistic therapies should look in this book under the heading *Alternative, Ayurvedic, Homeopathic, Natureopathic, and Other Holistic Healthcare.*

- Whatever choice a person makes in selecting a therapy for cancer, he should be aware that nutrition is very, very important in healing, and in maintaining health.
- When approaching developers of new cancer treatments, keep in mind that initial trials on humans usually involve severely ill patients who have not responded to other forms of treatment.
- A cancer patients' attitude often plays a major role in determining whether he will become a cancer statistic, or a cancer survivor. Support groups can play a major role in improving the attitude and hope of a cancer patient.

Action for Cancer Prevention Campaign, 845 Third Ave., 15th Flr., New York, New York 10022; (212)759-7982; E-mail: wedo@igc.apc.org

For a free booklet titled *Managing Cancer Pain, Patient Guide,* write the **Agency for Health Care Policy Research** , Publications Clearinghouse, Publication Number 94-0595 – Cancer Pain Guidelines, PO Box 8547, Silver Spring, MD 20907; (800)4-CANCER

American Bone Marrow Donor Registry: Search Coordinating Center, University of Massachusetts Medical Center, 55 Lake Ave., Worcester, MA 01655; (508)756-6444 or (800)726-2824

American Biologics-Mexico S.A Medical Center, 1180 Walnut Ave., Chula Vista, CA 91911; (619)429-8200 or (800)227-4458

American Brain Tumor Association, 2720 River Rd , Ste. 146, Des Plaines, IL 60018; (847)827-9910 or (800)886-2282

The American Cancer Society publishes a pamphlet titled *American with Disabilities Act — Legal Protection for Cancer Patients Against Employment Discrimination.* **American Cancer Society,** 1599 Clifton Rd., NE, Atlanta, GA 30329; (800) ACS-2345 or (800)422-6237

American Institute of Cancer Research Newsletter, 1759 R St., NW, Washington, DC 20009-2552; (202)328-7744 or (800)843-8114

American Society of Clinical Oncology, 435 N. Michigan Ave., Ste. 1717, Chicago, IL 60611; (312)644-0828

Association for Research of Childhood Cancer, PO Box 251, Buffalo, NY 14225-0251; (716)681-4433

Association of Community Cancer Centers, 11600 Nebel St., Ste. 201, Rockville, MD 20852; (301)984-9496

R.A. Bloch Cancer Support Center (for second opinions), (816)932-8453

Biological Therapy Institute Foundation, PO Box 681700, Franklin, TN 37068; (615)790-7535

Bone Marrow Transplant Family Support Network, PO Box 845, Avon, CT 06001; (800)826-9376

The Bone Marrow Transplant Newsletter is published 6 times a year. BMT also publishes a book titled *Bone Marrow Transplants: A Book of Basics for Patients.* **Bone Marrow Transplant Newsletter,** 1985 Spruce Ave., Highland Park, IL 60035; (847)831-1913; E-mail: bmtnews@transit.nyser.net

British Columbia Cancer Agency, 600 W. 10th Ave., Vancouver, British Columbia, Canada V5Z 4E6; (604)877-6000 ext. 2367

Bruce Medical-supply (sells supplies for cancer survivors), PO Box 9166, Waltham, MA 02254; (800)225-8446

Dr. Stanislov Burzynski is the doctor who uses antineoplaston to treat cancer. The treatment is not FDA approved, and is controversial. Many of his patients believe the treatments have saved their lives. Many people believe that antineoplastins do not do what Burzynski claims.

Dr. Stanislov Burzynski, 1200 Richmond Ave., Ste. 260, Houston, TX 77082-2431; (713)597-0111

Canadian Cancer Society, 565 W. 10th Ave., Vancouver, British Columbia V5Z 4J4 Canada; (604)877-4400

Cancer Care, Inc., 1180 Ave. of the Americas, New York, NY 10036; (212)302-2400

The Cancer Chronicles ($24 a year US, $40 Canada), 144 St. Johns Place, Brooklyn, NY 11217; (718)636-1679 or (800)929-WELL

Cancer Communication is a quarterly newsletter that provides information on prostate cancer.

Cancer Communication, **Patient Advocates for Advanced Cancer Treatments, Inc.,** 1143 Parmalee, NW, Grand Rapids, MI 49504; (616)453-9198

Cancer Conquerors Foundation, PO Box 238, Hershey, PA 17033; (717)533-6124 or (800)238-6479

CancerFax, Sends you information on cancer from the National Cancer Institute; (301)402-5874 You must dial from a fax machine and follow instructions.

Cancer Fund of America, 2901 Breezewood Lane, Knoxville, TN 37921-1099; (615)938-5281

The Cancer Letter, PO Box 15189, Washington, DC 20003; (203)543-7665

Cancernet, gopher://gopher.nih.gov:70/11/clin/cancernet

Cancer Pain, Net: http://www.stat.washington.edu/TALARIA.TALARIA.html

Cancer Prevention Coalition, (312)467-0600

For a copy of the Cancer Research Institute Help Book: *What to Do if Cancer Strikes*, send $2 with your name and address requesting the book to

Cancer Research Institute, PO Box 5199, New York, NY 10150-5199 — or — 681 Fifth Ave., New York, NY 10022-4209; (800)99CANCER

Cancer Support Network, Essex House, Ste. L10, Baum Blvd. at South Negley Ave., Pittsburgh, PA 15206; (412)361-8600

Cancervive, Inc., 6500 Wilshire Blvd., Ste. 500, Los Angeles, CA 90048; (310)203-9232

Candlelighters Childhood Cancer Foundation, 7910 Woodmont Ave., Ste. 460, Bethesda, MD 20814-3015; (301)657-8401 or (800)366-2223

Canhelp, 311 Paradise Bay Rd., Port Ludlow, WA 98365; (206)437-2291

CanSurvivors, 2106 NE 65th St., Fort Lauderdale, FL 33308

ChemoCare, 231 N. Ave. W., Westfield, NJ 07090-1428; (800)55-CHEMO

The Chemotherapy Foundation, 183 Madison Ave., Ste. 403, New York, NY 10016; (212)213-9292

Children's Leukemia Foundation, 29777 Telegraph Rd., Ste. 1651, Southfield, MI 48034; (810)353-8222 or (800)825-2536

Children's Oncology Camps of America, 4121 Jennifer St., NW, Washington, DC 20015; (301)402-0271

City of Hope National Medical Center, 1500 E. Duarte Rd., Duarte, CA 91010-3000; (818)359-8111

Designs for Comfort (Head coverings for chemo-caused hair loss), (800)443-9226

Exceptional Cancer Patients, 300 Plaza Middlesex, Middletown, CT 06457-3470; (203)343-5950

Families Against Cancer, PO Box 588, DeWitt, NY 13214; (315)446-5326 or 446-6385

Foundation for Alternative Cancer Therapies, PO Box 1242, Old Chelsea Station, New York, NY 10113; (212)741-2790

Fred Hutchinson Cancer Research Center, 1124 Columbia, Seattle, WA 98104; (206)667-5000

Friends Network, PO Box 4545, Santa Barbara, CA 93140

The Gerson Institute, PO Box 430, Bonita, CA 91908; (619)472-7450; E-mail: GersonInst@aol.com — or — Net: http://www.homepage.com/mall/gerson /gerson.html

The International Association of Cancer Victims and Friends concentrates on the work being done in the field of alternative, non-toxic therapies. These approaches include macrobiotics, herbal, homeopathic, and nutritional. There are associated chapters located throughout the US, Canada, and in Australia. The Association is not affiliated with any physicians, clinics, or healthfood stores. They publish a quarterly newsletter and maintain a referral list of other organizations, patients who have been treated with alternative therapies, and clinics and doctors who use holistic therapies. **International Association of Cancer Victims and Friends,** 7740 W. Manchester Ave., Ste. 203, Playa Del Rey, CA 90293; (310)822-5032

International Myeloma Foundation, 2120 Stanley Hills Dr., Los Angeles, CA 90046; (800)452-CURE

Jamaica Cancer Society, (809)927-4265

Jazz Up (Head coverings for chemo-caused hair loss), (800)497-1401

John Hopkins Pancreas Cancer Web Page, Net: http://www.med.jhu.edu/ pancreas/index.htm

Just In Time (Head coverings for chemo-caused hair loss), (215)247-8777

Komen Kids (friendship network for children of cancer patients), (800)462-9273

Leukemia Research Foundation, (708)480-1177

Leukemia Society of America, 600 3rd Ave., New York, NY 10016; (212)573-8484

Lymphedema Services, (800)848-1015 in New York, or (800)882-9498 in New Jersey

Lymphoma Research Foundation of America, Inc., 2318 Prosser Ave., Los Angeles, CA 90064; (310)470-4912

Make Today Count /Mid-America Cancer Center (support groups), 1235 E. Cherokee, Springfield, MO 65804-2263; (800)432-2273

Mathews Foundation for Prostate Cancer Research, 1010 Hurley Way, Ste. 195, Sacramento, CA 95825; (800)234-6284

The Mautner Project for Lesbians With Cancer, 1707 L St., Ste. 1060, Washington, DC 20036; (202)332-5536

Cancer Smart is a quarterly newsletter published by Memorial Sloan-Kettering Cancer Center. Subscriptions are $15.
Memorial-Sloan Kettering Cancer Center, 1275 York Ave., New York, NY 10021; (212)639-2000 or (800)525-2225; *Cancer Smart,* (800)996-7522

National Bone Marrow Transplant Link, 29209 Northwestern Hwy., Ste. 624, Southfield, MI 48034; (810)932-8483 or (800) LINK-BMT

National Brain Tumor Foundation, 785 Market St., Ste. 1600, San Francisco, CA 94103; (415)284-0208 or (800)934-CURE

The Cancer Information Service at the National Cancer Institute can provide information on experimental cancer treatments, referrals to local specialists, and addresses of cancer treatment centers. For a free booklet called *Cancer Tests You Should Know About: A Guide For People 65 And Over*, contact the
National Cancer Institutes, Office of Cancer Communications, Bldg. 31, Rm. 10A — 24, 900 Rockville Pike, Bethesda, MD 20892; (800)4-CANCER (422-6237)

National Cancer Institute, Net: http://biomed.Nus.SG/Cancer/welcome.html

National Cancer Survivors Day Foundation, PO Box 682285, Franklin, TN 37068-2285; (615)794-3006

National Children's Cancer Society, (800)882-6227

National Coalition for Cancer Research, 426 C St., NE, Washington, DC 20002; (202)544-1880

The National Coalition for Cancer Survivorship publishes a booklet titled *Working It Out: Your Employment Rights as a Cancer Survivor.*
National Coalition for Cancer Survivorship, 1010 Wayne Ave., Ste. 300, Silver Spring, MD 20910; (301)650-8868

National Familial Pancreas Tumor Registry, The Johns Hopkins Hospital Dept. of Pathology, 600 N. Wolfe St., Baltimore, MD 21287-6417; (410)955-9132; Fax (410)955-0115; E-mail: ffalatko@welchlink.welch.jhu.edu

National Family Caregivers Association, 9621 E. Bexhill Dr., Kensington, MD 20895; (800)896-3650

National Institute for Cancer Research, Net: http://www.ist.unege.it/

National Kidney Cancer Association, 1234 Sherman Ave., Ste. 200, Evanston, IL 60202; (708)332-1051

National Lymphedema Network, 2211 Post St., Ste. 404, San Francisco, CA 94115; (800)541-3259

National Marrow Donor Program, 3433 Broadway St., NE, Ste. 400, Minneapolis, MN 55413; (612)627-5860 or (800) MARROW-2

For a free booklet titled *Every Question You Need to Ask Before Selling Your Life Insurance Policy,* contact the
National Viator Representatives' Thinking Positive Newsletter, 56 W. 57th St., Flr. 4, New York, NY 10019; (800)932-0050; Net: http://www.nvrnvr.com

The Oley Foundation provides free information and emotional support to patients on enteral (tube) nutrition and parenteral (intravenous) nutrition.
Oley Foundation, 214 Hun Memorial, Albany Medical Center A-23, Albany, NY 12208-3478; (518)262-5079 or (800)776-OLEY

Oncology Nursing Society, 501 Holiday Dr., Pittsburgh, PA 15220-2749; (412)921-7373

Pediatric Oncology Group Page, Net: http://pog.ufl.edu/

People Against Cancer distributes books and other educational materials about non-toxic innovative forms of prevention, diagnosis, and therapy. They publish an international directory to alternative therapy centers and a newsletter called *Options: Revolutionary Ideas in the War on Cancer.* They are not affiliated with any physicians or clinics. They do not diagnose, prescribe, treat, or recommend treatment. For a catalog of the many books they sell, contact
People Against Cancer, PO Box 10, 604 E St., Otho, IA 50569; (515)972-4444; E-mail: nocancer@ix.netcom.com — or — Net: http://www.dodgenet.com/nocancer

The Physicians Data Query is a computerized listing of information for health professionals and their patients on the latest types of treatments and those involved in cancer treatment.
Physicians Data Query, (800)4-Cancer

Patient Advocates for Advanced Cancer Treatments (prostate cancer information), 1143 Parmelee, NW, Grand Rapids, MI 49504; (616)453-1477

R.A. Bloch Cancer Foundation (peer counseling & support groups), The Cancer Hotline, 4410 Main St., Kansas City, MO 64111; (816)932-8453

Radiation Research Society, 2021 Spring Rd., Ste. 600, Oak Brook, IL 60521; (708)571-2881

Reach to Recovery, American Cancer Society, (800) ACS-2345

Roswell Park Cancer Institute, Elm & Carlton St. Buffalo, NY 12463; (716)845-2300; Net: http://rpci.med.buffalo.edu

Skin Cancer Foundation, 245 — 5th Ave., Ste. 2402, New York, NY 10016; (212)725-5176

Society for Biological Therapy, PO Box 5630, Madison, WI 53705-0630; (608)276-6640

Society of Gynecologic Oncologists, 401 N. Michigan Ave., Chicago, IL 60611; (312)644-6610

Society of Surgical Oncology, 85 W. Algonquin Rd., Ste. 550, Arlington Heights, IL 60005; (708)427-1400

Support for People with Oral and Head and Neck Cancer, PO Box 53, Locust Valley, NY 11560-0053; (516)759-5333

John Wayne Cancer Institute, 2102 Santa Monica Blvd., Santa Monica, CA 90404; (310)315-6125

University of Pennsylvania OncoLink Cancer Information, Net: http://cancer.med.upenn.edu/

University of Texas Anderson Cancer Center, Houston, TX; For physician referrals (713)794-1392

University of Wisconsin Cancer Center, 3675 Medical Sciences Center, Madison, WI 53706; (608)262-2177 or 263-8090 or 263-7116

The Wellness Community is devoted to providing free psychological and emotional support to cancer patients and their families. To get a free copy of the pamphlet titled *Actions People With Cancer Can Take to Join With Their Physicians In the Fight for Recovery*, send a self-addressed stamped envelope to
The Wellness Community, 2716 Ocean Park, Ste. 1040, Santa Monica, CA 90405-5211; (310)314-2555

• CHILDBIRTH

Books:
- *Adopting the Hurt Child: Hope for Families with Special-Needs Kids*, by Gregory C. Keck and Regina M. Kupecky; Pinon Press, 1996
- *Birth as an American Rite of Passage*, by Robbie Davis-Floyd; University of California Press, 1992
- *The Fertility Sourcebook*, by M. Sara Rosenthal; Lowell House
- *Immaculate Deception: A New Look at Women and Childbirth in America*, by Suzanne Arms; Houghton Mifflin Company, 1975
- *The Infertility Book*, by Carla Harkness; Celestial Arts, 1995
- *The Natural Baby Food Cookbook*, by Margaret Kenda and Phyllis Williams; Avon Books, 1982
- *Natural Childbirth After Cesarean: A Practical Guide*, by Karis Crawford, PhD and Johanne C. Walters, BSN, RN; Blackwell Science ([800]215-1000), 1996
- *Nutrition for a Healthy Pregnancy; The Complete Guide to Eating Before, During, and After Pregnancy*, by Elizabeth Somer, MA, RD; Henry Holt and Company, 1995
- *Overcoming Infertility Naturally: The Relationship Between Nutrition, Emotions and Reproduction*, by Karen Bradstreet; Woodland Publishing ([800]777-2665), 1994
- *Pregnancy, Childbirth and the Newborn: A Complete Guide for Expectant Parents*, by Penny Simkin, Janey Whalley, and Ann Kepler; Meadowbrook, 1984
- *Vegetarian Pregnancy: The Definitive Nutritional Guide to Having a Healthy Baby*, by Sharon Yntema; McBooks Press ([800] 356-9315), 1994
- *The Well Pregnancy Book*, by Mike and Nancy Samuels; Summit Books, 1986
- *What Every Woman Needs to Know: Facts about Pregnancy, Childbirth and Womanhood*, by Penny Junior; Century Hutchinson, 1989
- *What to Expect When You're Expecting*, by Arlene Eisenberg, Heidi Murkoff, and Sandee Hathaway; Workman Publishing, 1991

- *When Pregnancy Isn't Perfect: A Layperson's Guide to Complications in Pregnancy*, by Laurie A. Rich; Penguin Books, 1991

Expectant mothers who are choosing an obstetrician may be introduced to or have appointments scheduled with all the doctors in the group practice. This will familiarize the patient with all the doctors who may be on call at the time of labor. Similar arrangements may be made when selecting a midwife.

> *The US ranks third in the world, behind Brazil (32% of births) and Puerto Rico (29% of births), in the number of cesareans performed each year. The US has held this notorious position for at least 15 years. Almost one million pregnant women in the US give birth by cesarean each year, one in four. Medical experts state that at least one-third and as many as one-half of these major abdominal operations are unnecessary, resulting in no improved outcome for mothers or their infants. The Centers for Disease Control estimates that the current number of unnecessary cesareans cost over a billion dollars in physician fees and hospital charges alone.*
> — Nicette Jukelevics, author of the forthcoming book *Cesarean Surplus: A Women's Guide to Avoiding the Most Common Operation in America*

If you are planning on becoming pregnant — and while you are pregnant:
- Eat nutritious foods and eliminate junk foods. The fetus receives nourishment from what the mother eats. Many birth defects are related to nutrient deficiencies.
- Take prenatal vitamins — special vitamin pills are available for pregnant women — check with your doctor and healthfood store.
- Avoid excess amounts of vitamin A early in pregnancy because too much increases the risk of birth defects.
- Avoid empty calorie foods, such as white sugar, white bread, white rice, soft drinks, and candy.
- Do not smoke.
- Avoid smoke-filled rooms.
- Do not drink alcohol.
- Do not take any drugs or medications without first asking a doctor and pharmacist if they are safe for a pregnant woman.
- Avoid x-rays.
- Find out if you have any sexually transmitted diseases (STDs).
- Educate yourself about pregnancy and childbirth by reading such publications as *Midwifery Today* and *Mothering Magazine*.
- Realize that pregnancy is a natural process and is *not* an illness.
- Know that the fetus is not a foreign substance, but *is* a part of you.

Adoption/Infertility Book Catalog, Net: http://webcom/~tapestry

American Academy of Husband-Coached Childbirth, PO Box 5224, Sherman Oaks, CA 91413; (818)788-6662 or (800)423-2397

American Academy of Natural Family Planning, 615 S. New Ballas Rd., St. Louis, MO 63141; (314)569-6495

American College of Home Obstetrics, PO Box 508, Oak Park, IL 60303; (708)383-1461

The American College of Nurse-Midwives administers a national certification exam, and accredits nurse-midwifery education programs.
American College of Nurse-Midwives (send $6.95 for a directory), 818 Connecticut Ave., NW, Ste. 900, Washington, DC 20006; (202)728-9860.

American College of Obstetrics and Gynecology, 409 — 12th St., SW, Washington, DC 20024; (202)638-5577

American Society for Reproductive Medicine, 1209 Montgomery Hwy., Birmingham, AL 35216-2809; (205)978-5000

American Society for Psychoprophylaxis in Obstetrics (Lamaze), 1101 Connecticut Ave., NW, Ste. 700, Washington, DC 20036; (800)368-4404

Atlanta Reproductive Health Clinic, Net: http://www.mindspring.com/~ mperloe/index.html

Association for Childbirth at Home, PO Box 430, Glendale, CA 91205

The Association of Labor Assistants and Childbirth Educators provides referrals to certified labor assistants/doulas and to certified childbirth educators, and offers a wide selection of books and videos on pregnancy, birth, breastfeeding, midwifery, and labor assisting. They provide information for parents on questions to ask a labor assistant/doula, and how to interview a midwife or doctor. The Association publishes a newsletter called *Special Delivery*. It provides information on choices in childbirth, women's health, and parenting. It is published quarterly and the yearly subscription rates are $20 in the US, and $23 in Canada or Mexico.

Association of Labor Assistants and Childbirth Educators, PO Box 382724, Cambridge, MA 02238; (617)441-2500; Fax (617)441-3167; E-mail: alacehq@aol.com — or — Net: http://www.alace.com

Association of Maternal and Child Health Programs, 1350 Connecticut Ave., NW, Washington, DC 20036; (202)775-0436

Cascade Birthing Supplies, 141 Commercial St., NE, Salem, OR 97301; (503)371-4445

Center for the Study of Multiple Births, 333 E. Superior St., Ste. 476, Chicago, IL 60611; (312)266-9093

Cesarean Support, Education, and Concern, 22 Forest Rd., Farmingham, MA 01701; (508)877-8266

Childbirth Education Association, PO Box 20048, Minneapolis, MN 55420; (612)854-8660

Childbirth Education Foundation, PO Box 5, Richboro, PA 18954; (215)357-2792

Childbirth Without Pain Education Association, 20134 Snowden, Detroit, MI 48235-1170; (313)341-3816

Consumer Advocates for the Licensure of Midwifery, PO Box 922, Davis, CA 95617; (916)756-5906

Cord Blood Banking Registry, 901 Mariners Island Blvd., Ste. 265, San Mateo, CA 94404; (800)588-6377

Depression After Delivery, PO Box 1282, Morrisville, PA 19067; (215)295-3994 or (800)944-4PPD

The Doula, PO Box 71, Santa Cruz, CA 95063-0071

Doulas of North America, E-mail: AskDona@aol.com — or — Net: http://www .dona.com/

Engel sells electric breast pumps and has a list of locations where a pump may be rented.

Engel, 765 Industrial Drive, Cary, IL 60013; (312)637-2900 or (800)323-8750

Healthy Mothers, Healthy Babies Coalition, 409 — 12th St., SW, Washington, DC 20024; (202)863-2552 or 863-2458

Homebirth Journal, (619)272-8474

Infertility Chat Group, Net: majordomo@acpub.duke.edu

Infertility Newsgroup, Net: alt.infertility

In the United States, Certified-Nurse Midwives (CNMs) can practice in every state. Most practice in hospitals, but an increasing number are opening birth centers, and some have homebirth practices. At present, women must first hold and RN degree, then take additional midwifery training, and pass the national boards of the American College of Nurse Midwives (ACNM); the 50 states have reciprocity in recognizing this certification.

— from *Becoming a Midwife*, a publication by Informed Homebirth/Informed Birth & Parenting

Informed Homebirth/ Informed Birth and Parenting provides information on alternatives in birth and parenting, as well as referrals to childbirth educators, birth assistants, and midwives. IH/IBP also sells books, booklets, and audio and videotapes. To obtain a brochure of the materials, send a self-addressed, stamped envelope to **Informed Homebirth/ Informed Birth and Parenting,** PO Box 3675, Ann Arbor, MI 48106; (313)662-6857

Intensive Caring Newsletter ($8 year) covers subjects related to high risk babies. It is published by
Intensive Caring Unlimited, 910 Bent Lane, Philadelphia, PA 19118; (215)233-4723

International Association of Parents and Professionals for Safe Alternatives in Childbirth (NAPSAC), Rte. 1, Box 646, Marble Hill, MO 63764; (314)238-2010

The International Cesarean Awareness Network works with chapters around the country that seek to educate women on the pros and cons of cesarean procedures and to lower the rate of unnecessary cesarean sections. ICAN agrees that, when necessary, cesareans can save lives, but an estimated half of the one million cesareans performed annually in the US are not medically required. ICAN supports itself through donations, membership fees, subscriptions to its newsletter named *CLARION,* and through the sale of videos and booklets that teach about cesarean prevention and vaginal birth after cesarean (VBAC).
International Cesarean Awareness Network, 1304 Kingsdale Ave., Redondo Beach, CA 90278; (310)542-6400; Fax (310)542-5368; E-mail: ican@fensende.com

International Childbirth Education Association, PO Box 20048, Minneapolis, MN 55420; (612)854-8660 or (800)624-4934

International Confederation of Midwives, 10 Barley Mow Passage, Chiswick, London, W4 4PH, United Kingdom; 44-081-994-6477

International Cord Blood Foundation, (800)747-3319

International Lactation Consultant Association, 200 N. Michigan Ave., Ste. 300, Chicago, IL 60601-3821; (312)541-1710

Breast-feeding is the best way to feed a baby and reduces the risk of a host of diseases. The United Nations Children's Fund estimated in 1994 that if all mothers were able to breast-feed for at least 12 weeks after giving birth, the US infant mortality rate — about 39,000 deaths per year — would decline by 4,000. The Fund encourages mothers to learn how to breast feed properly, and to give newborns no food or drink other than breast milk unless medically necessary.

La Leche League International is a world-renowned resource for breastfeeding information and offers mother-to-mother support through meetings and phone counseling. LLLI publishes its own professional literature, which presents the most current information regarding all aspects of breastfeeding. They can help find information on how to maintain breastfeeding through illness or medical procedures. They publish a quarterly journal called *Breastfeeding Abstracts* and a bimonthly magazine called *New Beginnings.* The LLLI catalog features many different educational pamphlets, brochures, videos, audio tapes, books, and other products, such as breast pumps, toys, and nursing stools. Membership is $30 and includes a subscription to *New Beginnings* and a 10% discount on LLLI books.
La Leche League International, 1400 N. Meacham Rd., PO Box 4079, Schaumburg, IL 60173-4840; (847)519-7730 or (800) LA-LECHE; Fax (847)519-0035; Net: http:// www.prairienet.org/llli/

Midwifery Communication and Accountability Project, PO Box 369, Newton Highlands, MA 02161; (617)630-8044

Midwifery Today publishes two (*Midwifery Today* and *International Midwife*) quarterly journals and one (*The Birthkit*) quarterly newsletter.
Midwifery Today, PO Box 2672, Eugene, OR 97402; (541)344-7438 or (800)743-0974; E-mail: Midwifery@aol.com — or — Net: http://www.efn.org/~djz/birth/home birth.html

Midwives Alliance of North America, PO Box 175, Newton, KS 67114-0175; (316)283-4543; E-mail: MANAinfo@aol.com

Subscriptions to *Mothering Magazine* are $18.95 per year. The company also publishes 6 books filled with articles and information on specific subjects that have appeared in the magazine. The titles of these books are: *Vaccinations; Circumcision; Being a Father; Teens: A Fresh Look; Midwifery and the Law;* and *The Way Back Home.*
Mothering Magazine, PO Box 1690, Santa Fe, NM 87504; (800)827-1061

National Adoption Center, 1500 Walnut St., Ste. 701, Philadelphia, PA 19102; (800)TO-ADOPT

The National Association of Childbearing Centers collects and disseminates information on freestanding birth centers. It sets national standards for birth center operation, promotes state regulation for licensure, and national accreditation by the Commission for the Accreditation of Freestanding Birth Centers. For a $1 donation they will send information on birth centers in your area, as well as information on how to select a birth center. They also publish a newsletter and sell other literature.
National Association of Childbearing Centers, 3123 Gottschall Rd., Perkiomenville, PA 18074-9546; (215)234-8068

National Maternal and Child Health Clearinghouse, 8201 Greensboro Dr., Ste. 600, McLean, VA 22102; (703)821-8955

Newborn Rights Society, PO Box 48, St. Peters, PA 19470-0048; (610)323-6061

North American Council on Adoptable Children, 970 Raymond Ave., Ste. 106, St. Paul, MN 55114-1149; (612)644-3036

The North American Registry of Midwives provides certification that validates mastery of entry-level skills and knowledge vital to responsible midwifery practice. The Registry has been issuing national certification for the Certified Professional Midwife (CPM) since October, 1994.
North American Registry of Midwives, Administration Offices, PO Box 15, Linn, WV 26384; (304)462-5617

Ontario Midwifery Consumer Network, Ontario, Canada; (905)648-0698

Peaceful Beginnings provides information on why circumcision should be avoided.
Peaceful Beginnings, 13020 Homestead Crt., Anchorage, AK 99516; (907)345-4813

For information on the damage fluorescent lighting can do to the eyes of premature infants, contact the
People's Medical Society, 462 Walnut St., Allentown, PA 18102

Postpartum Adjustment Support Service, PO Box 7282, Oakville, Ontario L6J-6C6, Canada; (905)844-9009

Postpartum Support International, 927 N. Kellog Ave., Santa Barbara, CA 93111; (805)967-7636

Public Citizen, the consumer awareness group, released a study in November of 1995 which concluded that women would have fewer Cesarean sections and their deliveries would be less expensive if they would rely more on nurse-midwives than on doctors. Public citizen publishes a guide to nurse-midwifery that is available for $15. The group also published two books on women's health — *Women's Health Alert: What Most Doctor's Won't Tell You* ($7.95) and *Unnecessary Cesarean Sections: Halting A National Epidemic* ($10). Include $2 for shipping per book.
Public Citizen Publications, 2000 P St., NW, Ste. 600, Washington, DC 20036; (202)833-3000

Resolve is a network of support groups for infertile couples. They also provide literature and therapy.
Resolve, 1310 Broadway, Somerville, MA 02144-1731; (617)623-0744 or (617)623-1156

Sidelines (Support for women with very high risk pregnancies), (714)497-2265

Substance Abuse Program for Pregnant Women, (202)574-2480

Unite provides grief support following the death of a baby, including miscarriage, ectopic pregnancy, stillbirth, and infant death. Unite provides support group meetings, a quarterly newsletter, and educational and training programs.

Unite, Inc., Grief Support, Jeanes Hospital, Social Services Dept., 7600 Central Ave., Philadelphia, PA 19111-2499; (215)728-3777; Fax (215)728-3914

ViaCord, 551 Boylston, Boston , MA 02116; (800)998-4226

Water Birth, Net: http://www.path.net:80/haril/

Whole Person Fertility Program, 22 Wyckoff St., Brooklyn, NY 11201; (718)625-4802 or (800)666-4325

• CHILDREN

Books:
- *Childhood Ear Infections: What Every Parent and Physician Should Know about Prevention, Home Care, and Alternative Treatment*, by Michael A. Schmidt; North Atlantic Press/Staying Well ([800]622-6309)
- *Childhood Symptoms: Every Parent's Guide To Childhood Illnesses*, by Edward R. Brace & John P. Pacanowski; Harper Collins, 1992
- *Dr. Mom*, by Dr. Marianne E. Neifert, Anne Price, & Nancy B. Dana; Signet, 1987
- *Homecare for the Chronically Ill or Disabled Child: A Manual and Service Book for Parents and Professionals*, by Monica Loose Jones; Harper and Row, 1985
- *Parenting the Overactive Child: Alternatives to Drug Therapy*, by Paul Lavin; Madison Books, 1989
- *Special Needs/Special Solutions: How to Get Quality Care for a Child With Special Health Needs*, by Georgianna Larson and Judith A. Kahn; Life Line Press (2500 University Ave., St. Paul MN 55141), 1990
- *Take Charge of Your Child's Health*, by Dr. George Wootan; Crown Books, 1992
- *Take This Book to the Pediatrician With You*, by Charles B. Inlander and J. Lynee Dodson; People's Medical Society (462 Walnut St., Allentown, PA 18102; [800] 624-8773), 1992
- *Vaccines: Are They Really Effective? A Parents Guide to Childhood Shots*, by Neil Z. Miller, New Atlantean Press, 1996
- *When Do I Call the Doctor?*, by Loraine M. Stern; Doubleday, 1993
- *Your Child's Health: A Pediatric Guide for Parents*, by Dr. Barton Schmitt; Bantam Books, 1991

Alliance to End Childhood Lead Poisoning, 227 Massachusetes Ave., NE, Ste. 200, Washington, DC 20007; (202)543-1147

The Alternative Therapy Network is an organization that focuses on nondrug approaches to Tourette syndrome, attention deficit disorder, hyperactivity, autism, and learning disabilities. Their newsletter is called *Latitudes*. Subscriptions are $24.

Alternative Therapy Network, 1120 Royal Palm Beach Blvd., Ste. 283, Royal Palm Beach, FL 33411; (407)798-0472; Fax (407)798-9820

American Association for Pediatric Ophthalmology and Strabismus, PO Box 193832, San Francisco, CA 94119; (415)561-8505

Ambulatory Pediatric Association, 6728 Old McLean Village Dr., McLean, VA 22101; (703)556-9222

American Academy of Pediatrics, PO Box 927, 141 Northwest Point Blvd., Elk Grove, IL 60007-0927; (708)228-5005 or (800)433-9016; Net: http://www.aap.org/dogl/dogl.html

American Board of Pediatrics, 111 Silver Cedar Crt., Chapel Hill, NC 27514; (919)929-0461

American Pediatric Society, 141 Northwest Point Blvd., Elk Grove Village, IL 60009-0675; (708)426-0205

Arkansas Children's Hospital, Net: http://www.ach.uams.edu/

The ACCH publishes a free catalog of books on the medical care of children.
Association for the Care of Children's Health, 7910 Woodmont Ave., Ste. 300,
Bethesda, MD 20814-3015; (301)654-6549

The Association of Birth Defect Children is a national clearinghouse that provides
parents and professionals with information about birth defects and services for children
with disabilities. The Association also sponsors the National Birth Defect Registry that
collects data on birth defects and developmental disabilities. They operate the parent
matching service to match families of children with similar birth defects for mutual
sharing and support. The Association publishes a quarterly newsletter and studies the
links between drugs, radiation, alcohol, chemicals, lead, mercury, dioxin, and birth
defects.
Association of Birth Defect Children, 827 Irma Ave., Orlando, FL 32803-3806;
(407)245-7035

Association of SIDS Program Professionals (sudden infant death syndrome),
Massachusettes Center for SIDS, Boston City Hospital, 818 Harrison Ave., Boston, MA
02118; (617)534-5742

Autism Research Institute, 4182 Adams Ave., San Diego, CA 92116

Building Blocks Pediatric Home Health Services, Newport Beach, CA; (714)650-1764

Center for Children With Chronic Illness and Disabilities, Box 721 — University of
Minnesota, Harvard St. at E. River Rd., Minneapolis, MN 55455

Center for Family Support, 386 Park Ave. S., New York, NY 10016; (212)481-1082

Center to Assist the Regulation of Enuresis, Division of Urology, The Children's
Memorial Hospital, 2300 Children's Plaza, Chicago, IL 60614; (312)880-4000

Center to Prevent Childhood Malnutrition, 7200 Wisconsin Ave., Ste. 204, Bethesda,
MD 20814; (301)986-5777

Child Health Alert Newsletter ($29 a year), PO Box 610228, Newton Highlands, MA
02161; (619)239-1762

Child Health Talk Newsletter provides information on health issues relating to African
American children. Subscriptions are $8.
Child Health Talk, **National Black Child Development Institute,** 1023 — 15th St.,
NW, Ste. 600, Washington, DC 20005; (202)387-1281

Children in Hospitals, Inc., 31 Wilshire Park, Needham, MA 02192; (617)482-2915

Children's Health, Net: gopher://mchnet.ichp.ufl.edu:70/1

Citizen's for Vaccination Liberation, 2101 Pallets Ct., Virginia Beach, VA 23454;
(804)486-3129

Daughters (newsletter for parents of adolescent daughters), 1808 Ashwood Ave.,
Nashville, TN 37212

Dear Dad (newsletter for single dads), 3135 — 4th St., Boulder, CO 80304

Determined Parents to Stop Hurting Our Tots (vaccine information), 915 S. University
Ave., Beaverdam, WI 53916; (414)887-1133

Developmental Delay Registry, (301)652-2263

Federation for Children with Special Needs, 95 Berkeley St., Boston, MA 02116;
(617)482-2915 or (800)331-0688

Federation of Families for Children's Mental Health, 1021 Prince St., Alexandria, VA
22314-2971; (703)684-7710

Florida Healthy Baby Hotline — Tallahassee Free-Net, Net: http://freenet3.sci
.fsu.edu:81/ht-free/fhbaby/html

Foundation for Nager and Miller Syndromes, 333 Country Lane, Glenview, IL 60025-
5104; (708)724-6449

Human Growth Foundation, 7777 Leesburg Pike, Falls Church, VA 22043; (703)883-1773 or (800)451-6434

Iowa SIDDS Alliance, (319)322-4870

March of Dimes Birth Defects Foundation, 1275 Mamaroneck Ave., White Plains, NY 10605; (914)428-7100

Mom's Advice, Net: http://www.cts.com/browse/crossink/online/Mom

National Association of Pediatric Nurse Associates and Practitioners, 1101 Kings Hwy. N., Ste. 206, Cherry Hill, NJ 08034; (609)667-1773

National Center for Education in Maternal and Child Health, 8201 Greensboro Dr., Ste. 600, McLean, VA 22101; (703)821-8955

National Clearinghouse on Child Abuse and Neglect Information, PO Box 1182, Washington, DC 20013-1182; (703)385-7576 or (800) FYI-3366

National Information Clearinghouse for Infants with Life-Threatening Conditions and Disabilities, University of Southern California, Center for Developmental Disabilities, Benson Bldg., 1st Flr., Columbia, SC 29208; (803)777-4435 or (800)922-9234 or 922-1107

National Parent to Parent Support & Information System matches families whose children have special healthcare needs, rare disorders, and children who have gone through similar surgeries. The organization is funded by a grant from the Maternal & Child Health Bureau and donations.
National Parent to Parent, PO Box 907, Blue Ridge, GA 30513; (706)632-8822 or (800)651-1151; Fax (706)632-8830; E-mail: nippsis@aol.com — or — Net: Judd103W @wonder.em.cdc.gov

Reye's Syndrome is a disease which affects all organs of the body, but most lethally the liver and the brain. It usually affects children from infancy to about 19 years of age. It is not contagious and the cause is unknown. The disease causes an abnormal accumulation of fat to develop in the liver and other organs of the body, along with a severe increase of pressure in the brain. Epidemiologic research has shown an association between the development of Reye's Syndrome and the use of aspirin for treating symptoms of influenza-like illness, chicken pox, and colds. Aspirin (acetylsalicylate) and combination medications that contain aspirin should not be given to children who are under 19 years of age during episodes of fever-causing illnesses. The Reye's Syndrome Foundation advises consulting with a doctor or pharmacist before giving any medication to a child.
National Reye's Syndrome Foundation, PO Box 829, 426 N. Lewis St., Bryan, OH 43506; (419)636-2679

National Vaccine Information Center, 512 W. Maple Ave., Vienna, VA 22180; (703)938-3783 or (800)909-7468; Fax (703)938-5768

National Vaccine Injury Compensation Program, Health Resources and Services Administration, Parklawn Bldg., Room 8A-35, 5600 Fisher Ln., Rockville, MD 20857; (800)338-2382

National Youth Crisis Hotline, (800)448-4663

Natural Immunity Information Network, 209 E. 7th St., New York, NY 10009; (212)979-7622

Ohio Parents for Vaccine Safety, 251 W. Ridgeway Dr., Dayton, OH 45459

Parenting Insights (newsletter for parents of adolescents), 16625 Redmond Wy., Ste. M, Redmond, WA 98052-4499

Parents Choice Book Center, 57 Stevens St., Stoneham, MA 02180; (617)438-8791 or (800)722-2939

Parents for Freedom of Choice (vaccine information), 7009 Caldwell Ln., Plano, TX 75025; (214)517-4282

Parents Helping Parents, Net: http://www.protal.com/~cbntmkr/php.html

Partnership for Individual Freedom, PO Box 685, Boontown, NJ 07005; (201)316-8142

Pediatric Rheumatology Homepage, Net: http://www.wp.com/pedsrheum

Pediatrics for Parents Newsletter ($18 year), 358 Broadway, Ste. 105, Box 1069, Bangor, ME 04401; (207)942-6212

Research Trust for Metabolic Diseases in Children/England, Golden Gate Lodge, Weston Rd., Crewe, Cheshire CWI IXN, England; 027-025-0221

Rubinstein-Taybe Parent Support Group, PO Box 146, Smith Center, KS 66967; (913)697-2984

Shriner's Hospital Referral Line, (800)237-5055

Siblings for Significant Change is and organization of brothers and sisters of people with disabilities.

Siblings for Significant Change, United Charities Building, 105 E. 22nd St., New York, NY 10010; (212)420-0776

SIDS Information Page, Net: http://q.continuum.net/~sidsnet

Single Mother (newsletter for single moms), PO Box 68, Midland, NC 28107

Society for Pediatric Research, 141 Northwest Point Blvd., PO Box 675, Elk Grove Village, IL 60009; (708)427-0205

Stickler Involved People, 53 Andelina, Agusta, KS 67010; (316)775-2993; E-mail: Houch@Southwind.net

St. Jude Children's Research Hospital, 501 St. Jude Place, PO Box 3704, Memphis, TN 38173-0704; (901)522-9733 or (800) USS-JUDE

Sudden Infant Death Syndrome Alliance, 1314 Bedford Ave., Ste. 210, Baltimore, MD 21208; (800)221-7437

Turner's Syndrome occurs in girls and is characterized by physical features, such as short stature, lack of sexual development, arms that turn out slightly at the elbow, low hairline on the back of the neck, prominent ears, soft fingernails that turn up at the end, and short fourth and fifth fingers.

Turner's Syndrome Society, 811 Twelve Oaks Ctr., 15500 Wayzata Blvd., Wayzata, MN 55391; (612)475-9944 or (800)365-9944; E-mail: tesc0016@maroon.tc.umn.edu

Vaccination Alternatives, PO Box 346, New York, NY 10023; (212)873-5051

Vaccine Research Institute, PO Box 4182, Northbrook, IL 60065; (847)564-1407

Your Child's Wellness Newsletter ($36 year US, $39.95 Canada), H/K Communications, 244 Madison Ave., New York, NY 10016; (800)638-2722

Your Grandchild (newsletter for grandparents), 1102 Grand, 23rd Flr., Kansas City, MO 64106

• CHIROPRACTIC

American Chiropractic Association, 1701 Clarendon Blvd., Arlington, VA 22202; (703)276-8800 or (800)637-6244

American Chiropractic Registry of Radiologic Technologists, 2330 Gull Rd., Kalamazoo, MI 49001; (616)343-6666

American College of Chiropractic Orthopedists, 1030 Broadway, Ste. 101, El Centro, CA 92243

Association for the History of Chiropractic, 1000 Brady St., Davenport, IA 52803; (800)722-2586

The Chiropractic Page, Net: http://www.mbnet.mb.ca/~jwiens/chiro/html

Federation of Chiropractic Licensing Boards, 901 — 54th Ave., Ste. 101, Greeley, CO 80634; (970)356-3500

Foundation for Chiropractic Education and Research, 1701 Clarendon Blvd., Arlington, VA 22209-2712; (703)276-7445

International Chiropractor's Association, 1110 N. Glebe Rd., Arlington, VA 22201; (800)423-4690

National Board for Chiropractic Examiners, 901 — 54th Ave. Greeley, CO 80634; (970)356-9100

World Chiropractic Alliance, 2950 N. Dobson Rd., Ste. 1, Chandler, AZ 85224; (800)347-1011

• COMA

Coma Recovery Association, 570 Elmont Rd., Ste. 104, Elmont, NY 11003; (516)355-0951

• DENTAL SPECIALISTS, AMERICAN BOARDS OF

American Board of Endodontics, 211 E. Chicago Ave., Ste. 1501, Chicago, IL 60611; (312)266-7310

American Board of Oral and Maxillofacial Surgery, 625 N. Michigan Ave., Ste. 1820, Chicago, IL 60611; (312)642-0070

American Board of Oral Pathology, 5401 W. Kennedy Blvd., PO Box 25915, Tampa, FL 33622-5915; (813)286-2444

American Board of Orthodontics, 225 S. Meramec Ave., Rm. 310, St. Louis, MO 63105; (314)727-5039

American Board of Pediatric Dentistry, Indiana University School of Dentistry, 1193 Woodgate Dr., Carmel, IN 46032; (317)573-0877

American Board of Periodontology, University of Southern California, School of Dentistry, 925 W. 34th St., Los Angeles, CA 90089; (213)743-2800

American Board of Prosthodontics, 4707 Olley Lane, Fairfax, VA 22032; (703)273-7323

• DIABETES

American Diabetes Association National Center, 1660 Duke St., Alexandria, VA 22314; (703)549-1500 or (800) DIABETES

Diabetes, Net: gopher://drinet.med.miami.edu:70/1

Diabetes Anonymous, PO box 60905, Sunnyvale, CA 94088-0905

Diabetes Insipidus and Related Disorders Network, Route 2, Box 198, Creston, IA 50801; (515)782-7838

Joslin Diabetes Center, 1 Joslin Place, Boston, MA 02215; (617)732-2400

Juvenile Diabetes Foundation, 432 Park Ave. S., New York, NY 10016; (212)785-9500 or (800)223-1138

• DIAGNOSTIC IMAGING

Book:
• X-rays: Health Effects of Common Exams, by John W. Gofman and Egan O'Connor; Sierra Club Books, 1985

The ability to photograph a persons' bones and other body structures by use of X-rays was discovered in November, 1895, by Wilhelm Konrad Roentgen, a physics professor a the University of Wurzburg in Bavaria. While x-rays remain the most popular form of diagnostic imaging, there are also many newer ways to obtain images of the internal structures and tissues of the body without using radiation. These other forms include magnetic resonance imaging and ultrasound.

American Association of Electrodiagnostic Medicine, 21 — 2nd St., SW, Ste. 306, Rochester, MN 55902

American Chiropractic Registry of Radiologic Technologists, 2330 Gull Rd., Kalamazoo, MI 49001; (616)343-6666

American College of Podiatric Radiologists, 169 Lincoln Rd., Ste. 308, Miami Beach, FL 33139

The American College of Radiology is the certifying organization for radiologists, accredits radiology facilities, and conducts a five-step accreditation process for mammography clinics.

American College of Radiology, 1891 Preston White Dr., Reston, VA 22091; (703)648-8900; Net: http://www.acr.org

American Healthcare Radiology Administrators, PO Box 334, Sudbury, MA 01776; (508)443-7591

American Registry of Diagnostic Medical Sonographers, 2368 Victory Pkwy., Ste. 510, Cincinnati, OH 45206-2810; (513)281-7111

American Registry of Radiologic Technologists, 1255 Northland Dr., St. Paul, MN 55120-1155; (612)687-0048

American Society of Clinic Radiologists, 300 Homer Ave., Palo Alto, CA 94301; (415)853-2955

American Society of Neuroimaging, 2221 University Ave., SE, Ste. 340, Minneapolis, MN 55414; (612)378-7240

American Society of Neuroradiology, 2210 Midwest Rd., Ste. 207, Oak Brook, IL 60521; (708)574-0220

The American Society of Radiologic Technologists is the national professional organization representing radiographers, radiation therapists, nuclear medicine technologists, and sonographers. The ASRT provides its members with continuing education opportunities and scholarly journals. Specialty areas of the radiography field include cardiovascular-interventional technology, computed tomography, and mammography. Magnetic, resonance Imaging is also included in the radiography field, even though MRI does not involve ionizing radiation.

American Society of Radiologic Technologists, 15000 Central Ave., SE, Albuquerque, NM 87123-3909; (505)298-4500

The American Society for Therapeutic Radiology and Oncology is a branch of the American College of Radiology. They publish a catalog of material that they sell to doctors. Some of the materials, such as pamphlets and videos, are meant for patient education. They also produce educational materials for doctors and those working in the field of radiation oncology.

American Society for Therapeutic Radiology and Oncology, 1891 Preston White Dr., Reston, VA 22091; (800)96-ASTRO; Publications E-mail: pub-sales@acr.org; American College of Radiology Headquarters' E-mail: info@acr.org; Mammography Accreditation E-mail: mamm-accred@acr.org

Brigham and Women's Hospital Dept. of Radiology, Net: http://count51.med.harvard.edu/BWH/BWHRad/html

Center for Biomedical Imaging Technology, Net: http://panda.uchc.edu/htbit/

The Committee for Nuclear Responsibility generates and distributes independent analyses of health effects from ionizing radiation, whether from medical usage (diagnostic x-rays and nuclear medicine), industrial/military usage, or from nuclear pollution.

Committee for Nuclear Responsibility, Inc., PO Box 421993, San Francisco, CA 94142; (415)776-8299; Net: http://www.ratical.com/radiation/CNR/

Journal of Medical Imaging, Net: http://jmi.gdb.org/JMI/ejourn.html

National Foundation for Non-Invasive Diagnostics, 103 Carnegie Center, St. 311, Princeton, NJ 08540; (609)520-1300

Northwestern University Dept. of Radiology, Net: http://pubweb.acns.nwu
.edu/~dbk675/nwu_radiology.html

Pennsylvania Radiological Society, Net: http//www.xray.hmc.psu.edu

Radiology Society of North America, Net: http://www.rsna.org/

University of Pennsylvania Medical Image Processing, Net: http://mipgsun.mipg.
upenn.edu/

Visible Human Project, Net: http://www.nlm.gov/factsheets.dir/visible_human
.html

• DIGESTION, UROLOGY, BOWEL DYSFUNCTION, AND INCONTINENCE

Book:
- *Managing Incontinence: A Guide to Living with Loss of Bladder Control*, Cheryle B. Gartley,
editor; The Simon Foundation ([709] 864-3913)

American Association of Genito-Urinary Surgeons, Baylor College of Medicine, 6560
Fannin St., Ste. 1004, Houston, TX 77030; (713)798-4001

American Board of Colon and Rectal Surgery, 20600 Eureka Rd., Ste. 713, Taylor, MI
48180; (313)282-9400

American Board of Urology, 31700 Telegraph Rd., Ste. 150, Bingham Farms, MI 48025;
(810)644-9720

American Celiac Society/Dietary Support Coalition, 58 Musano Court, W. Orange, NJ
07052; (201)325-8837

American College of Gastroenterology, 4900 B S. 31st St., Arlington, VA 22206-1656;
(703)820-7400

American Colon Therapy Association, 11739 Washington Blvd., Los Angeles, CA
90066; (310)390-5424

American Foundation for Urological Disease, 300 W. Pratt St., Ste. 401, Baltimore, MD
21201-2463; (410)727-2908 or (800)242-2383

American Gastroenterological Association, 7910 Woodmont Ave., 7th Flr., Bethesda,
MD 20814-3015; (301)654-2055

American Pediatric Gastroesophageal Reflux Association, 23 Acton St., Watertown,
MA 02172; (617)926-3586

American Society for Gastrointestinal Endoscopy, 13 Elm St., Manchester, MA 01944;
(508)526-8330

American Society of Colon and Rectal Surgeons, 85 W. Algonquin, Ste. 550, Arlington
Heights, IL 60005; (708)290-9184.

American Urological Association, 1120 N. Charles St., Baltimore, MD 21201; (410)727-
1100

Celiac Disease Foundation, 13251 Ventura Blvd., Ste. 3, Los Angeles, CA 91604-1838;
(818)990-2354

Celiac Spruce Association, PO Box 31700, Omaha, NB 68131-0700; (402)558-0600

Center to Assist the Regulation of Enuresis, Division of Urology, The Children's
Memorial Hospital, 2300 Children's Plaza, Chicago, IL 60614; (312)880-4000

Columbia University Gastroenterology Web, Net: http://cpmcnet.columbia.edu/
dept/gi/

Continence Restored, 407 Strawberry Hill Ave., Stamford, CT 06902; (203)348-0601 or
(914)285-1470

Crohn's and Colitis Foundation of America, 388 Park Ave. S., New York, NY 10016-
7374; (212)685-3440 or (800)932-2423 or 343-3637

Digestive Diseases National Coalition, 711 — 2nd St., NE, Ste. 200, Washington, DC 20002; (202)544-7497

Help for Incontinent People, Box 8310, Spartanburg, SC 29305; (803)579-5700 or (800)252-3337

International Foundation for Bowel Dysfunction, PO Box 17864, Milwaukee, WI 53217; (414)964-1799

Intestinal Disease Foundation, 1323 Forbes Ave., Ste. 200, Pittsburgh, PA 15219; (412)261-5888

National Digestive Diseases Information Clearinghouse, PO Box NDDIC, 9000 Rockville Pike, Bethesda, MD 20892-3570; (301)654-3810

Oley Foundation for Home Parenteral and Enteral Nutrition, Albany Medical Center, 214 Hun Memorial, A-23, Albany, NY 12208; (518)262-5079

The Simon Foundation for Continence publishes a newsletter, *The Informer*; sells a book titled *Managing Incontinence* that is available for $11.95 including postage; has a $15.00 annual membership fee; and sells reprints of articles about incontinence.
Simon Foundation for Continence, PO Box 835, Wilmette, IL 60091; (800)237-4666

Society for Surgery of the Alimentary Tract, 200 First St., SW, Rochester, MN 55901; (507)284-2870

Tri-State Incontinent Support Group, 51 Nassau Ave., Brooklyn, NY 11222; (718)599-0170

United Ostomy Association, 36 Executive Park, Ste. 120, Irvine, CA 92714-6744; (714)660-8624 or (800)826-0826

UCLA Digestive Disease Center, W. Los Angeles, CA 90024; (310)825-1597

• DISABILITIES INFORMATION

American Coalition of Citizens With Disabilities, 1012 Fourteenth St., NW, Ste. 901, Washington, DC 20005; (202)628-3470

A Newsletter called *Families and Disabilities* is published three times a year by the Beach Center on Families and Disabilities. There is no subscription charge.
Beach Center on Families and Disabilities, University of Kansas, Life Span Institute, 3111 Haworth Hall, Lawrence, Kansas 66045-7516; (913)864-7600; Net: http://kuhttp.cc.ukans.edu/cwls/units/LSI/b/beachhp.html

Center on Human Policy, 200 Huntington Hall, 2nd Floor, Syracuse, NY 132244-2340; (315)443-3851

Clearinghouse on Disability Information, US Department of Education, Office of Special Education and Rehabilitative Services, 330 C St. SW, Switzer Building, Room 3132, Washington, DC 20202-2524; (202)205-8241

Congress of Organizations of the Physically Handicapped, 16630 Beverly, Tinley Park, IL 60477-1904

The Council for Exceptional Children is a network of special educational professionals dedicated to improving educational outcomes for individuals with disabilities and/or who are gifted.
The Council for Exceptional Children, 1920 Association Dr., Reston, VA 22091-1589; (703)620-3660 or (800)8456CEC

Disabled Womyn's Educational Project, PO Box 8773, Madison, WI 53708-8773; (608)256-8883

Disability Rights Center, 2500 Q St., NW, Ste. 121, Washington, DC 20007; (202)337-4119

Disability Rights Education and Defense Fund, 2212 - 6th St., Berkeley, CA 94710; (510)644-2555

ERIC Clearinghouse on Disabilities and Gifted Education, (703)620-3660 or (800)328-0272; E-mail: Ericec@inet.ed.gov

The *Exceptional Parent Magazine* publishes a yearly annual directory of national support organizations for disabled children. To obtain a copy of the directory or to subscribe to the magazine, contact
Exceptional Parent Magazine, 209 Harvard St., Ste. 303, Bookline, MA 02146-5005; (800)247-8080

National Association of the Physically Handicapped, Bethesda Scarlet Oaks, #GA4, 440 Lafayette Ave., Cincinnati, OH 45220-1073; (513)961-8040; Fax (517)792-7549

National Center for Youth With Disabilities, University of Minnesota, PO Box 721, 420 DE St., SE, Minneapolis, MN 55455; (612)626-2825 or (800)333-6293

National Information Center for Children and Youth With Disabilities, PO Box 1492, Washington, DC 20013-1492; (202)884-8200 or (800)695-0285; E-mail: NICHCY @capcon.net

National Information Clearinghouse for Infants With Disabilities and Life-threatening Conditions, Columbia, SC; (800)922-9234 extension 201

National Parent Network on Disabilities, 1600 Prince St., Ste. 115, Alexandria, VA 22314; (703)684-6763

National Service for the Blind and Physically Handicapped, 1291 Taylor St. NW, Washington, DC 20542; (202)794-8650 or (800)424-8567

Society for the Advancement of Travel for the Handicapped, *Access Magazine,* 347 — 5th Ave., Ste. 610, New York, NY 10016; (212)447-7284

• DOCTOR ASSOCIATIONS (ALLOPATHIC)

American Association for Thoracic Surgery, 13 Elm St., Manchester, MA 01944; (508)526-8330

American Association for Women Radiologists, 1891 Preston White Dr., Reston, VA 22091; (703)648-8939

American Association of Hand Surgery, 435 N. Michigan Ave., Ste. 1717, Chicago, IL 60611; (312)644-0828

American Association of Immunologists, 9650 Rockville Pike, Bethesda, MD 20814; (310)530-7178

American Association of Neurological Surgeons, 22 S. Washington St., Ste. 100, Park Ridge, IL 60068; (708)692-9500

American Association of Neuropathologists, 204 Farber Hall, Dept. of Pathology, Buffalo Medical School, State University of New York, Buffalo, NY 14214

American Association of Plastic Surgeons, 2317 Seminole Rd., Atlantic Beach, FL 32233-5952; (904)359-3759

American Association of Plastic Surgery, 10666 N. Torrey Pines Rd., La Jolla, CA 92037; (619)554-9940

American Group Practice Association, 1422 Duke St., Alexandria, VA 22314; (703)838-0033

The American Medical Association is the largest allopathic physician organization in America and is very influential in Washington. It is composed of county and state medical societies along with representatives from specialty societies, hospitals, and other allopathic medical industry professionals.

The AMA publishes a yearly directory of officials and staff that lists various allopathic associations, boards, and other American healthcare worker groups. The Association also publishes the *Journal of the American Medical Association,* and the *Archives of Internal Medicine.*

The Physician Data Series, which is operated by the AMA, can provide you with some information on an allopathic doctor's professional history.

American Medical Association, Physician Data Series, 515 N. State St., Chicago, IL 60610; (312)464-5000 or 2000 or (800)621-8335; Net: http://2.umdnj.edu/~ama/ama.html

American Medical Women's Association, 801 N. Fairfax, Ste. 400, Alexandria, VA 22314; (703)838-0500

American Surgical Association, University of North Carolina, Dept. of Surgery, CB 7245, Chapel Hill, NC 27599-7245; (919)966-6320

Association of American Physicians and Surgeons, 1601 N. Tucson Blvd., Ste. 9, Tucson, AZ 85716; (602)327-4885

Association of Military Surgeons of the US, 9320 Old George Rd., Bethesda, MD 20814; (301)897-8800

Federal Physicians Association, PO Box 45150, Washington, DC 20026; (703)455-5947

• DOCTOR OF OSTEOPATHIC MEDICINE, SPECIALTY BOARDS OF

American Association of Osteopathic Specialists, 804 Main St., Ste. D, Forest Park, GA 30050; (800)447-9397

American Osteopathic Board of General Practice, 330 E. Algonquin Rd., Ste. 2, Arlington Heights, IL 60005; (708)635-8477

American Osteopathic Board of Anesthesiology, 17201 E. 40 Hwy., Ste. 204, Independence, MO 64055; (816)373-4700

American Osteopathic Board of Dermatology, 25510 Plymouth Rd., Detroit, MI 48239; (313)937-1200

American Osteopathic Board of Emergency Medicine, Philadelphia Osteopathic Medical Center, 4190 City Ave., Philadelphia, PA 19131; (215)871-2811

American Osteopathic Board of Family Physicians, Arlington Heights, IL; (708)640-8477

American Osteopathic Board of Internal Medicine, 5200 S. Ellis Ave., Chicago, IL 60615; (312)947-4880

American Osteopathic Board of Neurology and Psychiatry, 401 Haddon Ave., Camden, NJ 08103-1505; (609)757-7765

American Osteopathic Board of Nuclear Medicine, 5200 S. Ellis Ave., Chicago, IL 60615; (312)947-4490

American Osteopathic Board of Obstetrics & Gynecology, 5200 S. Ellis Ave., Chicago, IL 60615; (312)947-4630

American Osteopathic Board of Ophthalmology and Otorhinolaryngology, 405 Grand Ave., Dayton, OH 45405; (513)222-4213

American Osteopathic Board of Orthopedic Surgery, 5155 Raytown Rd., Ste. 103, Kansas City, MO 64133; (816)353-6400

American Osteopathic Board of Pathology, 13355 E. Ten Mile Rd., Warren, MI 48089; (313)759-7565

American Osteopathic Board of Pediatrics, Arlington Heights, IL; (707)640-8477

American Osteopathic Board of Preventive Medicine, 12535 Lt. Nichols Rd., Fairfax, VA 22033

American Osteopathic Board of Proctology, 2815 S. Pennsylvania Ave., Ste. 105-A, Lansing, MI 48910; (517)484-9885

American Osteopathic Board of Radiology, Route 2, Box 75, Milan, MO 63556

American Osteopathic Board of Rehabilitation Medicine, 9058 W. Church, Des Plaines, IL 60016; (312)699-0048

American Osteopathic Board of Surgery, 405 Grand Ave., Dayton, OH 45405; (513)226-2656

• DOCTOR SPECIALTY BOARDS (ALLOPATHIC)

American Board of Abdominal Surgery, 675 Main St., Melrose, MA 02176; (617)665-6101

American Board of Allergy and Immunology, University City Science Center, 3624 Market St., Philadelphia, PA 19104; (215)349-9466

American Board of Anesthesiology, 100 Constitution Plaza, Rm. 1668, Hartford, CT 06103; (203)522-9857

American Board of Colon and Rectal Surgery, 8750 Telegraph Rd., Ste. 410, Taylor, MI 48180; (313)295-1740

American Board of Dermatology, Henry Ford Hospital, Detroit, MI 48202; (313)871-8739

Doctors who specialize in emergency medicine are trained to detect symptoms that indicate the need for immediate attention. Emergency medicine became a board certified specialty in 1979. According to a report released in the fall of 1994 by Emory University in Atlanta, many hospital emergency rooms are staffed by doctors who have never been trained in trauma care and are unable to provide the best treatment when faced with serious medical emergencies. Only about half of the 25,000 positions in emergency medicine are staffed by doctors who are certified in the specialty of emergency medicine.

American Board of Emergency Medicine, 200 Woodland Pass, Ste. D, E. Lansing, MI 48823; (517)332-4800

American Board of Family Practice, 2228 Young Dr., Lexington, KY 40505; (606)269-5626

American Board of Internal Medicine, University City Science Center, 3624 Market St., Philadelphia, PA 19104; (215)243-1500

The Advisory Board of Medical Specialties was formed in 1933. In 1970, the name was changed to the American Board of Medical Specialties. The primary function of the ABMS is to maintain and improve the quality of allopathic medical care by assisting the member boards in their efforts to develop and use standards for the evaluation and certification of allopathic physician specialists.

The ABMS is the official medical certifying group responsible for administrating certification examinations to allopathic physician specialists. The intent of the certification process is to improve the quality of patient care. There are 23 allopathic specialties that are certified by the ABMS.

One way of checking to see if an allopathic doctor has been certified by the ABMS is to check in *The Official American Board of Medical Specialists Directory of Board Certified Medical Specialists*. This book is available in many public and university libraries. It shows whether an allopathic doctor has post-graduate education in the specialty he practices in. Because the book is a compilation of information from many sources, some of the information about the doctors listed in the directory may not be accurate.

American Board of Medical Specialties, 1007 Church St., Ste. 404, Evanston, IL 60201-5913; (708)491-9091; To find out if a doctor is certified: (800)776-2378 (CERT)

American Board of Neurological Surgery, Smith Tower, Ste. 2139, 6550 Fannin St., Ste. 2139, Houston, TX 77030-2701; (713)790-6015

American Board of Nuclear Medicine, 900 Veteran Ave., Rm. 12-200, Los Angeles, CA 90024; (310)825-6787

American Board of Obstetrics and Gynecology, 4225 Roosevelt Way, NE, Ste. 305, Seattle, Washington 98105; (206)547-4884

American Board of Ophthalmology, 111 Presidential Blvd., Ste. 241, Bala Cynwd, PA 19004; (215)664-1175

American Board of Orthopedic Surgery, 737 N. Michigan Ave., Ste. 1150, Chicago, IL 60611; (312)664-9444

American Board of Otolaryngology, 5615 Kirby Dr., Ste. 936, Houston, TX 77005; (713)528-6200

American Board of Pathology, 5401 W. Kennedy Blvd., Ste. 780, PO Box 25915, Tampa, FL 33622; (813)286-2444

American Board of Pediatrics, 111 Silver Cedar Court, Chapel Hill, NC 27514; (919)929-0461

American Board of Physical Medicine and Rehabilitation, Norwest Center, Ste. 674, 21 First St., SW, Rochester, MN 55902; (507)282-1776

American Board of Plastic Surgery, Seven Penn Center, Ste. 400, 1635 Market St., Philadelphia, PA 19103; (215)587-9322

American Board of Preventive Medicine, Dept. of Community Medicine, Wright State University School of Medicine, PO Box 927, Dayton, OH 45401; (512)278-6915

American Board of Psychiatry and Neurology, 500 Lake Cook Rd., Ste. 335, Deerfield, IL 60015; (312)945-7900

American Board of Radiology, 300 Park, Ste. 440, Birmingham, Michigan 48009; (810)645-0600

American Board of Surgery, 1617 John F. Kennedy Blvd., Ste. 860, Philadelphia, PA 19103-1847; (215)568-4000

American Board of Thoracic Surgery, One Rotary Center, Ste. 803, Evanston, IL 60201; (708)475-1520

American Board of Urology, 31700 Telegraph Rd., Ste. 150, Birmingham, MI 48010; (313)646-9720

- ## DOCTORS/PHYSICIANS, ROYAL COLLEGES OF (ALLOPATHIC)

Royal College of Physicians and Surgeons of Canada, 774 Promenade Echo Dr., Ottawa, Canada K1S 5NB; (613)730-8177 or 6212

Royal College of Physicians and Surgeons of the USA, 16126 E. Warren, Detroit, MI 48224; (313)882-0641

Royal College of Surgeons, Britain; 44-71-831-5161

- ## DOGS FOR DISABLED AND HANDICAPPED PERSONS

Assistance Dogs of America, 8806 State Rte. 64, Swanton, OH 43558; (419)825-3622

Canine Companions for Independence, PO Box 4568, Oceanside, CA 92052; (619)754-3300

Dogs for the Deaf, 10175 Wheeler Rd., Central Point, OR 97502; (541)826-9220

Guide Dogs for the Blind, PO Box 151200, San Rafael, CA 94915-1200; (415)499-4000

International Hearing Dog, 5901 E. 89th Ave., Henderson, CO 80640

National Education for Assistance Dog Service, PO Box 213, West Boylston, MA 01583; Voice or TTY (508)835-3304

National Service Dog Center, 289 Perimeter Rd. E., Renton, WA 98055-1329; (800)869-6898 or TDD (800)809-2714; E-mail: deltasociety@cis.compuserve.com.

Paws With a Cause, 4646 S. Division, Wayland, MI 49348; (800)253-7297

Support Dogs, 3958 Union Rd., St. Louis, MO 63125; (314)892-2554

Therapy Dogs International, Inc., 6 Hilltop Rd., Mendham, NJ 07945; (201)543-0888; Fax (201)543-0989; E-mail: tdi@gti.net

• EMERGENCY MEDICINE AND IDENTIFICATION BRACELETS

American Trauma Society, 8903 Presidential Pkwy., Upper Marlboro, MD 20772; (301)420-4189 or (800)556-7890

Medic Alert Foundation provides emblems that detail a person's health concerns as a precaution in case of an emergency. The emblem is worn similar to jewelry as a bracelet on the wrist, on a chain around the neck, or can be placed in the wallet or purse. They are now available in gold and silver to go along with other jewelry.

Reasons to wear a medical alert tag
- You are subject to seizures.
- You are on special medication.
- You are allergic to certain medications.
- You are on dialysis.
- You have a heart condition.
- You carry an infectious disease.
- You have a rare disease.
- You suffer from hemophilia or other bleeding disorders.
- You have had an organ transplant.
- You have some type of man-made implant.
- You have a living will or an advance directive for limits on medical treatment.
- Certain individuals need to be contacted if you experience an emergency.

Medic Alert Foundation, 2323 Colorado Ave., Turlock, CA 95380; (800)892-9211 or 422-2720; To enroll by phone (800)432-5378

National Emergency Medical Association, (800)332-6362

• EYES

Book:
- *A Guide to Independence for the Visually Impaired and Their Families,* by Vivian Younger and Jill Sardegna; Demos Publications ([212]683-0072), 1995

To protect the eyes, wear goggles whenever you are performing any task or participating in any activity where eye damage can occur. When you are out in the sun, wear sun glasses that protect against UV rays.

Affiliated Leadership League of and for the Blind of America, 1101 — 17th St., NW, Ste. 803, Washington, DC 20036; (202)833-0092

American Academy of Ophthalmology, 655 Beach St., San Francisco, CA 94109; (415)561-8500

American Academy of Optometry, 4330 E. W. Hwy., Ste. 1117, Bethesda, MD 20817; (301)718-6500

American Association for Pediatric Ophthalmology, PO Box 193832, San Francisco, CA 94119; (415)561-8505

American Association of Certified Orthoptists, Hermann Eye Center, 6411 Fannin, Houston, TX 77030-1697

American Association of the Deaf-Blind, 814 Thayer Ave., Rm. 300, Silver Springs, MD 20910

American Association of Eye and Ear Hospitals, 1350 New York Ave., NW, Ste. 200, Washington, DC 20005; (202)347-1990

American Council of the Blind, 1155 — 15th St., NW, Ste. 720, Washington, DC 20005; (202)467-5081 or (800)424-8666

American Foundation for the Blind, 15 W. 16th St., New York, NY 10011; (212)620-2000 or (800) AF-BLIND

American Foundation for Vision Awareness, 243 N. Lindbergh Blvd., St. Louis, MO 63141; (314)991-4100

American Optometric Association, 243 N. Lindbergh Blvd., St. Louis, MO 63121; (314)991-4100

American Optometric Foundation, 4330 E. W. Hwy., Ste. 1117, Bethesda, MD 20814; (301)718-6514

American Ophthalmological Society, Duke University Eye Center, Durham, NC 27710; (919)684-5365

American Printing House for the Blind, 1839 Frankfort Ave., PO Box 6085, Louisville, KY 40206-0085; (502)895-2405 or (800)223-1839; Fax (502)895-1509; E-mail: aph@iglou .com

American Society of Cataract and Refractive Surgery, 4000 Lugato Rd., Ste. 850, Fairfax, VA 22033; (703)591-2220

The Associated Blind, 135 W. 23rd St., New York, NY 10011; (212)255-1122

Associated Services for the Blind, 919 Walnut St., Philadelphia, PA 19107; (215)627-0600

Association of Macular Disorders, 210 E. 64th St., New York, NY 10021; (212)605-3719

Association of Radio Reading Services, 2100 Wharton St., Ste. 140, Pittsburgh, PA 15203; (412)488-3944

Better Vision Institute, 1800 N. Kent St., Ste. 904, Rosslyn, VA 22209; (703)243-1528 or (800)424-8422

Blind Children's Center, Net: http://www.primenet.com/bcc/

Blind Children's Fund, 2875 Northwind Dr., Ste. 211, E. Lansing, MI 48823-5040; (517)333-1725; Fax (517)333-1730

Blind Service Association, 22 W. Monroe, 11th Flr., Chicago, IL 60603; (312)236-0808

Blinded American Veterans Foundation, PO Box 65900, Washington, DC 20035-5900; (202)462-4430 or (800)284-2283

Blinded Veterans Association, 477 H St., NW, Washington, DC 20001; (202)371-8880 or (800)669-7079

Braille Revival League, 3841 Giles, Apt. 2N, St. Louis, MO 63116; (314)771-2338

Carrol Center for the Blind, 770 Centre St., Newton, MA 02158-2597; (617)969-6200

Council of Citizens With Low Vision, 1400 N. Drake Rd., Ste. 218, Kalamazoo, MI 49007; (616)381-9566

Council of Families With Visual Impairment, 26616 Rouge River Dr., Dearborn Heights, MI 48127; (800)424-8666

Doctors at the Dean A. McGee Eye Institute worked with the latest technologies to treat eye injuries inflicted by the Oklahoma City bomb.
Dean A. McGee Eye Institute, 720 Stanton L. Young, Oklahoma City, OK 73104; (405)271-6060

Eye Bank Association of America, 1001 Connecticut Ave., NW, Ste. 601, Washington, DC 20036-5504; (202)775-4999

Eye Bank for Sight Restoration, 210 E. 64th St., New York, NY 10021; (212)980-6700

Eye Donation Hotline, (800)638-1818, in Maryland phone (301)269-4031

E-zee Vision Prescription Eyeglasses, Net: http://www.eyeglass.com

Foundation Fighting Blindness, Executive Plaza I, Ste. 800, 11350 McCormick Rd., Hunt Valley, MD 21031-1014; (410)785-1414; TDD (410)785-9687 or (800)683-5555; TDD (800)683-5551; Fax (410)771-9470

Glaucoma Research Foundation, 490 Post St., Ste. 830, San Francisco, CA 94102; (415)986-3162 or (800)826-6693; Fax (415)986-3763; Net:: glaucoma@ucsfvm

.uscf.edu

A catalogue titled *Can-Do Products* specializing in products for visually impaired people can be ordered through
Independent Living Aids, 27 E. Mall, Plainview, NY 11803; (800)537-2118

International Eye Foundation, 7801 Norfolk Ave., Bethesda, MD 20814; (301)986-1830

Med Source Introduction to Vision Correcting Procedures, Net: http://www.ozark sol.com/medsource

National Association for Parents of the Visually Impaired, PO Box 317, Watertown, MA 02272-0317; (800)562-6265

The National Association for Visually Handicapped is devoted solely to serving the "hard of seeing" — not the totally blind. It does this by providing large-print materials and visual aids for sale and through a loaning library; emotional support; referrals; and educational outreach to the public and to professionals. They publish a catalog and a newsletter that are included in the yearly $40 membership fee.
National Association for Visually Handicapped, 22 W. 21st. St., New York, NY 10010; (212)889-3141 — or — 3201 Balboa St., San Francisco, CA 94121; (415)221-3201

National Center for the Blind, 1800 Johnson St., Baltimore, MD 21230; (410)659-9314 or (800)638-5555

National Children's Eye Care Foundation, 32100 Meadowlark Way, Pepper Pike, OH 44124; (214)407-0404

National Council of State Agencies for the Blind, 1232 — 29th St., NW, Washington, DC 20007; (202)298-8468

National Eye Care Project, PO Box 9688, San Francisco, CA 94101-9688; (800)222-EYES

National Eye Institute, 2020 Vision Place, Bethesda, MD 20892-3658; (301)496-5248

National Eye Research Foundation, 601 Driftwood Ln., Northbrook, IL 60062; (708)564-4641

National Glaucoma Research Report, American Health Assistance Foundation, 15825 Shady Grove Rd., Ste. 140, Rockville MD 20850; (301)948-3244

National Society to Prevent Blindness, 500 E. Remington Rd., Schaumburg, IL 60173; (708)843-2020 or (800)331-2020

New Eyes for the Needy collects used glasses and jewelry to use, or raise funds for helping poor people in all areas of the world see better by providing them with glasses.
New Eyes for the Needy, 549 Milburn Ave., PO Box 332, Short Hills, NJ 07078-0332; (201)376-4903

Outpatient Ophthalmic Surgery Society, PO Box 23220, San Diego, CA 92193; (619)692-4426

Prevent Blindness America, 500 E. Remington Rd., Schaumberg, IL 60173; (800)331-2020

Research to Prevent Blindness, 598 Madison Ave., New York, NY 10022; (212)752-4333

Seeing Eye, PO Box 375, Morristown, NJ 07963-0375; (201)539-4425

United Association of Blind Athletes, 33 North Institute St., Colorado Springs, CO 80903; (719)630-0422

Vision Foundation, 818 Mt. Auburn St., Watertown, MA 02172; (617)926-4232

Vision Impairments: A Guide for the Perplexed, Net: http://www.wimsey.com /~jlyon/index.html

Vision USA provides eye care to low-income, uninsured working people. The program is available in January and is operated by the American Optometric Association.
Vision USA , 243 N. Lindbergh Blvd., St. Louis, MO 63141; (800)766-4466

• FACIAL DEFECTS AND INJURIES

Books:
* *Children with Facial Differences: A Parent's Guide*, by Hope Charkins; Woodbine House ([800]843-7323), 1995
* *The Cleft Palate Story*, by Samuel Berkowitz, DDS, MS, FCID; Quintessence Publishing ([708] 682-3288)
* *Face Value: Coping With Facial Disfigurement*, by Linda R. Shafritz; Face Value (PO Box 45854, Los Angeles, CA 90045 — $10 + $2 S&H)

About Face (Canada), 99 Crown Lane, 4th Flr., Toronto, Ontario, M5R 3P4 Canada; (416)928-0888

About Face (US), PO Box 93, Limekiln, PA 19535; Phone (800)225-FACE; E-mail: abt FACE@AOL.com

American Cleft Palate — Craniofacial Association, 1218 Grandview Ave., Pittsburgh, PA 15211; (412)481-1376

The Belle Foundation was started to educate parents of children with cavernous hemangiomas about safe and effective treatments to remove these growths.
Belle Foundation, PO Box 385, Gracie Station, New York, NY 10028-0004

Carpenter Syndrome Network, PO Box 4215-48, 26661 Bear Valley Rd., Tehachapi, CA 93561; (805)821-1313

Center for Facial Restoration, 333 E. Virginia, Ste. 109, Phoenix, AZ 85004-1207; (602)258-3620

The Children's Craniofacial Association functions as a networking and referral service for healthcare professionals, for government officials, and for parents of craniofacially disfigured children.
Children's Craniofacial Association, 9441 LBJ Frwy., Ste. 115-LB 46, Dallas, TX 75243; (214)994-9902 or (800)535-3643

Children's Hospital, Dept. of Plastic Surgery, 111 Michigan Ave., NW, Washington, DC 20010-2970; (202)884-2157

Children's Hospital of Los Angeles, Plastic Surgery Dept., 4650 Sunset Blvd., Los Angeles, CA 90027; (213)660-2450

Craniofacial Center, 7777 Forest Lane, Suite C700, Dallas, TX 75230-9988; (800)443-3996

The Craniofacial Center of the University of Illinois sells literature and rents videotapes that cover various aspects of the special needs of babies and children with cleft lips and palates.
Craniofacial Center of the University of Illinois at Chicago Medical Center, M/C 588, 808 S. Wood St., Ste. 476, Chicago, IL 60612-7308; (312)996-7546

FACES provides financial assistance for expenses incurred while traveling away from home to a craniofacial medical center for reconstructive surgery and/or evaluation. The assistance is offered on the basis of financial and medical need and includes transportation, lodging, and food. Once a client is accepted, every attempt is made to continue aid for as long as it is needed. FACES publishes a quarterly newsletter.
FACES: The National Association for the Craniofacially Handicapped, PO Box 11082, Chattanooga, TN 37401; (423)266-1632 or (800)332-2373

Foundation for the Faces of Children, P.O. Box 1361, Brookline, MA 02146; (617)734-7576

Freeman-Sheldon Parent Support Group, 509 E. Northmont Way, Salt Lake City, UT 84103; (801)364-7060

Interplast is a group that sends volunteer medical teams to developing countries to perform cost-free reconstructive surgery on people who are suffering from various deformities caused by accidents and birth defects.
Interplast, 2458 Embarradera Way, Palo Alto, CA 94303; (415)424-0123

Let's Face It is an information and support network for people with facial disfigurement, their families, and professionals. Resources include newsletters, parent support training, books, videos, and a lending library. Publications for families include *Our Newborn has a Facial Disfigurement,* and *Your Child and the Craniofacial Team.* They publish the *Let's Face It Annual Resource List* once a year that includes phone numbers and addresses to health organizations, and information on books about the healthcare and emotional care of children with facial deformities and special needs.
Let's Face It, PO Box 29972, Bellingham, Washington 98228-1972; (360)676-7325

Moebius syndrome is a rare genetic disorder characterized by the inability to smile, frown, or do other facial movements. Some people with the syndrome cannot blink or move their eyes from side to side. In some instances the syndrome is also associated with physical problems in other parts of the body, such as missing or webbed fingers. For information on a quarterly newsletter for adults and parents of children with Moebius Syndrome, send a self-addressed, stamped envelope to the
Moebius Syndrome Foundation, PO Box 993, Larchmont, NY 10538; (914)834-6008

The National Foundation for Facial Reconstruction supports the Institute of Reconstructive Plastic Surgery at the New York University Medical Center. They maintain a patient-referral service for people suffering facial disfigurements caused by accidents, congenital malformations, and diseases. They also provide psychological and financial support services. They publish a book titled *Special Faces: Understanding Facial Disfigurement.*
National Foundation for Facial Reconstruction, 317 E. 34th St., Ste. 901, New York, NY 10016; (212)263-6656 or (800)422-FACE (3223)

The National Vascular Malformation Foundation has literature on various types of vascular malformations, such as hemangiomas, port wine stains, klippel-trenaunay, arteriovenous malformations, and Sturge-Weber. They publish a newsletter.
National Vascular Malformation Foundation, 8320 Nightingale St., Dearborn Heights, MI 48127; (313)274-1234; Fax (313)274-1234

Operation Smile International is a non-profit, volunteer medical organization that provides reconstructive surgery to needy children and adults who are born with cleft lips, other congenital deformities, disfigurement caused by facial tumors, and burns, club feet, and sometimes other injury- or disease-caused deformities. Operation Smiles' World Care Program identifies patients whose deformities and disfigurements are too severe for treatment in their home countries and brings them to the US for surgery. Operation Smile arranges for surgeons and other medical specialists to volunteer their services, and for the free hospitalization and care of the patients.
Operation Smile International, 717 Boush St., Norfolk, VA 23510-1501; (804)625-0375 or 622-7500 or 451-3799

Shadyside Maxillofacial and Cleft Palate Prosthetics Center, Shadyside Medical Center, Ste. 207, Pittsburgh, PA 15232; (412)661-2963

Sturge-Weber syndrome is characterized by a congenital facial birthmark and abnormalities, such as the development of excessive blood vessels on the surface of the brain (angiomas) on the same side as the port wine stain. These angiomas create abnormal condition for brain function in the regions. Other symptoms can include eye and internal organ irregularities. The Sturge-Weber Foundation publishes a newsletter called *Branching Out.* It is also a clearinghouse for information on all aspects of Sturge-Weber syndrome, Klippel Trenaunay Weber-Syndrome, and port wine stains.
Sturge-Weber Foundation, PO Box 418, Mt. Freedom, NJ 07970; (201)895-4445

Tennessee Craniofacial Center, Erlanger Medical Center, T.C. Thompson Children's Hospital, 975 E. Third St., Chattanooga, TN 37403; (800)418-3223

Wide Smiles Newsletter, Box 5153, Stockton, CA 95205-0153; (209)942-2812; E-mail: widesmiles@aol.com

• FEET

Academy of Ambulatory Foot Surgery, PO Box 2730, Ste. 263, Tuscaloosa, AL 35403; (205)758-3678

American Academy of Orthopaedic Surgeons, 6300 N. River Rd., Rosemont, IL 60018; (800)824-BONE (2663)

American Academy of Podiatric Sports Medicine, 1729 Glastonberry Rd., Potomac, MD 20854

American Association of Foot Specialists, PO Box 54, Union, NJ 07083

American Association of Hospital Podiatrics, 420 — 74th St., Brooklyn, NY 11209; (212)836-1017

American Board of Orthopedic Surgery, 737 N. Michigan Ave., Ste. 1150, Chicago, IL 60611; (312)664-9444

American College of Foot Orthopedists, 108 Orange St., Ste. 6, Redlands, CA 92373; (714)798-8910

American College of Foot Surgeons, 444 N. Northwest Hwy., Ste. 155, Park Ridge, IL 60068; (708)292-2237

American College of Podiatric Radiologists, 169 Lincoln Rd., Ste. 308, Miami, FL 33139

American College of Podopediatrics, 10515 Carnegie Ave., Cleveland, OH 44106; (216)231-3300

American Orthopedic Society for Sports Medicine, 6300 N. River Rd., Ste. 200, Rosemont, IL 60018; (708)292-4900

For free literature on foot care, call the
American Podiatric Medical Association, (800)366-8227

The One Shoe Crew provides free shoes to the foot-handicapped and matches shoe sizes with potential shoe partners by computer. About half of their clients wear two shoes of different sizes — these are frequently polio survivors, or those born with a club foot. The other half need only one shoe for reasons, such as amputation, stroke, and braces. The One Show Crew also has information about shoes and other items of interest to the handicapped. Services are free for US Veterans. All shoes are donated by individuals, retailers, or shoe manufacturers.
The One Shoe Crew, 86 Clavela Ave., Sacramento, CA 95828-4647; (916)364-SHOE; Send donated shoes to 920 S. River Rd., W. Sacramento, CA 95691. Shoes must be new.

• FINAL RELIEF (Also see *Hospice and Bereavement*, and *Living Wills*)

Book:
• *A Chosen Death: The Dying confront Assisted Suicide,* by Lonny Shavelson; Simon & Schuster, 1995

Many in the medical profession and those who counsel the terminally ill argue against assisted suicide. They point out that pain management with medication, treatment of depression, and family support services, such as counseling and hospice programs, are better ways of dealing with terminal illness, ensure patient comfort, and sufficiently enhance the quality of life to its end.

For those who find themselves in a situation where, because of terminal illness, their health is failing beyond the point at which they consider medical treatment worthwhile, or when medicine does nothing but prolong suffering, the sources listed below can provide information on painless, nonviolent final options that may be effective in terminating life before all interactive capacities are lost. Beware that these forms of self-deliverance do not always progress as planned. Also, people who assist with a suicide may find themselves charged with a felony.

As in any medical decision, the decision to relieve a dying patient through assisted suicide should only be the decision of the patient, and not a decision that was made under the pressure or the suggestion of others.

The following groups survive on financial donations and will provide information to anyone who sends a self-addressed, stamped envelope.

The stand of the organization called Death with Dignity is that hospice care should be expanded and promoted as the standard of care, available to all terminally-ill patients. Death with Dignity also believes that assisted dying should be the response of last resort, should be used infrequently, used only when requested by a competent patient, and should be subject to rigorous safeguards. The group seeks to inform and educate the public about physician aid-in-dying so they can make informed decisions regarding issues related to end-of-life choices.

Death with Dignity, PO Box 1238, San Mateo, CA 94401-0816; (415)594-9119 or (415)344-6489; (415)344-6489; E-mail: ddec@ail.com

Death with Dignity - Canada; 188 Eglinton Ave. E., Ste. 706, Toronto, Ontario, M4P 2X7 Canada; (416)486-3998; Fax (416)489-9010

Compassionate Friends, PO Box 3696, Oak Brook, IL 60522-3696; (708)990-0010

Compassion in Dying provides information and assistance to terminally ill patients in extreme suffering. This includes counseling about pain management, hospice care, and medications to hasten death in desperate cases. Volunteers can be with the patient and family as the patient succumbs. The organization is also challenging the constitutionality of laws which prohibit terminally ill patients from receiving medications with which to voluntarily hasten death.

Compassion in Dying, PO Box 75295, Seattle, WA 98125-0295; (206)624-2775

Dying With Dignity, Canada; (416)486-3998

The Hemlock Society advocates legalized voluntary physician aid-in-dying and is working to change laws that prohibit doctors from helping dying patients who request aid in hastening their deaths. The Society publishes and sells a newsletter called *Timelines*, pamphlets, and books. For a complimentary form letter that allows you to formally communicate your wishes regarding aid-in-dying to your physician, contact the

Hemlock Society, PO Box 11830, Eugene, OR 97440-4030; (503)342-5748 or (800)247-7421; E-mail: hemlock@efn.org

• GENETIC DISORDERS

Book:
• *Genetic Connections: A Guide to Documenting Your Individual and Family Health History,* by Danette L. Nelson-Anderson and Cynthia V. Waters; Sonters Publishing (PO Box 109 Washington, MO 63090), 1995

Alliance of Genetic Support Groups, 35 Wisconsin Circle, Ste. 440, Chevy Chase, MD 20815; (800)336-4363

American Association of Birth Defect Children, 827 Irma Ave., Orlando, FL 32803-3806

AT Children's Project, Boca Raton, FL; (407)395-2621

Dept. of Human Genetics, University of Pittsburgh, Pittsburgh, PA 15261; (412)624-9951; Fax (412)624-3020; E-mail bgettig@helix.hgen.pitt.edu

Genetic Disorders, Net: http://gdbwww.gdb.org/omimdoc/omimtop.html

Hereditary Disease Foundation, 1427 Seventh St., Ste. 2, Santa Monica, CA 90401

March of Dimes Birth Defects Foundation, 1275 Mamaroneck Ave., White Plains, NY 10605; (914)428-7100

Neurofibromatosis are genetic disorders of the nervous system which can cause tumors to form on the nerves anywhere in the body at any time. They are progressive genetic disorders and affect all races and both sexes.

Neurofibromatosis, Inc., 8855 Annapolis Rd., Ste. 110, Lanham, MD 20706-2924; (301)577-8984 or (800)942-6825

• HAIR

American Electrology Association (electrolysis = hair removal), 106 Oak Ridge Rd., Trumbull, CT 06611; (203)374-6667

American Hair Loss Council, 401 N. Michigan Ave., Chicago, IL 60611; (312)321-5128 or (800)274-8717

Bald-Headed Men of America, 102 Bald Dr., Morehead City, NC 28557

Council on Electrolysis Education, 46 S. Holmes St., Memphis, TN 38111; (901)458-1431

Daughters of Hirutism Association of America, 203 N. LaSalle St., Ste. 2100, Chicago, IL 60601; (312)558-1365

Hair Loss Handbook and Support Group Network, Net: http://www.mcny.com /hairloss

National Alopecia Areata Foundation, PO Box 150760, San Rafael, CA 94915-0760; (415)456-4644; E-mail: 74301.1642@compuserve.com

National Committee for Electrologist Certification, 96 Westminster Rd., W. Hempstead, NY 11552; (516)485-6309

• HANDS (Also see *Repetitive Motion Injuries*)

American Association for Hand Surgery, 435 N. Michigan Ave., Ste. 1717, Chicago, IL 60611-4067; (312)644-0828

American Society of Hand Therapists, 401 N. Michigan Ave., Chicago, IL 60611; (312)321-6866

• HEALTH RESEARCH GROUPS FOR HIRE

Canhelp, 3111 Paradise Bay Rd., Port Ludlow, WA 98365-9771; (360)473-2291

The Environmental Access Research Network can conduct medical and legal computer literature searches on any topic through the databases of the national Library of Medicine and Westlaw. EARN publishes a newsletter six times per year. The newsletter provides medical and legal information on the health effects of chemicals and other environmental issues that may effect health. The organization is affiliated with the Chemical Injury Information Network.
Environmental Access Research Network, PO Box 426, Williston, ND 58802-0426; (701)859-6363

Health Information Network, 4527 Montgomery Dr., Ste. E, Santa Rosa, CA 95409; (800)743-6996

The Health Resource, a medical information research service, was started by Janice Guthrie after she was angered by a discouraging doctor who told her she could "know too much" when she was suffering from a rare type of ovarian cancer. She spent hours in libraries scouring medical literature to find a treatment for her own condition. She found a more promising treatment than the one that her doctor prescribed.
The Health Resource, 564 Locust St., Conway, Arkansas 72032; (501)329-5272

Medical Data Exchange, 4730 Galice Rd., Merlin, OR 97532; (503)471-1627

Medical Information Foundation, 3000 Sand Hill Rd., Bldg. 2, Ste. 260, Menlo Park, CA 94025; (800)999-1999

Medical Information Service, Palo Alto Medical Foundation, 400 Channing Ave., Palo Alto, CA 94301; (415)853-6000

Palo Alto Medical Foundation, Palo Alto, CA; (800)999-1999

Planetree Health Research Center operates a consumer health library that concentrates on both conventional and holistic healthcare. They also conduct health research.

Planetree Health Resource Center, 2040 Webster St., San Francisco, CA 94115; (415)923-3680 or 923-3681

Schine Online Services, 39 Brenton Ave., Providence, RI 02906; (401)346-3287 or (800)FIND-CURE; Net: http://www.findcure.com

World Research Foundation, 15300 Ventura Blvd., Ste. 405, Sherman Oaks, CA 91403; (818)907-5483; Fax (818)907-6044

• HEARING

Book:
• *Life After Deafness: A Resource Book for Late-Deafened Adults,* by Bena Shuster; Canadian Hard of Hearing Association ([613]526-1584; Fax [613]526-4718), 1995

Academy of Dispensing Audiologists, 3008 Millwood Ave., Columbia, SC 29205; (803)252-5646

Academy of Rehabilitative Audiology, c/o Dr. Sharon Lesner, University of Akron, Dept. of Communication Disorders, Akron, OH 44325-3001; (216)972-7883

Acoustic Neuroma Association, PO Box 12402, Atlanta, GA 30355; (404)237-8023

Accoustic Neuroma Association of Canada, PO Box 369, Edmonton, Alberta T5J 2J6, Canada

Alexander Graham Bell Association for the Deaf, 3417 Volta Pl., NW, Washington, DC 20007; (202)337-5220

American Association of the Deaf-Blind, 814 Thayer Ave., Ste. 300, Silver Springs, MD 20910

American Association of Eye and Ear Hospitals, 1350 New York Ave., NW, Ste. 200, Washington, DC 20005; (202)347-1990

American Auditory Society, 1966 Inwood Rd., Dallas, TX 75236; (214)330-4203

American Hearing Research Foundation, 55 E. Washington St., Ste. 2022, Chicago, IL 60602; (312)726-9670

American Otological Society, Loyola University Medical School, 2160 S. 1st Ave., Bldg. 105, No. 1870, Maywood, IL 60153; (708)216-8526

American Professional Society of the Deaf, 35 Rainbow Trail, Mountain Lakes, NJ 07046; (908)730-1546

American Tinnitus Association, Box 5, Portland, OR 97207; (503)248-9985

Better Hearing Institute, 5021B Backlick Rd., Annandale, VA 22003; (703)642-0580 or (800)327-9355; Fax (703)750-9302

Children of Deaf Adults, PO Box 30715, Santa Barbara, CA 93130; (805)682-0997

Cochlear Implant Club International, PO Box 464, Buffalo, NY 14223-0464; v/tty/fax (716)838-4662; E-mail: 76207,3114@compuserve.com

Deafness Research Foundation, 9 E. 38th St., New York, NY 10016; (212)684-6556 or (800)535-3323

Deafpride, 1350 Potomac Ave., SE, Washington, DC 20003; (202)675-6700

Deaf Reach, 3521 — 12th St., NE, Washington, DC 20017; (202)832-6681

Deaf World Web, Net: http://deafworldweb.org/deafworld/

Ear Structure CT Images, Net: http://www.sbu.ac.uk/SAS/dirt/EAR_CT.html

Hearing Is Priceless Campaign, House Ear Institute, 2100 W. 3rd St., 5th Flr., Los Angeles, CA 90057; (213)483-4431

House Ear Institute, 2100 W. 3rd, 5th Flr., Los Angeles, CA 90057; (213)483-4431

Houston Ear Research Foundation, 7737 SW Freeway, Ste. 630, Houston, TX 77074; (713)771-9966 or (800)843-0706

International Association of Sports Vision, 200 S. Progress Ave., Harrisburg, PA 17109; (717)652-8080

Massachusetts Eye and Ear Infirmary, 243 Charles St., Boston, MA 02114; (617)573-3711

Meniere's Network, 2000 Church St., Ste. 111, Nashville, TN 37236-0001; (615)329-7807 or (800)545-HEAR

National Hearing Aid Society, 20361 Middlebelt, Livonia, MI 48152; (800)521-5247

National Information Center on Deafness, 800 Florida Ave., NE, Washington, DC 20002

National Institute on Deafness and Other Communication Disorders Information Clearinghouse, 1 Communication Ave., Bethesda, MD 20892-3456; (800)241-1044 or TTY (800)241-1055

National Temporal Bone, Hearing, and Balance Pathology Resource Registry, 243 Charles St., Boston, MA 02114-3096; (617)573-3711 or (800)822-1327; TDD (617)573-3888

Self Help for Hard of Hearing People, 7910 Woodmont Ave., Ste. 1200, Bethesda, MD 20814; (301)657-2248 or TTY (301)657-2249; E-mail: 71162.634@compuserv.com

Telecommunications for the Deaf, 8719 Colesville Rd., Ste. 300, Silver Spring, MD 20910; voice (301)589-3786 or TTY (301)389-3797; E-mail: sonnytdi@aol.com

Tripod, 2901 N. Keystone St., Burbank, CA 91504-1620; V/TTY (US) (800)352-8888 or V/TTY (California only) (800)2-TRIPOD; E-mail: Tripodla@aol.com

Vestibular Disorders Association, PO Box 4467, Portland, OR 97208; (503)229-7705 or (800)837-8428; E-mail: veda@teleport.com — or — Net: http://www.tele port.com/~veda

• HEART

Books:
- *Avoiding the Heart Surgery Trap: What Everybody with a Heart Problem Needs to Know to Stay Out of the Hospital,* by Julian M. Whitaker, MD; Regency Publishing, Inc., 1994
- *Dr. Dean Ornish's Program for Reversing Heart Disease,* by Dean Ornish; Ballintine Books/Random House, 1990
- *8 Steps To A Healthy Heart,* by Robert S. Kowalski; Warner Books, 1992
- *Is Heart Surgery Necessary?: What Your Doctor Won't Tell You,* by Julian Whitaker, MD; Regency Publishing, 1995
- *Mayo Clinic Heart Book,* by the Mayo Clinic staff; Morrow, William and Company, 1993
- *The McDougall Plan,* by John A. McDougall & Mary McDougall; New Win Publishing, 1983
- *The McDougall Program: 12 Days to Dynamic Health,* by John A. McDougall, MD; Penguin Books, 1990
- *The Pritikin Program for Diet and Exercise,* by Nathan Pritikin & Patrick McGrady; Bantam Books, 1984
- *The Yale University School of Medicine Heart Book,* by Barry L. Zaret, Laurence S. Cohen, Marvin Moser & Genell Subak-Sharpe, Eds.; Morrow, William, & Company, 1992

Since December 3, 1967, when Dr. Christiaan Barnard performed the first human heart transplant in Capetown, South Africa, there have been many advancements in heart surgery. According to a National Hospital Discharge Survey, in 1991 there were 839,000 heart surgeries including bypass and angioplasty. Additionally there were 2,132 heart transplants. While new medications developed to treat heart disease have helped some potential heart surgery patients avoid surgery, more and more people are turning to nutrition and exercise to improve heart health.

Keeping the heart healthy:
- Stay active.
- Exercise daily to relieve stress and condition the body.
- Go for a walk every day.
- Do not smoke.
- Keep your weight under control. Loose any extra weight.
- Eat small meals. Large meals place a strain on the heart.
- Avoid salty foods and do not add salt to your food.
- Avoid, or greatly limit, your intake of meat, dairy, and egg products.
- Maintain a diet that is rich in fiber. You can get fiber from eating whole grain foods, beans, fruits, and vegetables. Meat and dairy products do not contain fiber and should be avoided.
- Potassium helps the body maintain healthy blood pressure. Leafy green vegetables, tomatoes, potatoes, oranges, cantaloupe, and bananas all contain potassium.
- The mineral magnesium is beneficial to maintaining a healthy heart. It is found in fresh dark green vegetables, soybeans, whole grains, figs, apples, corn, and almonds.
- Avoid saturated fats. These are found in meat, eggs, and dairy products including chicken and turkey. In other words, eat a strict vegetarian diet to help reverse your heart disease.
- Learn about the benefits of essential fatty acids. Take flax seed supplements – available at healthfood stores.
- Get an adequate supply of antioxidants, which include vitamins A, C and E, beta-carotene, and various flavonoids.
- Drink plenty of water to replenish the fluids in your system.
- Drinking alcohol lightly or moderately, especially red wine, lowers the risk of experiencing a heart attack (*New England Journal of Medicine*, May 11, 1995). However, though light drinking may be beneficial to the heart, alcohol is related to many other serious health problems. Alcohol consumption increases the risk of cancers of the breast, head, mouth, larynx, esophagus, neck, and pancreas, and also increases the risk of nutritional deficiencies and cirrhosis of the liver. Alcohol alters brain function, increases the risk of brain hemorrhage, constricts blood vessels, increases triglycerides, and destroys an enzyme necessary for contraction. Heavy drinking can lead to a serious heart condition called alcoholic cardiomyopathy — a weakening of the heart muscles (*Journal of the American Medical Association*, July 12, 1995). Women are more susceptible to the damaging effects of alcohol because they have a smaller amount of the substance called alcohol dehydrogenase, which breaks down alcohol in the stomach and liver. Older people become intoxicated easier and their body tissues can be harmed my smaller amounts of alcohol. Alcohol interferes with the absorption of nutrients and can have an effect on medication.
- Garlic helps the body maintain a healthy cholesterol level. Take garlic supplements every day — unless otherwise instructed by your doctor. Unscented garlic tablets are available in many healthfood stores.
- Some kinds of fish have a polyunsaturated fat called eicosapentaneac acid (EPA). This fat thins the blood and reduces the risk of experiencing a blood clot that may hasten a heart attack. The problem with taking fish oil supplements is that the oil is derived from the liver of the fish. The liver is the detoxification center of the body. Livers and tissues of fish often contain man made chemical and industrial pollutants, such as PCBs, mercury, DDT, arsenic, and lead.
    Better sources of EPAs are flaxseed oil, soybeans and soybean products, walnuts, and wheat germ oil.
- Oats have been proven to be helpful in bringing cholesterol to healthy levels.
- Purchase mistletoe (viscum album) abstract at your healthfood store and take this to help lower your blood pressure.
- Experience humor to help release stress.
- Massage your spouse, and have your spouse massage you.

Signs and symptoms of heart and circulatory system disease can include:
• Arm or leg pain.
• Sudden changes in vision.
• Fainting.
• Light-headedness.
• Shortness of breath.
• Constant fatigue.
• Heart palpitations.
• Chest pain.
• Unexplainable skin sores.
• Swollen ankles.

Classic symptoms of a heart attack may include (Many people report no symptoms):
• Persistent pain, pressure, or tightness in the center of the chest.
• Chest discomfort radiating to the neck, jaw, shoulder, or arms.
• Shortness of breath.
• Numbness in the left arm.
• Tingling in the inner part of the left arm.
• Dizziness.
• Cold sweat.
• Nausea and vomiting.

Some people have normal-appearing cardiograms for several hours into their heart attacks. In a study that was performed at the Cleveland Mayo Clinic, only 29 of 67 patients who were experiencing heart attacks were identified through their EKGs.

There is nothing more beneficial to the health of a heart than a healthy, low-cholesterol, and lowfat diet that includes plenty of fresh fruits and vegetables along with sufficient exercise, and abstinence from tobacco products.

American Association of Cardiovascular and Pulmonary Rehabilitation, 7611 Elmwood Ave., Ste. 201, Middletown, WI 53562

American College of Advancement in Medicine, PO Box 3427, Laguna Hills, CA 92653; (714)583-7666

American College of Cardiology, 9111 Old Georgetown Rd., Bethesda, MD 20814; (301)897-5400 or (800)253-4636

American Heart Association (offices in nearly every state), 7272 Greenville Ave., Dallas, TX 75231-4596; (214)373-6300 or (202)822-9380 or (800)242-8721; Net: http://www.amhrt.org — or — gopher://gopher.amhrt.org./

Arizona Heart Institute & Foundation, (800)835-2920

Canadian Cardiovascular Society, 360 Victoria Ave, Ste. 401, Westmount, Quebec H3Z 2N4 Canada; (514)482-3407

Cardiac Alert, Phillips Business Information, 7811 Montrose Rd., Potomac, MD 20854; (301)340-2100 or (800)722-9000

Cardiomyopathy and Transplant Center, Division of Cardiac Surgery, Brigham and Women's Hospital, 75 Francis St., Boston, MA 02115; (617)732-7678

Cardiovascular Institute of the South, Net: http://www.cardio.com/

Cholesterol, Net: http://nearnet.gnn.com/wic/nutrit.02.html

Cleveland Clinic, 9500 Euclid Ave., Cleveland, OH 44195; (216)444-2200

Congenital Heart Anomalies Support, Education and Resources, 2112 N. Wilkins Rd., Swanton, OH 43558; (419)825-5575

Garlic Information Center, Cornell University Medial Center, 515 E. 71st St., Ste. 904, New York, NY 10021; (800)330-5922

Health and Healing Newsletter, Phillips Publishing, 7811 Montrose Rd., Potamic, MD 20854

For a free brochure titled *Living with Heart Disease: Is it Heart Failure?*, write or call
Heart Failure Guidelines, US Public Health Services Agency for Healthcare Policy, PO Box 8547, Silver Spring, MD 20907; (800)358-9295

The Heart Health Newsletter, Heart and Stroke Foundation of Canada, 160 George St., Ste. 200, Ottawa, Ontario, K1N 9M2 Canada; (613)237-4361

Heart Mind Body Institute, Net: http://www.power.net/hbm/hbm1.html

The Heart Preview Gallery, Net: http://sln.fi.edu/tfi/preview/heartpreview.html

High Blood pressure Information Center, 2121 Wisconsin Ave., NW, Ste. 410, Washington, DC 20036; (301)251-1222

The Mayo Clinic has the largest cardiovascular staff of any medical clinic in the world.
Mayo Clinic, 200 S. W. First St., Rochester, MN 55905; (507)284-2511

John McDougall writes books about how to improve health through diet, including reversing heart disease. He and his wife work together on the health books, cook books, videos, and a newsletter.
The McDougalls, PO Box 14039, Santa Rosa, CA 95402; (707)576-1654

National Institutes of Health, High Blood pressure Information Center, Bethesda, MD 20892; (301)496-1809

National Heart, Lung and Blood Institute Information Center, National Institutes of Health, PO Box 30105, Bethesda, MD 20824-0105; (301)251-1222 or (800)575-WELL

The Preventative Medicine Research Institute offers one-week residential retreats where heart patients are taught how to reverse the progression of cardiovascular disease through stress management, exercise, and diet. Dr. Dean Ornish, the author of books on reversing heart disease, is associated with the PMRI.
Preventative Medicine Research Institute, 900 Bridgeway, Ste. 1, Sausalito, CA 94965; (415)332-2525 or (800)775-PMRI

Preview of the Heart, Net: http://sln.fi.edu/tfi/preview/heartpreview.html

Pritikin Longevity Center, 1910 Ocean Front Walk, Santa Monica, CA 90405; (310)450-5433 or (800)421-9911 — or — 5875 Collins Ave., Miami Beach, FL 33140; (305)866-2237 or (800)327-4914

Society for Cardiac Angiography and Intervention, PO Box 40279, San Francisco, CA 94150; (415)647-1668

To locate a wide variety of health spa hotels where guests are taught nutritional eating and effective exercises, call
Spa Finders, (800)255-7727 or in New York call (212)924-6800

Telectronics Pacing Systems; Implant recipients' information line (800)349-9446

UCLA Cardiomyopathy Center, 10833 La Conte, Los Angeles, CA 90024; (310)825-8811

University of Pittsburgh Heart Institute, Pittsburgh, PA; (412)647-8762

Wakunago produces organically grown garlic that is sold in pill form.
Wakunago of America, 23501 Madero, Mission Viejo, CA 92691; (800)421-2998

Whitaker Wellness Institute, 4321 Birch St., Ste. 100, Newport Beach, CA 92660; (714)851-1550

• HERBS AND PLANT-BASED (BOTANICAL) MEDICINES/THERAPIES

(Also see Alternative and Holistic Healthcare, and Oriental Medicine)

Books:
• *Chinese Herb Medicine and Therapy*, by Hong yen Hsu PhD and William G. Preacher MC; Keats Publishing, 1982

- *Chinese Herbal Therapy: A Guide to it's Principles & Practice,* by Takahide Kuwaki, MD; Oriental Healing Arts Institute, 1990
- *The Complete Woman's Herbal: A Manual of Healing Herbs and Nutrition for Personal Well-Being and Family Care,* by Anne McIntyre; Henry Holt, 1995
- *Herbal Medicine: The Natural Way to Get Well and Stay Well,* by Dian Dincin Buchman; Wings Books, 1979
- *The Little Herb Encyclopedia: The Handbook of Nature's Remedies for a Healthier Life,* by Jack Ritchason; Woodland Books, 1994
- *Herb's for Common Ailments,* by Anne McIntyre; Fireside Books, 1992
- *Herb's that Heal: Prescription for Herbal Healing,* by Michael A. Weiner, PhD & Janet A. Weiner; Quantum Books, 1994
- *Medical Botany: Plants Affecting Man's Health,* by Walter H. Lewis and Memory P.F. Elvin-Lewis; John Wiley & Sons, 1977
- *The New Age Herbalist: How to Use Herb's for Healing, Nutrition, Body Care, and Relaxation,* by Richard Mabey, Michael McIntyre, Pamela Michael, Gail Duff, and John Steven; Collier Books, 1988
- *Prescription for Nutritional Healing: A Practical A-Z Reference to Drug-Free Remedies Using Vitamins, Minerals, Herb's, and Food Supplements,* by James F, Balch MD and Phyllis A. Balch CNC; Avery Publishing Group, 1990

American Botanical Council, PO Box 201660, Austin, TX 78720-1660; (512)331-8868

American Herbalist Guild, PO Box 1683, Soquel, CA 95073; (408)464-2441

American Herb Association, PO Box 1673, Nevada City, CA 95959

Aphrodisia, 282 Bleeker St., New York, NY 10014; (212)989-6440

Avena Botanicals, 219 Mill St., Rockport, ME 04856; (207)594-0694; Fax (207)594-2975

Back-2-Nature, Net: http://netmar.com/~back2nat/TTOIndex.html

Dragon Herbarium, Net: http://www.teleport.com/~seahorse/dragon/

East Earth Herbs, P.O. Box 2082, Eugene, OR 97402; (541)687-0155 or (800)827-HERB; Fax (541)485-7347

Ellon Traditional Flower Remedies, 644 Merrick Rd., Lynbrook, NY 11563-2332; (516)593-2206 or (800)423-2256; E-mail: rbrody01@interserv.com — or — Net: http://cybershopping.com/ellon

Frontier Cooperative Herbs, PO Box 299, Norway, IA 52318; (800)786-1388

Health Center for Better Living (herb catalog), 1414 Rosemary Lane, Naples, FL 33940-4283; (800)544-4225

The Herbal Green Pages, The Herb Growing and Marketing Network, PO Box 245, Silver Spring, PA 17575-0245; (717)393-3295

Herbal Hall, Net: http://www.crl.com/~robbee/herbal.html

Interweave Press is the publisher of *Herb Companion Magazine.* Subscriptions are $24 per year. The magazine features articles on both herbs for cooking (culinary) and herbs for healing (medicinal).
The Herb Companion, Interweave Press, 201 E. 4th St., Loveland, CO 80537; (970)669-7672; E-mail: HC@IWP.Compuserve.Com

Herb Hypercard, Net: gopher://nic.lth.se

Herb Information, Net: http://www.healthcraze.com — or — http://sunsite.unc.edu/herbs

Herb'n Outfitters, Net: http://204.213.234.53/

The Herb Quarterly, PO Box 689, San Anselmo, CA 94960-9810; (415)455-9540 or (800)371-HERB

Herb Research Foundation, 1007 Pearl St., Ste. 200, Boulder, CO 80302; (303)449-2265 or (800)748-2617; Net: http://sunsite.unc.edu/herbs

Herbs for Kids, PO Box 837, Bozeman, MT 59771; (406)587-0180

The Herb, Spice and Medicinal Plant Digest, Lyle E. Craker, Dept. of Plant and Soil Sciences, University of Massachusetts, Amherst, MA 01003; (413)545-2347

Indiana Botanic Gardens, 3401 East Ridge Rd., Hobart, IN 46342; (219)947-4040

Kwan Yin Herb Company, PO Box 18617, Spokane, WA 99208

Motherlove Herbal Company, 280 Stratton Park, Bellvue, CO 80512; (303)493-2892

Mountain Rose Herbs, PO Box 2000, Redway, CA 95560; (800)879-3337

My Life International, Net: http://www.cashflow.com/mylife

Native Essense Herb Company, 216M N. Pueblo Rd., Ste. 301, Taos, NM 87571; (800)358-0513

Nature's Bounty, PO Box 9001, Oakdale, NY 11769; (800)645-1030

Northeast Herbal Association, PO Box 146, Marshalfield, VT 05658-0146

Penn Herb Co., 603 N. 2nd St., Philadelphia, PA 19123-3098; (800)523-9971

Traditional Medicinals, 4515 Ross Rd., Sebastopol, CA 95472

Vital Herb/Everyoung Herbs, 1850 S. Sepulveda Blvd., Ste. 203, Los Angeles, CA 90025; (310)479-8862

Wish Garden Herbs, PO Box 1304, Boulder, CO 80306; (303)665-9508

ZAND Herbal Formulas, PO Box 5312, Santa Monica, CA 90409; (310)822-0500

• HOSPICE AND BEREAVEMENT (Also see *Living Wills*, and *Final Relief*)

Books:
- *Everybody Dies: A Guide to Final Arrangements*, by Partridge Publications (1651 W. Foothill Blvd., Ste. F-105, Upland, CA 91786)
- *Final Choices: To Live or Die in an Age of Medical Technology*, by George M. Burnell; Insight Books/Plenum Press, 1993
- *Letting Go: Death, Dying & the Law*, by Melvin I. Urofsky; Charles Scribner's Sons/Macmillan Publishing Co., 1993
- *National Directory of Bereavement Support Groups and Services*, by Mary M. Wong; ADM Publishing (PO Box 751155, Forest Hills, NY 11375-8755; [718]657-1277; E-mail: adm pub@internetmci.com — or — Net: http://www.ReadersNdex.com/ADMpub)
- *The Other Mid-Life Crisis: Everything You Need to Know About Wills, Hospitals, Life-and-Death Decisions, and Final Matters*, by Adeline Rosemire (arosemire@aol.com); Meridian Publishing ([800]270-2116), 1996
- *Planning for Incapacity: A Self-Help Guide*, by the American Association of Retired Persons. (To obtain a copy, send $5 to Legal Counsel for the Elderly, PO Box 96474, Washington, DC 20090-6474)
- *Saying Good-bye to Daniel: When Death Is the Best Choice*, by Juliet Cassuto Rothman; Continuum Publishing, 1995
- *When There Are No Words: Finding Your Way to Cope With Loss and Grief*, by Charlie Walton; Pathfinder Publishing, 1996

Hospices are organized to give assistance to dying people during their remaining months or weeks, and to the families of dying people to cope with the transition both before and after the death. The focus of hospice care is on pain relief and the comfort (palliative care) of the dying person. A hospice provider can help determine what a dying person needs, and arrange for necessary equipment and supplies for the person to remain at home, or in a hospice environment. Beside the family that can help care for a dying person, the hospice can assist with a team that may include doctors, nurses, social workers, counselors, home health aides, clergy, therapists, and volunteers. Hospice care is covered by many insurance plans. Other financial coverage can be provided for people who do not have insurance.

Bereavement Magazine is published six times per year. The company also publishes booklets on bereavement.

Bereavement Magazine, 8133 Telegraph Dr., Colorado Springs, CO 80920-7169; (719)282-1948; Fax (719)282-1850; E-mail grief@usa.net

Center for Loss & Life Transition, 3735 Broken Bow Rd., Ft. Collins, CO 80526; (970)226-6050

Children's Hospice International, 1850 M St., NW, Ste. 900, Washington, DC 20036; (703)684-0330

Compassionate Friends (for parents who have had children die), PO Box 3696, Oak Brook, IL 60522-3696; (708)990-0010

For information on laws governing funeral homes, contact the
Federal Trade Commission, Public Reference Branch, 6th St. and Pennsylvania Ave., Rm. 130, NW, Washington, DC 20580; (202)326-2502

Foundation for Hospice and Home Care, 519 C St., NE, Stanton Park, Washington, DC 20002; (202)547-6586

For referrals to hospices and palliative care programs nationwide, contact the
Hospice Education Institute, 190 Westbrook Rd., Essex, CT 06426; (203)767-1620 or (800)331-1620 or (800)544-2213

In Loving Memory (support for parents who have had children die), 1416 Green Run Ln., Reston, VA 22090; (703)435-0608

Life After Repeated Grief: Options (newsletter for parents who have had children die), 1192 S. Uvalda St., Aurora, CO 80013; (303)745-1799

National Association for Home Care, 519 C St., NE, Washington, DC 20002-5809; (202)547-7424; Fax (202)547-3540; Net: http://www.nahc.org

National Center for Grieving Children and Families, The Dougy Center, PO Box 86852, Portland, OR 97286; (503)775-5683

National Hospice Foundation, 1901 N. Moore St., Ste. 901, Arlington, VA 22209-1714; (703)516-4928; Fax (703)525-5762

National Hospice Organization, 1901 N. Moore St., Ste. 901, Arlington, VA 22209; (703)243-5900 or (800)658-8898

National Institute for Jewish Hospice, 8723 Alden Dr., Ste. 652, Los Angeles, CA 90048; (213)467-7423 or (800)446-4448

National Organization for Victim Assistance (information for victims and survivors of violent crime and disaster), 1757 Park Rd., NW, Washington, DC 20010' (202)232-6682 or (800)879-6682

Parents of Murdered Children, 100 E. 8th St., Cincinnati, OH 45202; (513)721-5683

Rainbows (support for children and adults who are grieving),1111 Tower Rd., Schaumburg, IL 60173; (708)310-1880

Society of Military Widows, 5535 Hempstead Wy., Springfield, VA 22151; (703)750-1342

• HOSPITALS, STATE LICENSING OF

Alabama Hospital Licensing Office, Dept. of Public Health, Environmental Health Service Standards Division, Bureau of Licensing and Certification, State Office Bldg., 434 Monroe St., Montgomery, AL 36130-1701; (205)242-2883

Alaska Hospital Licensing Office, Alaska Dept. of Health and Social Services, Division of Medical Assistance, Health Facilities Licensing and Certification, 4433 Business Park Blvd., Bldg. M, Anchorage, AK 99503; (907)561-2171

Arizona Hospital Licensing Office, Dept. of Health Services, Division of Emergency Medical Services and Health Care Facilities, 701 E. Jefferson, Phoenix, AZ 85304; (602)255-1177

Arkansas Hospital Licensing Office, Arkansas Dept. of Health, Bureau of Health Resources, Division of Health Facility Services, 4815 W. Markham St., Little Rock, AR 72205-3867; (501)661-2201

California Hospital Licensing Office, California Health and Welfare Agency, Dept. of Health Services, Division of Licensing and Certification, 714 P St., Sacramento, CA 95814-2070; (916)445-3045

Colorado Hospital Licensing Office, Colorado Dept. of Health, Office of Health Care and Prevention, Division of Health Facilities Regulation, 4210 E. 11th Ave., Denver, CO 80220; (303)331-6690

Connecticut Hospital Licensing Office, Connecticut Dept. of Health Services, Hospital and Health Care Division, Licensure and Certification, 1049 Asylum Ave., Hartford, CT 06106-2435; (203)566-3880

Delaware Hospital Licensing Office, Delaware Dept. of Health and Social Services, Office of Health Facilities Licensing and Certification, 3000 Newport Gap Pike, Bldg. C, Wilmington, DE 19808; (302)995-6674

District of Columbia Hospital Licensing Office, District of Columbia Dept. of Consumer and Regulatory Affairs, Service Facility Regulation Administration, Health Facility Division, 614 H St., NW, Washington, DC 20001; (202)727-7194

Florida Hospital Licensing Office, Florida Dept. of Health and Rehabilitative Services, Office of Regulation and Health Facilities, 1317 Winewood Blvd., Tallahassee, FL 32399-0700; (904)487-2513

Georgia Hospital Licensing Office, Georgia Dept. of Human Resources, Office of Regulatory Services, Standards and Licensure Section, 47 Trinity Ave., SW, Atlanta, GA 30334; (404)894-5144

Hawaii Hospital Licensing Office, Hawaii Dept. of Health, Hospital and Medical Facilities Branch, PO Box 3378, Honolulu, HI 96801; (808)548-5935

Idaho Hospital Licensing Office, Idaho Health Facilities Authority, 1655 Fairview Avenue, Ste. 206, Boise, ID 83702; (208)342-8772

Illinois Hospital Licensing Office, Illinois Dept. of Public Health, Office of Health Regulation, Health Facilities Standards Division, Hospital Licensing Section, 525 W. Jefferson St., Springfield, IL 62761; (217)782-4977

Indiana Hospital Licensing Office, Indiana State Board of Health, Division of Acute Care Services, 1330 W. Michigan St., Box 1964, Indianapolis, IN 46206; (317)633-8472

Iowa Hospital Licensing Office, Iowa Dept. of Inspections and Appeals, Division of Health Facilities, Lucas State Office Bldg., Des Moines, IA 50319; (515)281-4233

Kansas Hospital Licensing Office, Kansas Dept. of Health and Environment, Division of Health, Bureau of Adult and Child Care Facilities, Hospital Program, London State Office Bldg., 900 SW Jackson, Topeka KS 66612; (913)296-1240

Kentucky Hospital Licensing Office, Kentucky Human Resources Cabinet, Office of Inspector General, Division of Licensing and Regulation, 275 E. Main St., Frankfort, KY 40601; (502)564-2800

Louisiana Hospital Licensing Office, Louisiana Dept. of Health and Hospitals, Health Standards Section, Division of Licensing and Certification, 1201 Capitol Access Road, PO Box 3767, Baton Rouge, LA 70821; (504)342-0138

Maine Hospital Licensing Office, Maine Dept. of Health Services, Bureau of Medical Services, Division of Licensing and Certification, Statehouse Station 11, Augusta, ME 04333; (207)289-2606

Maryland Hospital Licensing Office, Maryland Dept. of Health and Mental Hygiene, Licensing and Certification Division, 4201 Patterson Avenue, Baltimore, MD 21215; (410)764-2750

Massachusetts Hospital Licensing Office, Massachusetts Executive Office of Human Services, Dept. of Public Health, Bureau of Health Care Systems, Division of Health Care Quality, 150 Tremont St., 2nd Flr., Boston, MA 02111; (617)727-5860

Michigan Hospital Licensing Office, Michigan Dept. of Public Health, Health Facilities Bureau, Division of Health Facilities, Licensing and Certification, 3423 N. Logan, PO Box 30195, Lansing, MI 48909; (517)335-8505

Minnesota Hospital Licensing Office, Minnesota Dept. of Health, Health Resources Bureau, 717 Delaware St., SE, Box 9441, Minneapolis, MN 55440; (612)643-2171

Mississippi Hospital Licensing Office, Mississippi Dept. of Health, Division of Licensure and Certification, 2688 Insurance Center Drive, Jackson, MS 39216; (601)981-6880

Missouri Hospital Licensing Office, Missouri Dept. of Health, Health Resources Division, Bureau of Hospital Licensing and Certification, PO Box 570, Jefferson City, MO 65102; (314)751-6302

Montana Hospital Licensing Office, Montana Dept. of Health and Environmental Sciences, Division of Health Services, Licensing, Certification and Construction Bureau, Cogswell Bldg., Rm. C214, Helena, MT 59620; (406)444-2037

Nebraska Hospital Licensing Office, Nebraska Dept. of Health, Health Facilities Standards Bureau, 301 Centennial Mall S., PO Box 95007, Lincoln, NE 68509; (402)471-2946

Nevada Hospital Licensing Office, Nevada Dept. of Human Resources, Division of Health, Bureau of Regulatory Health Services, 505 E. King St., Rm. 600, Carson City, NV 89710; (702)687-4475

New Hampshire Hospital Licensing Office, New Hampshire Dept. of Health and Human Services, Division of Public Health Services, Bureau of Health Facilities Administration, 6 Hazen Dr., Concord, NH 03301; (603)271-4592

New Jersey Hospital Licensing Office, New Jersey Dept. of Health, Health Facilities Evaluation and Licensing Division, 300 Whitehead Rd., CN-367, Trenton, NJ 08625; (609)588-7725

New Mexico Hospital Licensing Office, New Mexico Dept. of Health and Environment, Division of Public Health, Licensing and Certification Bureau, 1190 St. Francis Dr., Santa Fe, NM 87501; (505)827-2409

New York Hospital Licensing Office, New York State Dept. of Health, Office of Health Systems Management, Bureau of Health Standards and Surveillance, Corning Tower, Empire State Plaza, Albany, NY 12237-0001; (518)473-3517

North Carolina Hospital Licensing Office, North Carolina Dept. of Human Resources, Division of Facility Services, Council Bldg., 701 Barbour Drive, Raleigh, NC 27603; (919)733-2342

North Dakota Hospital Licensing Office, North Dakota Dept. of Health and Consolidated Laboratories, Health Resources Section, Health Facilities Division, 600 E. Boulevard, Bismark, North Dakota 58505; (701)224-2352

Ohio Hospital Licensing Office, Ohio Dept. of Health, Bureau of Medical Services, Division of Licensure and Certification, 246 N. High St., PO Box 118, Columbus, OH 43266-0588; (614)466-7857

Oklahoma Hospital Licensing Office, Oklahoma Dept. of Health, Medical Facilities Services, 1000 NE 10th St., PO Box 53551, Oklahoma City, OK 73152; (405)271-6868

Oregon Hospital Licensing Office, Oregon Dept. of Human Resources, Division of Health, Office of Environment and Health Systems, Health Facilities Section, State Office Bldg., Rm. 608, PO Box 231, Portland, OR 97207; (503)229-5686

Pennsylvania Hospital Licensing Office, Pennsylvania Dept. of Health, Office of Planning and Quality-assurance, Bureau of Quality-assurance, Division of Hospitals, 532 Health and Welfare Bldg., Harrisburg, PA 17108; (717)783-8980

Rhode Island Hospital Licensing Office, Rhode Island Dept. of Health, Family Health Services, Division of Facilities Regulation, 3 Capitol Hill, Providence, RI 02908; (401)277-2827

South Carolina Hospital Licensing Office, South Carolina Dept. of Health and Environmental Control, Division of Health Regulation, Health Facilities Regulation Bureau, 2600 Bull St., Columbia, SC; (803)734-4842

South Dakota Hospital Licensing Office, South Dakota Dept. of Health, Licensure and Certification Program, Foss Bldg., 523 E. Capitol, Pierre, SD 57501; (605)773-3364

Tennessee Hospital Licensing Office, Tennessee Dept. of Health and Environment, Manpower and Facilities Bureau, Division of Health Care Facilities, 344 Cordell Hull Bldg., Nashville, TN 37247-0101; (615)367-6303

Texas Hospital Licensing Office, Texas Dept. of Health, Health Facility Licensure and Certification Division, 1100 W. 49th St., Austin, TX 78756; (512)458-7245

Utah Hospital Licensing Office, Utah Dept. of Health, Community Health Services Division, Health Facilities Licensing Bureau, 288 N. 1460 W., Salt Lake City, UT 84116; (801)538-6152

Vermont Hospital Licensing Office, Vermont Agency of Human Services, Dept. of Aging and Disabilities, Licensing and Protection Division, 19 Commerce St., PO Box 536, Williston, VT 05495; (802)836-7250

Virginia Hospital Licensing Office, Virginia Dept. of Health, Office of Planning and Regulatory Services, Division of Licensure and Certification, 3600 W. Broad St., Ste. 216, Richmond, VA 23230; (804)367-2102

Washington Hospital Licensing Office, Washington Dept. of Social and Health Services, Health and Rehabilitative Services, Health Services Division, Health Facilities Survey Section, Mail Stop OB-44, Olympia, WA 98504; (206)753-5851

West Virginia Hospital Licensing Office, West Virginia Dept. of Health and Human Resources, Administration and Finance Bureau, Health Facilities Licensure and Certification Section, Bldg. 3, Rm. 265, State Capitol Complex, Charleston, WV 25305; (304)558-0050

Wisconsin Hospital Licensing Office, Wisconsin Dept. of Health and Social Services, Division of Health, Bureau of Quality Compliance, One W. Wilson Street, PO Box 7850, Madison, WI 53707; (608)267-7185

Wyoming Hospital Licensing Office, Wyoming Dept. of Health, Division of Health and Human Services, Medical Facilities, Hathaway Bldg., Cheyenne, WY 82002; (307)777-7123

• HYPNOSIS

American Academy of Medical Hypnoanalysts, 5587 Murray Rd., Memphis, TN 38119

American Association of Professional Hypnotherapists, PO Box 29, Boones Mill, VA 24065; (540)334-3035

American Hypnosis Association, 18607 Ventura Blvd., Ste. 310, Tarzana, CA 91356; (818)344-4464

American Society for Clinical Hypnosis, 2250 E. Devon, Ste. 336, Des Plaines, IL 60018-5434; (708)297-3317

National Guild of Hypnotists, PO Box 308, Merrimack, NH 03054-0308; (603)429-9438

Society for Clinical and Experimental Hypnosis, 6728 Old McLean Village Dr., McLean, VA 22101-3906; (703)556-9222

• INSURANCE

Book:
* *Insuring National Health Care: The Canadian Experience — What Americans can learn from one of the most successful health care programs in the world,* by Malcolm G. Taylor, University of North Carolina Press, 1990

Getting insurance
Group insurance is less expensive and is likely to have more benefits than an individual insurance plan. Joining an HMO may also be a wiser choice than purchasing an individual insurance plan. Before you purchase insurance coverage for yourself, check to see if you may be eligible for health insurance through:
* Your union.
* An association, such as the Chamber of Commerce or a professional association.
* Your bank.
* Your credit card company.
* Another insurance plan that you already carry.
* Your school.
* An alumni association.
* Medicare.
* Medicaid.

You and your insurance coverage
1. Do you know what type of insurance plan you have and what it covers?
   * A managed care plan or other form of insurance plan, such as an indemnity plan, a health maintenance organization (HMO), individual practice association (IPA), or a preferred provider organization (PPO).
   * Accident insurance: covers care needed because of an accident.
   * Comprehensive insurance: a package that may cover a selection of the following: accident, all diseases, dental, disability, hospital care, long-term care, major medical, surgical, and healthcare needs during travel
   * Dental insurance: covers regular dental care as well as a variety of other dental needs.
   * Disability and income insurance: provides income when a person is not able to work because of an accident or illness outside of those ailments covered by state disability insurance.
   * Disease-specific insurance: covers limited number of health problems.
   * Hospital insurance: covers inpatient and outpatient hospital services.
   * Long-term care insurance: covers care needed for a long period of time, such as nursing home care, or home care.
   * Major medical insurance: covers care needed for serious illnesses or because of an accident.
   * Medical/surgical insurance: covers doctor visits in the hospital or the office, lab tests, x-rays, prescriptions, surgeon's fees, and anesthesia.
2. Get a copy of your insurance policy and read it so you understand its terms and conditions.
3. Does the insurance plan have a 30-day trial period when you can cancel and receive a refund it you have decided it is not right for you?
4. Do you pay your insurance premium on a yearly or quarterly basis? Paying on a yearly basis may be less expensive.
   Find out what the grace period is. You may be required to pay the premium before a specific date, or they may allow you to be late a certain number of days without recourse.
5. Is your insurance company financially stable?
   You may want to check the rating of your insurance company in publications at your local library. Publications that have insurance ratings include those by A.M. Best, Duff & Phelps, Moody's, and Standard & Poor.

You may also want to find out if the insurance company is authorized to sell insurance in your state by calling the state insurance commissioner's office in your state capital.

6. Are you supposed to notify the insurance company before seeing a doctor?
   The insurance company may need to provide you with an approval code that you would then include on any paperwork you send them concerning treatment for that particular ailment.

7. Are you required to turn in paperwork by a certain date?

8. When you have an emergency and are treated by a doctor or at a hospital that is not in your insurance plan, are you required to visit a doctor from the insurance company's approved list to confirm that the treatment you received was indeed an emergency?

9. Is the deductible on a yearly basis, or is it a per-incident basis?
   A yearly deductible may be anywhere from $100 to more than $1,000. After you have paid this amount in medical bills every year, you are then required to cover a small portion of your bill, such as 20%.
   Know what your deductible is, and if you can change it.

10. Is there a total out-of-pocket limit on what you have to pay for your healthcare each year?
    After your medical bills have reached a certain dollar amount (stop-loss amount), the insurance company may cover all your bills up to a maximum limit. This way you may pay up to $1,000 a month or several thousand a month. Your insurance may have a lifetime limit of $1 million or more.

11. Does the plan require a deductible and copayments? You may want to choose a plan where basic services are covered.

12. Are there any waiting periods before certain insurance benefits become available to you?

13. Does your insurance policy not cover certain health conditions? Does the policy consider any of your health problems to be "preexisting conditions?"
    The company may not cover any preexisting conditions, or may cover them after a certain number of months. Find out what is excluded.

14. Does the insurance cover what is already covered in your automobile insurance, life insurance, homeowner insurance, or other insurance plan?

15. Does the insurance cover prescription drugs?

16. Does the insurance cover mental health needs, such as psychotherapy and family therapy?

17. Does the insurance cover alternative therapies, such as chiropractic, acupuncture, nutritional counseling, or special preventative care?

18. Does the insurance cover emergency care while you are traveling?

19. Can the insurance company change the benefits at its will?

20. Does the insurance plan have a conversion clause that allows you to purchase insurance coverage individually in the event that the group policy is terminated?

21. How much will it cost you to keep your insurance if you were to lose your job?

22. Is the insurance policy renewable?
    A guaranteed-renewable plan is preferable. The policy may only be written for a year. A guaranteed-renewable clause will allow you to keep the insurance and may also guarantee the price of the premium. A conditional-renewal clause may state that you may renew the plan under certain conditions, such as until you reach a certain age. An optionally renewable clause may state that the company can cancel the insurance on the anniversary date.

23. How much does the plan cover toward visits you receive from a doctor when you are in a hospital? Does it limit the number of doctor visits that are covered when you are in the hospital?

24. How many hospitalization days does the insurance cover?

25. Does the plan cover visits the doctor makes to your home?

26. How much does the plan cover when you visit a doctor in his office?

27. Does the policy cover diagnostic tests that are performed in the doctor's office?

28. Does the policy cover laboratory tests?

29. Does the plan cover second opinions?

30. Does the plan cover surgery as it is priced in your area, or does it provide a limited cost for surgery?

31. Does the plan cover the cost of consultants that your doctor may need to handle your case?

32. Does the policy cover the fee of more than one surgeon if an assistant surgeon is needed?

33. What hospitals and ambulatory surgery centers in your community accept your insurance plan?

34. What doctors in your community accept your insurance?

35. Are you supposed to choose one doctor as your primary physician ("gatekeeper"), or can you go to any doctor you like?

    Gatekeeper physicians are usually general physicians, family physicians, internists, or, if you are a woman, OB/GYNs. Some insurance plans allow women to have two primary care doctors, a gynecologist and a family doctor.

    Some insurance plans allow you to go to any doctor you like, but you have to pay a much higher premium if you choose a doctor outside the list of member doctors.

    Just because a doctor you want to see is not listed in the insurance company directory does not mean he is not under contract with the insurance plan. The doctor may have been signed with the insurance company after the directory was published. Some doctors who have unusual areas of training also may not be listed in the directory even though they are under contract with the insurance plan. The doctor may be limiting his practice to very unusual cases.

36. What are the requirements that need to be met before you can visit a specialist doctor?

37. Do you need to see your primary doctor to get approval for each visit to a specialist doctor for treatment of a chronic illness, or does one referral for a specialist last for a year or more (blanket referral)?

38. Does your insurance cover mental health needs, such as visiting with marriage and family counselors, or psychologists?

    Some insurance plans do not cover visits to mental health specialists. A patient may find the insurance company only covers prescriptions to risky psychoactive drugs, and only if the drugs are prescribed by the primary doctor (who likely has little training in mental health).

39. Does your insurance cover eye/vision care? If so, does it charge more to visit an ophthalmologist than it does to visit an optometrist?

40. What is the phone number of your health insurance company, and what department are you supposed to call when you have questions?

    • Always try to talk to the same person at your insurance company and always be polite to this person.

    • Keep a record of the time and date of all the phone calls you had with the insurance company, the name and title of the person you spoke with, and what was said.

- When you speak to the insurance company representative, ask if there is anything you are not doing that you should be doing to speed up the reimbursement process.

- All insurance companies have a formal procedure to deal with grievances. If you have a problem with the insurance company, ask to speak to a supervisor with the company. If the supervisor cannot help you, or refuses to help you, find out how to make a formal complaint with the company. Many insurance companies have an appeals process that you can use to clear up problems.

  If your insurance is part of your job benefits, check with the person at your workplace who handles the insurance work and see if he can help you with any problems you are having with the insurance company.

  In California there is a law that came into existence in 1996 where the California State Department of Corporations was required to begin handling complaints state residents have with their insurance companies. The CSDC set up a toll-free number, (800) 400-0815, where people who have grievances with their health insurance coverage may register complaints.

  Find out what laws exist in your state that will help you when you have problems with your insurance company. Your state insurance commissioner's office or other state agency may be able to help you.

- Keep a copy of all letters, completed forms, and other paperwork that you send to the insurance company.

- Keep all your medical records and your health insurance information in a file or drawer. You may want to invest in a small fireproof safe for storing these materials.

Alternative Health Insurance Services, (800)966-8467

American Managed Care and Review Association, 1227 — 25th St., NW, Ste. 610, Washington, DC 20037; (202)728-0506

Clinton Healthcare Security Act, Net: gopher://mchnet.ichp/ufl/edu

Communicating for Seniors, PO Box 677, Fergus Falls, MN 56538; (800)432-3276

Group Health Association of America, 1129 — 20th St., NW, Ste. 600, Washington, DC 20036; (202)778-3200

Health Insurance Association of America, 1025 Connecticut Ave., NW, Ste. 1200, Washington, DC 20036-3998; (202)223-7780

Joint Commission on the Accreditation of Healthcare Organizations, One Renaissance Blvd., Oakbrook Terrace, IL 60181; (708)916-5600

National Association of Insurance Commissioners, 120 W. 12th St., Kansas City, MO 64105; (816)842-3600

National Committee for Quality-assurance, 2000 L St., NW, Ste. 500, Washington, DC 20036; (202)955-3500

National Health Security Plan, Net: http:sunsite.unc.edu/ngs/NHSToC

National Insurance Consumer Helpline, American Council of Life Insurance, Health Insurance Association of America, Insurance Information Institute, 1001 Pennsylvania Avenue, NW, Washington, DC 20004; (800)942-4242

The Consolidated Omnibus Budget Reconciliation Act (COBRA) was passed in 1986 to allow for terminated employees who lose insurance coverage because of their termination, and for those who lose insurance coverage because of reduced work hours to purchase group health insurance through the employers insurance plan for themselves and their dependents and spouses who were covered by the insurance. Depending on the reason for the loss in insurance coverage, and who the insurance is covering, the insurance may be continued for 18 to 36 months. The law does not cover churches, the federal government, the District of Columbia, or employers with fewer than twenty employees. For more information on COBRA, contact the

Unites States Dept. of Labor, Pension and Welfare Benefits, Administration, Division of Technical Assistance and Inquiries, 200 Constitution Ave., NW, Rm. N-5619, Washington, DC 20210

White House Health Plan, Net: gopher://gopherinform.umd.edu

• INSURANCE — GOVERNMENT HEALTH PLANS

To find out if you are eligible for coverage under Medicare or Medicaid, contact your local Social Security office as it is listed in the phone book of your town.

To register a complaint against a doctor, hospital, or other health professional working under the Medicare sanctions program operated under the Department of Health and Human Services, contact the

Dept. of Health and Human Services, Office of the Inspector General, PO Box 17303, Baltimore, MD 21203-7303; (301)597-5779 or (800)368-5779

Healthcare Financing Administration, Office of Public Affairs, US Dept. of Health Services, Hubert H. Humphrey Bldg., Rm. 435-H, 200 Independence Ave. SW, Washington, DC 20001; (202)690-6113; Medicare hotline (800)638-6833

Health Resources and Services of the Federal Government; (301)443-2086

Inspector General's Medicare Fraud Line, (800)368-5779

Medicare Information Hotline, US Dept. of Health and Human Services, Health Care Financing Administration, Washington DC 20201; (800)888-1770 or (800)888-1998

Medicare Medigap Insurance Fraud Line, US Dept. of Health and Human Services, Health Care Financing Administration, Washington, DC 20201; (800)638-6833

The United States Government Printing Office prints a yearly *Medicare Information Report.* It is available in some libraries, or can be purchased through the

United States Government Printing Office; (202)783-3238

• KIDNEYS

The American Association of Kidney Patients publishes a magazine twice a year called *Renalife.*

American Association of Kidney Patients, 100 S. Ashley Dr., Ste. 280, Tampa, FL 33602; (813)223-7099 or (800)749-2257

American Kidney Fund, 8110 Executive Blvd., Rockville, MD 20852; (301)881-3052 or (800)638-8299

Cystinuria Support Network, 22814 NE 21st Pl., Redmond, WA 98053

IgA Nephropathy Support Network, 234 Summit Ave., Jenkintown, PA 19046

The Kidney Stones Network Newsletter ($25 a year), Four Geez Press, 1911 Douglas Blvd., Ste. 85-131, Roseville, CA 95661; (800)2-KIDNEYS; E-mail: ggolomb@NS.NET — or — Net: http://www.readersndex.com/fourgeez

National Kidney and Urologic Diseases Information Clearinghouse, 3 Information Way, Bethesda, MD 20892-3580; (301)654-4415 or (800)891-5390

National Kidney Cancer Association, 1234 Sherman Ave., Ste. 203, Evanston, IL 60202-1375; (708)332-1051; Fax (708)328-4425; Net: nkca@merle.acns.nwu.edu

National Kidney Foundation, 30 E. 33rd St., New York, NY 10016; (212)889-2210 or (800)622-9010

Oxalosis and Hyperoxaluria Foundation, 37 R Thompson St., Maynard, MA 01754; (508)461-0614; E-mail: OHF@OHF.Ultranet.com — or — Net: http://www.ultra net.com/~ohf/

Polycystic Kidney Research Foundation, 4901 Main St., Ste. 320, Kansas City, MO 64112-2674; (816)753-2873 or (800)753-2873; E-mail: 75713.2275@Compuserve.com — or — Net: http:www.kumc.edu/pkrf/

Positive Renal Outreach Program, PO Box 311, Maryknoll, NY 10545-0311

Renalnet, Net: http://ns.gamewood.net//renalnet.html

• LEGAL ASSISTANCE

Books:

- *The Consumer Reports Law Book,* Consumer Reports Books (PO Box 10637, Des Moines, IA 50336; [515]237-4903)
- *The Consumer's Legal Guide to Today's Healthcare: Your Medical Rights and How to Assert Them,* by Stephen L. Isaacs, JD & Ava C. Swartz, MPH; Houghton Mifflin Co., 1992
- *The Criminal Elite: The Sociology of White Collar Crime,* by James William Coleman; St. Martin's Press, 1985
- The Complete Book of Victims' Rights, by Debra J. Wilson, JD; ProSe Associates, 1995
- *Doctors from Hell,* by Fred Rosen; Windsor Publishing, 1993
- *Galileo's Revenge: Junk Science in the Courtroom,* by Peter Huber; Basic Books, 1993
- *The Girl Who Died Twice: The Libby Zion Case and the Hidden Hazards of Hospitals,* by Natalie Robins; Delacorte Press, 1995
- *Kiplinger's Handbook of Personal Law: Protect Yourself From Everyday Legal Problems that Could Cost You Plenty,* by Jill Rachlin; Kiplinger Books, 1994
- *The Lawyer Book: A Nuts and Bolts Guide to Client Survival,* by Wesley J. Smith; Price, Stern, Sloan, 1986
- *A Measure of Malpractice: Medical Injury, Malpractice Litigation, and Patient Compensation,* by Paul C. Weiler, Howard H. Hiatt, Joseph P. Newhouse, William G. Johnson, Troyen A. Brennan, and Lucian L. Leape; Harvard University Press, 1993
- *Medical Malpractice on Trial,* by Paul C. Weiler; Harvard University Press, 1991
- *Representing Yourself: What You Can Do Without a Lawyer,* published by Public Citizen's Health Research Group ([202]833-3000)
- *The Rights of Patients: The Basic ACLU Guide to Patient Rights,* by George Annas; Humana Press, 1992
- *Silent Violence, Silent Death: The Hidden Epidemic of Medical Malpractice,* by Harvey Rosenfield; Essential Books ([202]387-8030), 1994
- *Wrongful Death: A Medical Tragedy,* by Sandra M. Gilbert; W.W. Norton & Company, 1995
- *You Must Be Dreaming,* by Barbara Noel and Kathryn Watterson; Simon & Schuster, 1992

The 8-volume *Martindale-Hubbell Law Directory* (630 Central Ave., New Providence, NJ 07974) lists attorneys in the US. Many public libraries carry a copy of it. The American Trial Lawyer's Association also publishes a directory of lawyers.

Courthouse records of medical malpractice cases may point you in the direction of a lawyer who can handle your case. Newspaper articles about medical malpractice are also a good way to find the lawyers in your area who are experienced in medical malpractice.

Check your local courthouse to see what books, pamphlets, and other resources they have on hand that may help you in your legal decisions.

The American Academy of Hospital Attorneys is an association of attorneys who represent, or are employees of, hospitals or other healthcare facilities and organizations. **American Association of Hospital Attorneys,** American Hospital Association, 840 N. Lake Shore Dr., Chicago, IL 60611; (312)280-6601

American Association of Legal Nurse Consultants, PO Box 3616, Phoenix, AZ 85030-3616; (602)495-2899

American Association of Medico-Legal Consultants, The Barclay, Rittenhouse Square, Philadelphia, PA 19103; (215)545-6363

The American Association of Nurse Attorneys is made up of attorneys who are in nursing school, nurses who are in law school, and nurses who are attorneys.

The American Association of Nurse Attorneys, 720 Light St., Baltimore, MD 21230-3816; (410)752-3318

The American Association of Testifying Attorneys was founded in 1948. It was formerly known as the "Insurance company Doctors Council." The Association provides information and publishes literature (*Malpractice/Torts Emergency Reports, Effective Testimony Bulletin*, and *Cross Examination Comprehender*)that can train a doctor to testify in court.
American Association of Testifying Attorneys, 2330 S. Brentwood Blvd., St. Louis, MO 63144-2096; (314)961-2300

American Bar Association, 740 — 15th St., NW, Washington, DC 20005; (312)988-5000; Net: http://www.abanet.org/ABA/aba.html — or — the ABA Commission on Legal Problems of the Elderly; (202)662-8690; Net: abaelderly@attmail.com

American College of Legal Medicine, 611 E. Wells St., Milwaukee, WI 53202; (414)276-1881

American College of Trial Lawyers, (714)727-3194

American Trial Lawyer's Association, 1050 – 31st St., NW, Washington, DC 20007-4499; (800)424-2725 or 2727

Canadian Law Notes, Net: http://www-bprc.mps.ohio-state.edu/cgi-bin/hpp?Mur Co.html

To find if someone has done time in prison, call the
Inmate Locator Service of the Federal Bureau of Prisons in Washington DC, (202)307-3126

International Academy of Trial Lawyers, (408)275-6767

The International Society of Barristers does not refer people to attorneys. However, the group will confirm if a lawyer is a member of the society.
International Society of Barristers; (313)763-0165

Law.Net, Net: http://law.net/

Law-Related Gophers and Web Servers, Net: http://riskweb.bus.utexas.edu/legal /html

Lawyers Weekly USA, 41 West St., Boston, MA 02111; (617)451-7300

Legal Indexes, Net: http://tarlton.law.utexas.edu/library/netref/law_search.html

Legal Information Institute at Cornell, Net: http://www.law.cornell.edu

Legal.Net, Net: http://www.lgal.net

Michigan Lawyers Weekly, 333 S. Washington Ave., Ste. 300, Lansing, MI 48933; (800)678-5297

National Academy of Elder Law Attorneys, 655 N. alvernon Wy., Ste. 108, Tucson, AZ 85711; (602)881-4005

Since 1969, the National Health Law Program has served as a legal services national support center specializing in health issues for low-income people, minorities, the disabled, and the elderly. NHeLP communicates with a variety of Washington-based groups on healthcare access issues. NHeLP has published numerous guides on a variety of health issues including Medicaid, Medicare, state and local indigent healthcare programs, maternal and child health, and civil rights and healthcare.
National Health Law Program, 2639 S. LaCienega Blvd., Los Angeles, CA 90034; (310)204-6010

National Women's Law Center, 11 Dupont Circle, NW, Ste. 800, Washington, DC 20036; (202)588-5180

National Senior Citizen's Law Project, (202)887-5280 or (213)482-3550

Nolo Press publishes books on legal matters for consumers. Call them for a catalog.
Nolo Press, (510)549-1976 or (800)992-6656; E-mail: NOLOSUB@NOLOPRESS.com

Several books put out by the People's Medical Society deal with medical rights.
People's Medical Society, 462 Walnut St., Allentown, PA 18102; (215)770-1670

Pike Institute on Law and Disability, Harry Beyer, Esq, Director, Boston University School of Law, 765 Commonwealth Ave., Boston, MA 02215; (617)353-2904

Public Citizen Books publishes a book titled *Representing Yourself: What You Can Do Without a Lawyer.* The book tells how to solve routine legal problems without a lawyer, how to decide if you do need a lawyer, and how to make sure you are adequately represented.
Public Citizen Books, 2000 P St., NW, Ste. 605, Washington, DC 20036; (202)833-3000

St. Louis University Center for Health Law Studies, Net: http://lawlib.slu.edu /centers/hlthlaw.htm

Victims of Crime Resource Center, (800)842-8467

Women's Legal Resources, Net: http://asa.ugl.lib.umich.edu/chdocs/womenpolicy /women/lawpolicy.html

World Wide Web Virtual Library — Law, Net: http://www.law.indiana.edu/law /lawindex.html

• LITTLE PEOPLE

Billy Barty Foundation, 929 W. Olive Ave., Ste. C, Burbank, CA 91506; (818)953-5410

Little People of America, 7238 Piedmont Dr., Dallas, TX 75227-9324; (214)388-9576 or (800)24-DWARF

• LIVER

American Association for the Study of Liver Disease, 6900 Grove Rd., Thorofare, NJ 08086; (609)848-1000

American Liver Foundation, 1425 Pompton Ave., Cedar Grove, NJ 07009; (201)256-2550 or (800)223-0179; Net: http://sadieo.ucsf.edu/alf/alffinal/homepagealf .htm/

Wilson's Disease Association, PO Box 75324, Washington, DC 20013

• LIVING WILLS (also see *Final Relief,* and *Hospice*)

Books:
* *The Beneficiary Book,* by Martin Kuritz, John Sampson and David Sanchez; Active Insights ([800]222-9125)
* *Beyond the Grave: The Right Way and the Wrong Way of Leaving Money to Your Children and Others,* by Gerald M. Condon and Jeffrey L. Condon; Harper Business, 1995
* *Easing the Passage: A Guide for Prearranging and Ensuring a Pain-Free and Tranquil Death via a Living Will, Personal Medical Mandate, and Other Medical, Legal, and Ethical Resources,* by David E. Outerbridge and Alan R. Hersh, MD; Harper Collins, 1991
* *The Essential Guide to a Living Will: How to Protect Your Right to Refuse Medical Treatment,* by B.D. Colen; Prentice Press, 1991
* *Living Wills and More: Everything You Need to Ensure that All Your Medical Wishes are Followed,* by Terry Barnett; Published by John Wiley & Sons, Inc., 1992
* *The Other Mid-Life Crisis: Everything You Need to Know About Wills, Hospitals, Life-and-Death Decisions, and Final Matters,* by Adeline Rosemire (arosemire@aol.com); Meridian Publishing ([800]270-2116), 1996
* *Planning for Uncertainty: A Guide to Living Wills and Other Advance Directives for Healthcare,* by David John Doukas, MD, and William Reichel, MD; The Johns Hopkins University Press ([800]537-5487), 1994

Though a doctor may consider it a failure when a patient dies, and a doctor may be morally opposed to withdrawing life support, keeping a patient alive by all means possible may not be what is best for the patient. Because the ability of medical science to prolong life artificially by taking what some people refer to as "heroic measures" sometimes amounts to what can be considered medical torture, many people have recognized the need for dying patients, their families, and doctors to be in control of and have the legal ability to make the final choice when the prognosis of a patient is extremely poor, such as when a patient enters a persistent vegetative state.

Probably the most popular case that demonstrated the need for people to fill out a living will was that of Karen Ann Quinlan. In 1975, the New Jersey teenager fell into a persistent vegetative state after a mixture of drugs and alcohol caused her to stop breathing. Her father allowed the medical team treating her to connect her to life-supporting machinery. When the parents realized the brain damage was so extensive that their daughter had no chance of waking up and healing, they had to go to court to get permission to have the machinery disconnected. Much of the case dwelt on what she herself would have wanted done. When testimony was given that she had once said she would not want to be kept alive on medical machinery, it was decided that she should be disconnected.

Two types of documents known as "advance directives" that can guide the treatment people receive when they are incapacitated are the living will and durable power of attorney for healthcare. Sometimes an advance directive is a combination of both.

A living will is a document that may or may not give direct permission to terminate medical assistance on a person who does not choose to be kept alive by all medical means possible when his ability to heal and carry on a meaningful existence has passed. The action of allowing the disease process to take its course without intervention or assistance is known as "passive euthanasia"— the word euthanasia means "good death." During this time the patient may desire to take medication that alleviates physical discomfort.

A living will allows a dying person to have some control over the ending to his life and can spell out specific conditions under which treatment (oxygen, food, and hydration devices that support life) should be continued, stopped, or avoided (CPR, medications, transfusions, dialysis, diagnostic tests, implantation of a pacemaker, or other surgery). A living will may also include instructions for hospice care to be administered.

A living will often includes a DNR (Do Not Resuscitate) order. Some states require a special document for this with a physician's signature, or notarization. A DNR order should include instructions detailing what circumstances would need to be present before the order is carried out. It may include instructions on what measures should be taken, such as if electric shock should be administered, or if a respirator should be used. It may also include instructions permitting the use of pain medications and antibiotics. When a patient is in the hospital, or a long-term facility, the DNR order is placed on the front of the patient's chart.

A durable power of attorney (DPA) is a document in which a patient names a specific person (known as the agent) to make decisions, should the hospitalized individual be unable to do so. The document can include instructions for this agent to follow. Most people choose a spouse, sibling, parent, adult child, other relative, or a close friend to serve as their agent. Within reason, the more details the instructions include, and the more scenarios of conditions and treatment that are covered, the easier it will be for the agent to make decisions that correspond with the patient's wishes. In the event the agent does not want the responsibility, the patient and the agent should discuss the DPA well in advance of necessity. The living will documents may also determine the patient's desire to donate his organs and tissues for transplantation or other uses.

A living will helps to avoid situations in which expensive procedures are performed on patients who will die or become brain dead regardless of treatment, which can leave families financially and emotionally stressed. A doctor's risk of legal liability is also reduced when he carries out the preferences expressed in an advance directive. Patients should discuss their living will with their doctor to make sure the doctor will obey the instructions given.

When a person writes out a living will he should consider the possibilities of:
- An incurable cancer.
- Illness that causes loss of memory and inability to recognize family members.
- Becoming mentally incompetent.
- Not being able to feed himself, and of being reliant on others for basic needs.
- Being in a persistent vegetative state (PVS). The *British Medical Journal* (July 6, 1996) published a study that found 17 of 40 patients diagnosed as being in a PVS were later found to be alert, aware, and often able to express a simple wish. A person in a PVS is confined to bed, goes through a waking and sleeping period, and is unable to talk or care for himself. A person in a coma does not exhibit a sleep-wake cycle.
- Pain, how it should be treated, and what measures should be taken to keep him comfortable.
- What medications should, and should not, be given.
- What medical machinery should be used, or avoided.
- What medical machinery can and cannot do, and how it may cause discomfort.
- Where he would like to live out his remaining days.
- Conflicts within the family and how this may interfere with his comfort.
- The benefits of a healthcare proxy/person who he will determine to make healthcare decisions for him in case he may no longer be able to do so.
- The insurance company deciding to deny payments for his care.

Ongoing good health is always uncertain — something can go wrong with the human body at any time. Above all, death is a sure thing for everyone. Anyone wishing to avoid the possibility of being kept alive by medical machinery should fill out a living will and advance directive as soon as possible while no one can doubt that the patient made the decision while of a sound mind. This can save thousands of dollars in medical costs and avoid legal fights, difficult choices for family members, suffering of the patient, and heartache for the family and friends who are left behind. These documents may actually help the family cope better with and accept the decisions that have been made. (A pregnant woman may want to include special instructions in her living will that would cover the possibility of catastrophic illness or injury during the time of her pregnancy.)

Death has occurred when:
- The pupils do not respond to light.
- There is no response to pain.
- The person cannot breath without assistance.

Your doctor, lawyer, hospital, nursing home, local hospice, library, bar association, medical society, or legal stationery store may also have information on living wills and sample copies for you to consider. Whatever form is used, it is important that it is worded correctly so that you are legally protected. As B.D. Colen says in his book, *The Essential Guide to a Living Will*, "Preparing a Living Will now will not guarantee that your family members or attorney will not have to go to court to enforce your wishes, but it will certainly make that eventuality far less likely." Consulting with a doctor, an attorney, or one of the groups below may clear up your concerns regarding the specific wording you should include on your advance directive to ensure correct interpretation of your preferences.

According to a study that examined 180 hospital admissions of elderly patients in New York, doctors and hospital staff often do not know that patients have living wills. (*Journal of the American Medical Association*, August 9, 1995)

There have been times where doctors and medical workers have ignored a living will. In 1995 a North Carolina court ruled that a patient in a nursing home was not liable for medical bills incurred after the facility ignored the living will of the patient. In February of 1996 a Michigan court awarded $16.6 million to a patient whose living will was ignored.

The Patient Self-Determination Act that went into effect on December 1, 1991, requires hospitals, nursing homes, home healthcare agencies, and hospices that are certified by Medicare or Medicaid, and for managed care organizations to make adult patients aware of their rights to accept or refuse treatment, and obligates hospitals to inform patients of their right to sign an advance directive. Federal law also prohibits medical facilities from requiring patients to sign an advance directive. The law also states that a person cannot be discriminated against because they have not signed an advance directive.

For a pamphlet titled *A Consumer's Guide to Advance Directives*, send a letter of request along with a self-addressed, stamped envelope to
American Health Information Management Association, Professional Practice Division, 919 N. Michigan Ave., Ste. 1400, Chicago, IL 60611

Association for Death Education and Counseling, 638 Prospect Ave., Hartford, CT 06105-4298; (203)232-4825

Choice in Dying, Inc., 200 Varick St., 10th Flr., New York, NY 10014-4810; (212)366-5540 or (800)989-9455; Fax (212)366-5337

The Harvard Medical Schools' Health Letter sells a Medical Directive form that you can fill out. It gives instructions on what treatments you may and may not want. To obtain copies, send a check or money order for $6 for two copies or $11 for five copies to **Medical Directive,** Harvard Medical School's Health Letter, PO Box 6100, Holliston, MA 01746-6100

National Electronic Archive of Advance Directives, 11000 Cedar Ave., Cleveland, OH 44106-3052; (800)379-6866

National Hospice Hotline, (800)658-8898

To get a free copy of a booklet titled *Estate Planning Through Trusts* that explains the types of trusts and the problems of not setting them up properly, write to **Neuberger & Berman Trust Co.,** 605 — 3rd Ave., New York, NY 10158

Widowed Persons Services, American Association of Retired Persons, 601 E. St., NW, Washington, DC 20049

• **LUNGS** (Also see *Smoking Cessation*)

American Lung Association, 1740 Broadway, New York, NY 10019-4374; (212)315-8700 or (800) LUNG-USA

Asbestos Victims of America, PO Box 559, Capitola, CA 95010; (408)476-3646

Black Lung Association, PO Box 872, Crab Orchard, WV 25827; (304)252-9654

Brown Lung Association, PO Box 7583, Greenville, SC 29610; (803)269-8048

Comprehensive Lung Center of the University of Pittsburgh Medical Center, Net: http://www.clc.upmc.edu/

Congenital Central Hypoventilation Syndrome Family Support Network, 71 Maple St., Oneonta, NY 13820; (607)432-8872

Cystic Fibrosis, Net: LISTSERV@YALEVM.CISYALE.EDU

Cystic Fibrosis Foundation, 6931 Arlington Rd., Bethesda, MD 20814; (301)951-4422 or (800)344-4823

Environmental Protection Agency, National Radon Hotline, (800) SOS-RADON

Indoor Air Quality Information Clearinghouse, PO Box 37133, Washington, DC 20013; (800)438-4318

International Ventilator Users Network, 4207 Lindell Blvd., Ste. 110, St. Louis, MO 63108-2915

Life & Breath Newsletter, **Saskatchewan Lung Association,** 1231 — 8th St. E., Saskatoon, SK, S7H 0S5 Canada; (306)343-9511

Lifecare International manufactures portable respiratory equipment for homes, hospitals, long-term care facilities, and transport worldwide.
Lifecare International, 1401 W. 122nd Ave., Westminster, CO 80234; (303)457-9234

National Jewish Center for Immunology and Respiratory Medicine, Denver, CO; (800)423-8891; Lungfacts (800)552-LUNG; Lungline (800)222-LUNG

National Radon Hotline, (800)SOS-RADON

National Safety Council's Radon Program, 1019 Nineteenth St., NW, Washington, DC 20036; (800)55-RADON

Take a Breather Newsletter, 573 King St. E, Ste. 201, Toronto, Ontario, Canada M5A-1M5; (416)864-1112

Tuberculosis Research Center at Stanford, Net: http://molepi.stanford.edu

White Lung Association, PO Box 1483, Baltimore, MD 21203; (410)243-5864

• LUPUS

American Lupus Society, 260 Maple Ct., Ste. 123, Ventura, CA 93003; (805)339-0443 or (800)331-1802

Bay Area Lupus Foundation, 2635 N. First St., Ste. 206, San Jose, CA 95134; (408)954-8600 or (800)523-3363

Lupus Erythematosus Support Club, 8039 Nova Court, N. Charleston, NC 29420; (803)764-1769

Lupus Foundation of America, 4 Research Pl., Ste. 180, Rockville, MD 20850-3226; (301)670-9292 or (800)558-0121

Lupus Network, 230 Ranch Dr., Bridgeport, CT 06606; (203)372-5795; E-mail: RJxF85A@prodigy.com

• LYME DISEASE

Book:
• *Coping With Lyme Disease: A Practical Guide to Dealing with Diagnosis & Treatment,* by Denise Lang; Henry Holt & Co., 1993

American Lyme Disease Foundation, Royal Executive Park, 3 International Dr., Rye Brook, NY 10573; (914)934-9155

Lyme Aid, (800)886-LYME

Lyme Disease Foundation, 1 Financial Plaza, Hartford, CT 06103; (203)525-2000 or (800)886-LYME

Lyme Disease Network, 43 Winton Rd., E. Brunswick, NJ 08816; (908)390-5027

• MARIJUANA AS MEDICINE

Books:
• *Ain't Nobody's Business if You Do: The Absurdity of Consensual Crimes in a Free Society,* by Peter McWilliams; Prelude Press, 1996
• *Smoke and Mirrors: The War on Drugs and the Politics of Failure,* by Dan Baum; Little, Brown, 1996

Even though criminal penalties nor treatment programs have successfully deterred marijuana use, possessing, selling, and growing marijuana is currently against the law and the government spends billions of dollars to try and control marijuana use. A marijuana offense may result in a jail term, fine, property confiscation, or probation. Companies that test employees for drug use may suspend or fire an employee who is found to have used marijuana.

Alliance for Cannabis Therapeutics and Marijuana AIDS Research, PO Box 21210, Kalorama Station, Washington, DC 20009; (202)483-8595

Californians for Compassionate Use, (310)314-4049; Net: http://www.medical marijuana.org

Cannabis Patient Registry, 1801 Tippah Ave., Charlotte, NC 28205; (704)358-0518; Fax (704)358-1650; E-mail: cpr@maps.org

Citizens Foundation for Medical Marijuana, 201 Maple St., Santa Cruz, CA 95060; (408)429-8819

Help End Marijuana Prohibition, (310)392-1806

Hemp BC, 324 W. Hastings, Vancouver, BC, Canada; (800)330-HEMP; Net: http://www.hempbc.com

Hemptech, PO Box 820, Ojai, CA 93204; (805)646-4367; Net: http://www.hemptech .com

Hempworld, E-mail: hemplady@crl.com — or — Net: http://hempworld.com/

High Times, Net: http://www.hightimes.com/~hightimes

International Cannabis Alliance of Researchers and Educators (I-CARE), (Send $15 for a video) Fish Pond Plantation, 1472 Fish Pond Rd., Howardsville, VA 24502; (804)263-4484; E-mail: MLM45@VIRGINIA.EDU — or — Net: Mary_Lynn@PATIENT .WIN.NET

Patients Out of Time, Fish Pond Plantation, 1472 Fish Pond Rd., Howardsville, VA 24562; (804)263-4484; Net: AL_BYRNE@PATIENT.WIN.NET

National Organization for the Reform of Marijuana Laws, 1001 Connecticut Ave., NW, Ste. 1010, Washington, DC 20036; (202)265-8070 or (900)97-NORML; E-mail: NATLNORML@aol.com

New Yorkers for Drug Policy Reform, 226 W. 4th St., Ste. 4, New York, NY 10014; (212)691-5112

Roxane is the pharmaceutical company that makes Marinol, a synthetic form of THC.
Roxane, (800)327-4865

San Francisco Cannabis Buyers Club, 1444 Market St., San Francisco, CA 94102; (415)621-3986

• MASSAGE, REFLEXOLOGY, AND YOGA

Books:
* *The Alexander Technique,* by Judith Leibowitz and Bill Connington; Harper Collins, 1990
* *Body Work: What Type of Massage to Get and How to Make the Most of It,* by Thomas Claire; Morrow, 1995
* *Yoga for Health and Healing: From the Teachings of Yogi Bhajan,* by Alice B. Clagett and Kirsten Meredeth; 1995

Manipulative therapies are those that are done by adjusting the body, positioning the body, massaging, or applying pressure to one area that corresponds to other areas or regions to tone the body systems, to help in the treatment of various physical and mental ailments, and to increase healing.

The Accupressure Institute publishes a catalog which features books, instructional yoga, and massage video and audio tapes, reference charts, and massage devices.
Acupressure Institute, 1533 Shattuck Ave., Berkeley, CA 94709; (510)845-1059 or (800)442-2232

American Center for the Alexander Technique, 129 W. 67th St., New York, NY 10023; (212)799-0468

American Massage Therapy Association, 820 Davis St., Ste. 100, Evanston, IL 60201; (708)864-0123 or (312)761-2682

Associated Bodywork & Massage Professionals, 28677 Buffalo Park Rd., Evergreen, CO 80439-7347; (303)674-8478

Bonnie Prudden Pain Erasure, Bonnie Prudden School for Physical Fitness and Myotherapy, 7800 E. Speedway, Tucson, AZ 85710; (800) 221-4634

Feldenkrais Guild (movement therapy), PO Box 489, Albany, OR 97321; (503)926-0981 or (800)775-2118

Institute of Conscious Body Work, 100 Shaw Dr., San Anselmo, CA 94960; (415)258-0402

Yoga has been practiced for thousands of years in India and is done to maintain physical vitality and flexibility. There are several types of yoga, including Hatha, Ashtanga, Iyengar, Kripalu, Kundalini, Integral, and Tri.

International Association of Yoga Therapists, 109 Hillside Ave., Mill Valley, CA 94941; (415)383-4587; E-mail: yoganet@aol.com

International Institute of Reflexology, PO Box 12642, St. Petersburg, FL 33733; (813)343-4811

International Rolf Institute, PO Box 1868, Boulder, CO 80306; (303)449-5903

Jin Shin Do Foundation for Bodymind Acupressure, PO Box 1097, Felton, CA 95018; (408)338-9454

Massage Magazine, PO Box 1500, Davis, CA 95617; (800)872-1282

North American Society of Teachers of the Alexander Technique, PO Box 517 Urbana, IL 61801; (217)367-6956

Radiance Technique Association International, PO Box 40570, St. Petersburg, FL 33743-0570

Reiki Alliance, PO Box 41, Cataldo, ID 83810; (208)682-3535

Rolfing and Massage, Net: http://www.bnt.com/~rolfer/

The Rolf Institute of Structural Integration provides pamphlets and referral listings upon request, publishes a quarterly journal, and offers a number of books and pamphlets for sale.

Rolf Institute of Structural Integration, 205 Canyon Blvd., Boulder, CO 80302; (303)449-5903 or (800)530-8875; E-mail: RolfInst@aol.com

The Touch Research Institute concentrates on the sense of touch and how it can be applied to medicine and the treatment of disease. The institute publishes a quarterly newsletter, *Touchpoints,* that is available for $10, and a book, *Advances in Touch,* that is also available for $10.

Touch Research Institute, Dept. of Pediatrics, D-820, University of Miami School of Medicine, PO Box 016820, Miami, FL 33101; (305)243-6781

Yoga International, RR 1, Box 407, Honesdale, PA 18431; (800) 586-1777 or (800)821-YOGA

Yoga Journal, 2054 University Ave., Ste. 600, Berkeley, CA 94704; (800)359-YOGA

• MEDICAL LEAVE FROM EMPLOYMENT, LAWS GOVERNING

The following may provide you with information regarding laws that govern employees taking time off from work for medical reasons.

AFL-CIO, Dept. of Occupational Safety, Health, and Social Security, 815 — 16th St., NW, Washington, DC 20006; (202)637-5000

The *Human Resources Focus Guide to the Family and Medical Leave Act* is available for $19.95 from the

American Management Association, (800)538-4761

Association of Occupational and Environmental Clinics, 1010 Vermont Ave., NW, Washington, DC 20005; (202)347-4976

Coalition of Labor Union Women, 1126 — 16th St., NW, Washington, DC 20036; (202)466-4610 or 4615

National Coalition of Injured Workers, 12 Rejane St., Coventry, RI 02816; (401)828-6520

National Institute for Occupational Safety and Health, 4676 Columbia Pkwy., Cincinnati, OH 45226; (800)35-NIOSH

National Labor Relations Board, 1717 Pennsylvania Ave., NW, Washington, DC 20570

National Safety Council, 1121 Spring Lake Dr., Itasca, IL 60143; (800)621-7615

Occupational Safety and Health Administration, US Dept. of Labor, Rm. N-3647, Washington, DC 20210; (202)219-8148

A Sample Policy for Family or Medical Leave is available for $10 from the **Society for Human Resource Management,** (703)548-3440

US Dept. of Labor, Employment Standards Administration Office of Public Affairs, 200 Constitution Ave., NW, Washington, DC 20210; (202)219-8743 or (202)576-7100

• MEDICAL TRANSCRIBERS

Medical transcriptionists translate the records of patients from the oral tape-recorded "dictation" of the doctor into typewritten form. Some medical facilities employ their own medical transcriptionists; other smaller medical groups and individual doctors may hire transcriptionists on a freelance basis through a transcription agency.

American Association for Medical Transcriptionists, PO Box 576187, Modesto, CA 95357; (209)551-0883

• MEN'S HEALTH

Books:
* *How I Survived Prostate Cancer . . . and So Can You: A Guide for Diagnosing and Treating Prostate Cancer,* by James Lewis, Jr., PhD; Health Education Literary Publisher ([616] 453-1477), 1994
* *My Prostate and Me: One Man's Experience with Prostate Cancer,* by William Martin; Cadell & Davies, 1994
* *The Male Body: A Physician's Guide to what Every Man Should Know,* by Abraham Morgantaler; Simon & Schuster, 1993
* *Prostate: Questions You Have . . . Answers You Need,* by Sandra Salmans; People's Medical Society ([800]624-8773), 1995

Prostate cancer (adenocarcinoma of the prostate) strikes about 317,000 American men yearly and results in over 41,000 deaths (American Cancer Society 1996 estimate). Prostate cancer is the most frequently diagnosed malignancy and second leading cause of cancer death in men (*Cancer Communication Newsletter,* June 1996).

Three ways to diagnose prostate cancer are through Digital (finger) Rectal Examination (DRE), TransRectal Ultrasound (TRUS), and a blood test called Prostate Specific Antigen (PSA). The American Cancer Institute recommends PSA screening for all men over fifty, and earlier for men in high-risk groups (black men are twice as likely as white men to get prostate cancer).

For every prostate cancer death, only $1,200 is spent on research, for each breast cancer death, $10,000 is spent on research; for AIDS it is $50,000.
— Senator Diane Watson who introduced a bill in California to add two cents a pack to cigarette sales for the benefit of prostate cancer research and screening.

- In figures derived from autopsies, it is known that approximately one-third of men over fifty years old have cancerous cells in the prostate, but only 10% of men will experience serious health problems from prostate cancer.
- Digital rectal examination (DRE) is done by inserting a finger into the rectum to feel for prostate gland abnormalities.
- Transrectal ultrasound or echography of the prostate (TRUS) uses the echo of soundwaves during ultrasound to create an image of the prostate on a television monitor.
- A PSA (prostate-specific antigen) blood test may be helpful in detecting prostate cancer before it has spread. The prostate normally produces the PSA protein to carry sperm. High levels of PSA may be a sign of prostate cancer, but may also only be caused by an infected or an enlarged prostate. Some people in the medical field say that the PSA test is overrated, and is often inaccurate.
- The blood test that can help detect the spread of prostate cancer was developed at Columbia-Presbyterian Medical Center in New York City.
- The test called enhanced reverse transcriptase-PCR for PSA can tell if prostate cancer has spread beyond the prostate gland. The test is made by Dianon Systems of Stratford, Connecticut.
- Dr. Gary R. Pasternack of Johns Hopkins University developed a test that searches for a genetic marker in cells obtained from the prostate tumor. The presence of the marker, called pp32, can help identify a tumor that has the potential of spreading rapidly.
- Imaging procedures, such as CAT scans and MRI, may be helpful in determining if prostate cancer has spread (metastasized) beyond the prostate.
- Surgery, hormonal therapy, and radiation treatments are the three most common allopathic ways to treat prostate cancer.
- Before a man undergoes treatment for prostate cancer, he should consider the possibility that the therapy may interfere with the ability to produce sperm. Storing sperm in a sperm bank is one option.
- Two problems that may be experienced after prostate cancer therapy are incontinence (loss of bladder control) and impotence (inability to maintain an erection).
- Recent advances in surgical techniques, such as cryosurgery, have lowered the chances of incontinence and impotence after prostate surgery.
- Dr. Patrick Walsh of the Brady Urological Institute at Johns Hopkins University is credited with devising surgical techniques that reduce blood loss during prostate surgery, and "nerve sparing techniques" that increase the likelihood of preserving sexual function.
- Two surgeries done to relieve impotence are by inserting a manufactured penile implant, or by performing a penile bypass where an abdominal artery is connected to one or both of the arteries serving the penis.
- Suction pumps and injectable drugs may also be used to treat impotence.
- Impotence, difficulty with ejaculations, and loss of sexual desire are sometimes caused by medications or diabetes. Smoking is also a risk factor.
- Impotence may also be caused by emotional difficulties, such as esteem issues or a history of childhood sexual abuse.

American Association of Sex Educators, Counselors and Therapists, 435 N. Michigan Ave., Ste. 1717, Chicago, IL 60611; (312)644-0828

American Medical Systems (manufactures penile implants), Minneapolis, MN 55440; (800)543-9632

American Prostate Society, 1340 Charwood Rd., Ste. F, Hanover, MD 21076; (410)859-3735 or (800)678-1238

The urology department at the Boston University Medical Center offers comprehensive treatment for male infertility and sexual dysfunction.
Boston University Medical Center, Boston, MA; (617)638-6767

Brady Urological Institute, Baltimore, MD; (410)955-6707

Continence Restored, 407 Strawberry Hill Dr., Stamford, CT 06902; (203)348-0601 or (914)285-1470

Cryobiology, Inc. is a company that can preserve a man's sperm before he undergoes surgery.
Cryobiology, 4830 Ste. D, Knights Bridge Blvd., Columbus, OH 43214; (800)359-4375

Duke University Medical Center is known for its treatment of prostate cancer, male fertility, and dysfunction.
Duke University Medical Center, Durham, NC; (919)684-2033

Econugenics sells Ecogen and Pecta-Sol, supplements that contain isoflavones. These plant chemicals have proven helpful in strengthening the ability of the body to fight prostate cancer.
Econugenics, (415)927-1088 or (800)308-5518

The Geddings D. Osborn Foundation provides booklets and other information that explain treatment options for impotence.
Geddings D. Osbon Sr. Foundation, Impotence Resource Center, 1246 Jones St., PO Box 1593, Augusta, GA 30903-1593; (800) 433-4215 or (800) 821-8011

Extract of Saw Palmetto berries is helpful in reducing enlarged prostates. A high-quality form of the extract can be purchased through
Klabin Marketing, 2067 Broadway, Ste. 700, New York, NY 10023; (212)877-3632 or (800)933-9440

Impotence Information Center, PO Box 9, Minneapolis, MN 55440; (800)843-4315

Impotence Institute International, 119 S. Ruth St., Maryville, TN 37803-5746; (423)983-6064

Impotence Institute of America, 8201 Corporate Dr., Ste. 320, Landover, MD 20785; (301)577-0650 or (800)669-1603

Mathews Foundation for Prostate Cancer Research, 1010 Hurley Way, Ste. 195, Sacramento, CA 95825; (916)567-1400 or (800)234-6284

Men's Confidential Newsletter ($24 a year), Rodale Press, 33 E. Minor St., Emmaus, PA 18098; (800)666-2160

The National Kidney and Urologic Disease Information Clearinghouse will send you a free booklet on treatment options for benign prostatic hyperplasia.
National Kidney and Urologic Disease Information Clearinghouse, (301)654-4415

National Men's Resource Center, PO Box 800, San Anselmo, CA 94979-0800

National Organization for Men, 11 Park Pl., New York, NY 10007

National Organization of Circumcision Information Research, PO Box 2512, San Anselmo, CA 94979-2512; (415)488-9883

National Organization to Halt the Abuse and Routine Mutilation of Males, PO Box 460795, San Francisco, CA 94146; (415)826-9351

NECC is a company that can preserve a man's sperm before he undergoes surgery.
NECC, Boston, MA; (617)262-3311

The urology department at the Cornell Medical Center is known for their advanced surgical techniques in treating men who need penile reconstruction.
New York Hospital—Cornell Medical Center, New York, NY; For physician referral service (800)822-2694

Patient Advocates for Advanced Cancer Treatments is devoted to helping prostate cancer patients understand new and emerging treatments. They provide information packets on request and publish a newsletter six times per year called *Prostate Cancer Report.* Ask for a copy of the booklet titled *The Saw Palmetto Story* by Dr. Michael Murray, ND.

PAACT encourages patients to maintain personal medical files and provides a pamphlet containing charts that may be used to record medical treatment. PAACT also has a 24 hour recorded touch-tone activated message menu of prostate-related informative recordings. To access this system, dial (616)453-1351.

Patient Advocates for Advanced Cancer Treatments, 1143 Parmelee, NW, PO Box 141695, Grand Rapids, MI 49514-1695; (616)453-1477

Prostate Discussion Group, Net: http://www.sci.med.prostate.bph

Recovery of Male Potency, 27211 Lahser Rd., No. 208, Southfield, MI 48034; (810)357-1314 or (800) TEL-ROMP

St. Luke's Hospital has one of the most well-known male-fertility clinics in the country.

St. Luke's Hospital, St. Louis, MO; (314)576-1400

Stanford University Medical Center's urology department is known for its "wait and see" approach to the treatment of prostate cancer. This has helped to prevent unnecessary surgeries.

Stanford University Medical Center, Stanford, CA; (415)723-6024

Star Center, 27211 Lahser Road, Ste. 208, Southfield, MI 48034; (313)357-1314 or (800)835-7667

Theragenics manufactures radioactive pellets used by allopathic doctors in interstitial radiation therapy treatments of prostate cancer.

Theragenics Corporation, 5325 Oakbrook Pkwy., Norcross, GA 30093; (404)381-8338 or (800)458-4372

US TOO is sponsored by the American Foundation for Urologic Diseases, and is a prostate cancer information source with over 400 support group chapters that meet once or twice per month.

US TOO International, 930 N. York Rd., Ste. 50, Hinsdale, IL 60521-2993; (708)323-1002 or (800)808-7866

• MENTAL HEALTH, PSYCHOLOGICAL COUNSELING, AND THERAPY

Books:
- *Darkness Visible: A Memoir of Madness,* by William Styron; Random House, 1990
- *Dead Serious: A Book for Teenagers About Teenage Suicide,* by Jane Mersky Leder; Atheneum Books, 1994
- *On The Edge Of Darkness: Conversations About Conquering Depression,* by Kathy Cronkite; Doubleday, 1994
- *You Are Not Alone: Words of Experience & Hope for the Journey Through Depression,* by Julia Thorn & Larry Rothstein; HarperCollins, 1993

American Academy of Psychotherapists, PO Box 607, Decatur, GA 30031

American Association of Behavioral Therapists, PO Box 767156, Roswell, GA 30076-7156

American College of Psychoanalysts, 2006 Dwight Way, Ste. 304, Berkeley, CA 94704

American Family Therapy Association, 2020 Pennsylvania Ave., Ste. 273, Washington, DC 20006; (202)994-2776

American Mental Health Counselors Association, 5999 Stevenson Ave., Alexandria, VA 22304; (703)823-9800 ext. 383

American Psychological Association, 750 First St., NE, Washington, DC 20002-4242; (202)336-5700 or 5500

American Psychosomatic Society, 6728 Old McLean Village Dr., McLean, VA 22101; (703)556-9222

Committee for Truth in Psychiatry, PO Box 76925, Washington, DC 20013

The Complete Guide to Psychology-Related Sites on the Net, Net: http://pegasus
.acs.ttu.edu/~civelek/thanatos.html

Depression Awareness, Recognition and Treatment Program, The National Institute
of Mental Health, Rm. 15—C—05, 5600 Fishers Lane, Rockville, MD 20857

For a free copy of a brochure developed to help people with depression recognize
symptoms and seek treatment options, send a self-addressed, stamped envelope to
Depression Guidelines, PO Box 8547, Silver Spring, MD 20907

Emotional Health Anonymous, PO Box 63236, Los Angeles, CA 90063-0236

Federation of Families for Children's Mental Health, 1021 Prince St., Alexandria, VA
22134-2971; (703)684-7710

Gift From Within, (posttraumatic stress disorder information) 1 Lily Pond Dr., Camden,
ME 04843; E-mail: JoyceB3955@aol.com — or — Net: http://www
.sourcemaine.com/gift

International Association of Psychosocial Rehabilitation Services
Sterrett Place, Ste. 214, Columbia, MD 21044-2626; (410)730-7190

Manic Depressive Illness Foundation, 2723 P St., Washington, DC 20007

Mental Health Consumer Initiative, PO Box 1276, Melrose, MA 02176-0009

National Alliance for the Mentally Ill, 2101 Wilson, Ste. 302, Arlington, VA 22201;
(703)524-7600 or (800)950-NAMI

National Depression and Manic Depressives Association, 730 N. Franklin, Ste. 501,
Chicago, IL 60610; (312)642-0049 or (800)826-2632

National Foundation For Depressive Illness, Inc., PO Box 2257, New York, NY 10116;
(212)268-4260 or (800)248-4344

National Institute of Mental Health, Information Resources and Inquiries Branch,
5600 Fishers Lane, Rm. 15C—05, Rockville, MD 20857; (800)421-4211

National Mental Health Consumers' Self-Help Clearinghouse, 1211 Chestnut St.,
Philadelphia, PA 19107; (215)751-1810

Project Overcome was formed in 1977 by a group of mental health care consumers
to help eliminate the stigma surrounding mental illness.
Project Overcome, PO Box 385226, Minneapolis, MN 55438-5226; (612)820-0464

• MINORITY HEALTHCARE

Books:
- *Bad Blood: The Tuskegee Syphilis Experiment,* by James Jones; Free Press, 1994
- *Black Women's Health Book: Speaking for Ourselves,* by Evelyn White; Seal Press, 1994
- *Body and Soul: The Black Women's Guide to Physical-health and Emotional Well Being,*
  edited by Linda Villarosa; Harper-Perennial, 1994
- *Momma Might be Better off Dead: The Failure of Health Care in America,* by Laurie Kaye
  Abraham; University of Chicago Press, 1993

American Black Chiropractors Association, 1918 E. Grand Blvd., St. Louis, MO 63107;
(314)531-0615

Arise (low income rights), 718 State St., Springfield, MA 01109; (413)734-4948

Association of American Indian Physicians, 1235 Sovereign Row, Ste. C-7, Oklahoma
City, OK 73108

Association of Asian/Pacific Community Health Organizations, 1212 Broadway, Ste.
730, Oakland, CA 94612; (510)272-9536

Office of Minority Health Resource Center, PO Box 37337, Washington, DC 20013-
7337; (800)444-6472 or TDD (301)589-0951

The National Black Child Development Institute publishes a newsletter titled *Child Health Talk* that focuses on the health issues of African American children. It is available for $8.00 a year.

National Black Child Development Institute, 1023 — 15th St. NW, Ste. 600, Washington, DC; (202)387-1281

National Black Men's Health Network, 250 Georgina Ave., Ste. 321, Atlanta, GA 30312; (404)524-7237

National Black Nurses Association, 1660 L St., NW, Ste. 907, Washington, DC 20036; (202)673-4551

The National Black Women's Health Project publishes *Vital Signs Newsletter* which covers the health concerns of black women.

National Black Women's Health Project, 1237 Ralph D. Abernathy Rd., Atlanta, GA 30310; (404)758-9590 or (800) ASK-BWHP

National Center for the Black Aged, 1424 K St., NW, Ste. 500, Washington, DC 20005; (202)637-8400

National Coalition of Hispanic Health and Human Services Organizations, 1501 — 16th St., NW, Washington, DC 20036; (202)387-5000

National Indian Health Board, 1385 S. Colorado Blvd., Ste. A-708, Denver, CO 80222; (303)759-3075

Office of Minority Health Resource Center, US Dept. of Health and Human Services, PO Box 37337, Washington, DC 20013; (301)587-1938 or (800)444-6472

• MOUTH, TEETH, JAW, DENTAL AND ORAL HEALTH

(Also see *Dental Specialists, American Boards of*)

Books:
• *It's All In Your Head: The Link Between Mercury Amalgams and Illness,* by Dr. Hal A. Huggins; Avery Publishing, 1993
• *Root Canal Cover-Up,* by George E. Meinig, DDS, FACD; Bion Publishing, 1994

Academy of Dentistry for the Handicapped, 211 E. Chicago Ave., 17th Flr., Chicago, IL 60611; (312)440-2661

Academy of General Dentistry, 211 E. Chicago Ave., Ste. 1200, Chicago, IL 60611; (312)440-4300

Academy of Operative Dentistry, 643 Broadway, Menomonie, WI 54751; (715)235-7566

Academy of Oral Diagnosis Radiology and Medicine, 43 Blenheim Rd., Manalapan, NJ 07726; (908)536-2501

American Academy of Cosmetic Dentistry, 2711 Marshall Ct., Madison, WI 53705; (608)238-6529 or (800)543-9220

American Academy of Crown and Bridge Prosthodontics, 3302 Gaston Ave., Rm. 330, Dallas, TX 75246

American Academy of Dental Electrosurgery, PO Box 374, Planetarium Station, New York, NY 10024

American Academy of Dental Radiology, PO Box 31162, Aurora, CO 80041

American Academy of Esthetic Dentistry, 500 N. Michigan St., Ste. 1400, Chicago, IL 60611; (312)661-1700

American Academy of Fixed Prosthodontics, 3302 Gaston Ave., Rm. 330, Dallas, TX 75246

American Academy of Gnathologic Orthopedics, 1723 N. Hearthside Court, PO Box 548, Richmond, TX 77406-0548

American Academy of Head, Facial and Neck Pain and TMJ Orthopedics, Atlantic Bldg., Ste. 1310, 260 S. Broad St., Philadelphia, PA 19102

American Academy of Implant Dentistry, 6900 Grove Rd., Thorofare, NJ 08086; (312)335-1550

American Academy of Implant Prosthodontics, 5555 Peachtree-Dunwoody Rd., NE, Ste. 140, Atlanta, GA 30342; (404)847-9200

American Academy of Maxillofacial Prosthetics, MCG School of Dentistry, Dept. of Prosthodontics, Augusta, GA 30912

American Academy of Oral Medicine, 4143 Mischive, Houston, TX 77025

American Academy of Orofacial Pain, 10 Joplin Court, Lafayette, CA 94549

American Academy of Orthodontics for the General Practitioner, 3953 N. 76th St., Milwaukee, WI 53222

American Academy of Orthotists and Prosthetists, 717 Pendleton St., Alexandria, VA 22314

American Academy of Pediatric Dentistry, 211 E. Chicago Ave., Ste. 1036, Chicago, IL 60611; (312)337-2169

American Academy of Periodontology, 211 E. Chicago Ave., Ste., 1400, Chicago, IL 60611; (312)787-5518

American Academy of Restorative Dentistry, 1235 Lake Plaza Dr., Colorado Springs, CO 80906; (719)576-8840

American Association for Functional Orthodontics, 106 S. Kent St., Winchester, VA 22601; (703)662-2200

American Association of Dental Examiners, 211 E. Chicago Ave., Ste. 844, Chicago, IL 60611; (708)699-7900

American Association of Dental Victims, 3316 E. 7th St., Long Beach, Chicago, IL 60611; (312)440-2661

American Association of Endodontists, 211 E. Chicago Ave., Ste. 1501, Chicago, IL 60611

American Association of Oral and Maxillofacial Surgeons, 9700 W. Bryn Mawr Ave., Rosemont, IL 60018-5701; (708)768-6200, toll-free (800)822-6637 or (800)467-5268

American Association of Orthodontists, 401 N. Lindbergh Blvd., St. Louis, MO 63141-7816; (314)993-1700 or (800)222-9969

American Association of Women Dentists, 401 N. Michigan Ave., Chicago, IL 60611-4267; (312)644-6610

American College of Dentists, 7315 Wisconsin Ave., Ste. 352N, Bethesda, MD 20814

American College of Oral and Maxillofacial Surgeons, 1100 NW Loop 410, Ste. 500, San Antonio, TX 78213-2260; (210)344-5674

American Dental Association, 211 E. Chicago Ave., Chicago, IL 60611

American Dental Society of Anesthesiology, 211 E. Chicago Ave., Ste. 948, Chicago, IL 60611; (312)664-8270

American Endodontic Society, 1440 N. Harbor Blvd., Ste. 719, Fullerton, CA 92635; (714)870-5590

American Equilibration Society (TMJ), 8726 Ferris Ave., Morton Grove, IL 60053; (708)965-2888

American Society for Dental Aesthetics, 635 Madison Ave., New York, NY 10022; (212)751-3263

American Society of Dentistry for Children, 211 E. Chicago Ave., Ste. 1430, Chicago, IL 60611; (312)943-1244

Centers for Disease Control and Prevention, Division on Oral Health; 1600 Clifton Rd., F10, Atlanta, GA 30337; (404)639-8375

Dental Assisting National Board, 216 E. Ontario St., Chicago, IL 60611; (312)642-3368

Dental Links, Net: http://www.nyu.edu/Dental

Dental Net, Net: http://www.dentalnet.com/dentalnet/

Foundation for Toxic-free Dentistry, PO Box 608010, Orlando, FL 32860-8010 (For information, send a business-sized SASE)

General Dentistry, Net: http://www.iquest.net/denstisry/index.html

Holistic Dental Association, PO Box 5007, Durango, CO 81301; (303)259-1091

International Academy of Oral Medicine and Toxicology, PO Box 608531, Orlando, FL 32860-8531

International Congress of Oral Implantologists, 248 Lorraine Ave., 3rd Flr., Upper Montclair, NJ 07043; (201)783-6300

Jaw Joints & Allied Musculo-Skeletal Disorder Foundation, Forsyth's Research Institute, 140 The Fenway, Boston, MA 02115-3799; (617)266-2550

National Association of Dental Assistants, 900 S. Washington St., Ste. G-13, Falls Church, VA 22046; (703)237-8616

National Foundation for Ectodermal Dysplasias, 219 E. Main St., PO Box 114, Mascoutah, IL 62258-0114; (618)566-2020

National Oral Health Information Clearinghouse, Box NOHIC, 9000 Rockville Pike, Bethesda, MD 20892-3500; (301)402-7364; Net: nidr@aeri.com

Orthodontics, Net: http://www.unique.ch/smd/orthotr.html

TMJ Association, 6418 W. Washington Blvd., Wauwatosa, WI 53213; (800)818-8652

TMJ Hotline, (800)554-5297

• NURSES, MEDICAL ASSISTANTS, AND MEDICAL TECHNOLOGISTS

The medical community cannot function without nurses. They are the supporting structure of the medical industry and outnumber doctors three to one. They are there when the doctors are gone, when emergencies arise, when procedures are performed, when patients vent their frustrations, and when patients leave to go home. Nurses are often the only ones who are present when a patient dies. At times, especially when a nurse has had more contact with a patient than a doctor, a nurse can be more important than a doctor toward recognizing the needs of a patient.

Since Florence Nightingale trudged through the fields of the Crimean War to care for soldiers there and went on to reform the nursing industry of 19th century Europe by founding the St. Thomas Hospital Training School for Nurses in 1860, the nursing industry has flourished in many ways. Somewhere along the line the status of nursing was overshadowed by doctors, and nurses were placed in a subordinate role where they were treated like servants.

The nursing profession is currently experiencing many changes as specialty nurses and advanced practice nurses (in opposition to some doctors' groups) are filling positions once held by general practitioners. This change is the result of the diminishing number of doctors entering into the general practitioner area of medicine as it is becoming popular for medical students to enter into better paying specialized fields of medicine. Giving well educated nurses more power is also part of the growing popularity of managed care and HMO insurance plans that look for ways to cut costs.

Along with this trend toward advanced care nurses who specialize in obstetrics and gynecology, pediatrics, and adult medicine, some medical and nursing schools are introducing programs to train more nurses in more advanced forms of medicine than had been taught in the past. These nurse practitioners work independently but often in cooperation with doctors.

Some medical groups now prefer to have a nurse practitioner on staff. The arrangement of using nurses in positions where doctors once served can be financially beneficial to medical centers because the nurses make less than doctors (nurse practitioners average about $40,000 a year). This is also where criticism is focused by some who say that giving nurses more responsibility as a way to cut costs also sacrifices quality because nurses' training is not as extensive as doctors' and they may not recognize a potentially serious health problem that would be obvious to someone with a more thorough knowledge of medicine.

Of course not everyone in the nursing profession continues with their education to become a nurse practitioner. There are still nurse's aides, practical nurses, and registered nurses who perform many important duties.

The American Nurses Credentialing Center Certification Catalog lists 24 specialized areas of certification for Registered Nurses. These are listed under the *Professional Titles* heading in this book.

In addition to the nurses who care for patients, some nurses continue with schooling to obtain an MBA (masters in business administration) and seek employment as nursing managers who deal with the budgeting, bookkeeping, and supply-ordering area of the nursing profession.

Accreditation Review Committee on Education for Physician Assistants, 515 N. State St., Chicago, IL 60610; (312)464-4623

American Academy of Ambulatory Nursing Administration, Box 56, N. Woodbury Rd., Pitman, NJ 08071; (609)582-9617

American Academy of Nurse Practitioners, Capitol Station, LBJ Bldg., PO Box 12846, Austin, TX 78711; (512)442-4262

American Academy of Nursing, 2420 Pershing Rd., Kansas City, MO 64108; (816)474-5720

American Academy of Physician Assistants, 950 N. Washington St., Alexandria, VA 22314-1552; (703)836-2272

American Assembly for Men in Nursing, PO Box 31753, Independence, OH 44131

American Association for the History of Nursing, PO Box 90803, Washington, DC 20090-0803; (202)543-2127

American Association of Colleges of Nursing, 1 Dupont Circle, NW, Ste. 530, Washington, DC 20036; (202)463-6930

American Association of Critical Care Nurses, 101 Columbia, Aliso Viejo, CA 92656; (714)362-2000 or (800)899-2226

The American Association of Medical Assistants was founded in 1956. The membership of the Association consists of doctor assistants, secretaries, receptionists, bookkeepers, nurses, laboratory personnel, and other individuals who work in medical facilities. The Association publishes a bi-monthly publication called *Professional Medical Assistant.* The Association's certification programs consist of an exam which, when passed, entitles the person to a certificate as a Certified Medical Assistant. The Association also conducts one- and two-year programs in medical assisting in conjunction with the Committee on Allied Health Education and Accreditation of the American Medical Association.

American Association of Medical Assistants, 20 N. Waker Dr., Ste. 1575, Chicago, IL 60606-2903; (312)899-1500

American Association of Neuroscience Nurses, 218 N. Jefferson St., Ste. 204, Chicago, IL 60606

American Association of Nurse Anesthetists, 222 S. Prospect, Park Ridge, IL 60068-4001; (708)692-7050

American Association of Pathologists Assistants, 229 Ocean Ave., Malverne, NY 11565; (516)596-0078

American Association of Surgeon Assistants, 1730 N. Lynn St., Ste. 502, Arlington, VA 22209; (703)525-1191

American Board of Post Anesthesia Nursing Certification, 11512 Allecingie Pkwy., Richmond, VA 23235; (804)378-4936

American College of Nurse-Midwives, 818 Connecticut Ave., NW, Ste. 900, Washington, DC 20006; (202)289-0171

American Journal of Nursing, Net: http://www.ajn.org:80

American Licensed Practical Nurses Association, 1090 Vermont Ave., NW, Ste. 1200, Washington, DC 20005; (202)682-5800

American Medical Technologists maintains a registry of certified medical laboratory technologists, medical laboratory technicians, phlebotomy technicians, medical assistants, and dental assistants.
American Medical Technologists, 710 Higgins Rd., Park Ridge, IL 60068-5765; (708)823-5169

American Nephrology Nurses Association, Box 56, N. Woodbury Rd., Pitman, NJ 08071; (609)589-2187

American Nurses Association, 600 Maryland Ave., SW, Ste. 100 W., Washington, DC 20024-2571; (202)554-4444 or (800)274-4ANA

American Nurses Credentialing Center, 600 Maryland Ave., SW, Ste. 100 W., Washington, DC 20024-2571; (800)284-CERT

American Nurses in Business Association, PO Box 741384, Houston, TX 77274-1384; (713)771-6619

American Nursing Assistants Association, PO Box 103, Ottawa, KS 66067-0103

American Organization of Nurse Executives, American Hospital Association Bldg., 840 N. Lake Shore Dr., Chicago, IL 60611; (312)280-5213

American Psychiatric Nurses' Association, 6900 Grove Rd., Thorofare, NJ 08086; (609)848-7990

American Registry of Medical Assistants, 69 Southwick Rd., Ste. A, Westfield, MA 01085-4729; (413)562-7336

American Society of Post Anesthesia Nurses, 11512 Allecingie Pkwy., Ste. C, Richmond, VA 23235; (804)379-5516

American Society of Plastic and Reconstructive Surgical Nurses, Box 56, N. Woodbury Rd., Pitman, NJ 08071; (609)589-6247

Ask-A-Nurse, (800)535-1111

Association of Pediatric Oncology Nurses, 11512 Allecingie Pkwy., Richmond, VA 23235; (804)379-9150

Association of Women's Health, Obstetric and Neonatal Nurses, 700 — 14th St., NW, Ste. 600, Washington, DC 20005-2019; (202)662-1600

College of Nursing at the University of Tennessee, Knoxville, Net: http://nightin gale.con.utk.edu:70/0/homepage.html

Commission of Graduates of Foreign Nursing Schools, 3600 Market St., Ste. 400, Philadelphia, PA 19104; (215)222-8454

Emergency Nurses Association, 216 Higgins Rd., Park Ridge, IL 60068; (708)698-9400

National Association of Pediatric Nurse Associates and Practitioners, 1101 Kings Hwy. N., Ste. 206, Cherry Hill, NJ 08034; (609)667-1773

National Association of Registered Nurses, 11508 Allecingie Pkwy., Ste. C, Richmond, VA 23235; (804)794-6513

National Black Nurses Association, 1660 L St., NW, Ste. 907, Washington, DC 20036; (202)673-4551

National Commission on Certification of Physicians Assistants, 2845 Henderson Mill Rd., NE, Atlanta, GA 30341; (404)493-9100

National League of Nursing, 350 Hudson St., New York, NY 10014; (212)989-9393

Oncology Nursing Certification Corporation, 501 Holiday Dr., Pittsburgh, PA 15220-2749; (412)921-8597

Oncology Nursing Society, 501 Holiday Dr., Pittsburgh, PA 15220-2749; (412)921-7373

Physicians Assistant Web Page, Net: http://www.halcyon.com/physasst/

Society of Pediatric Nurses, (800)723-2902

• NURSING HOME AND LONG-TERM CARE

Books:
- *Choosing a Nursing Home,* by Seth B. Goldsmith; Prentice Hall Press, 1990
- *Choosing Medical Care in Old Age: What Kind, How Much, When to Stop,* by Muriel R. Gillick, MD; Harvard University Press, 1994
- *How to Evaluate and Select a Nursing Home,* published by People's Medical Society (215)770-1670
- *The Medical Planning Handbook: A Guide to Protecting Your Family's Assets from Catastrophic Nursing Home Costs,* by Arthur A. Bove; Little, Brown, 1992
- *Patients, Pain & Politics: Nursing Home Inspector's Shocking True Story & Expert Advice for You and Your Family (on what to look for when selecting a nursing home),* by Mary Richards Rollins RN, BSN; New Century Publishing (PO Box 9861, Fountain Valley, CA 92708), 1994

American Association of Children's Residential Centers, 440 — 1st St., NW, Ste. 310, Washington, CD 20001; (202)638-1604

American Association for Continuity of Care, 1730 N. Lynn St., Arlington, VA 22209; (703)525-1191

American Association of Homes and Services for the Aging, 1129 — 20th St. NW, Washington, DC 20036; (202)783-2242 or 296-5960

American Baptist Homes and Hospitals Association, PO Box 851, Valley Forge, PA 19482-0851

American Disabled for Attendant Program Today, 201 S. Cherokee, Denver, CO 80203; (303)733-9324

American Federation of Home Health Agencies, 1320 Fenwick Lane, #100, Silver Spring, MD 20910; (301)588-1454

American Health Care Association, 1201 L St., NW, Washington, DC 20005; (202)842-4444

Assisted Living Facilities Association of America, 9401 Lee Hwy., Fairfax, VA 22031; (703)691-8100

The American Society of Consultant Pharmacists is made up of registered pharmacists who consult with nursing homes and other healthcare facilities on pharmaceutical matters.
American Society of Consultant Pharmacists, 1321 Duke St., Alexandria, VA 22314-3563; (703)739-1300

Beverly Foundation, 70 S. Lake Ave., Ste 750, Pasadena, CA 91101; (818)792-2292

Bretheren Homes and Older Adult Ministries, 1451 Dundee Ave., Elgin, IL 60120; (708)742-5100 or (800)323-8039

Care for Life, 1018 W. Diversey Parkway, Chicago, IL 60614; (312)883-1018

Caregiver's Catalog, c/o Creative Christian Ministries, Box 12624, Roanoke, VA 24027-2624

Children of Aging Parents, 1609 Woodbourne Rd., Levittown, PA 19057; (215)345-5104

Concerned Relatives of Nursing Home Patients, PO Box 18820, Cleveland Heights, OH 44118; (216)321-0403

Consultant Dietitians in Health Care Facilities, A Dietetic Group of the American Dietetic Association, 216 W. Jackson Blvd., Ste. 800, Chicago, IL 60606; (412)283-7025

National Association of Boards of Examiners for Nursing Home Administrators, 808 - 17th St., NW, Ste., 200, Washington, DC 20006; (202)223-9750

National Citizen's Coalition for Nursing Home Reform, 1224 M St. NW, Ste. 301, Washington, DC 20005-5183; (202)393-2018

National Institute on Adult Daycare, c/o National Institute on the Aging, 409 - 3rd St., SW, 2nd Flr., Washington, DC 20024; (202)479-6680

• NURSING, STATE BOARDS OF

National Council of State Boards of Nursing, 676 N. St. Clair, Ste. 550, Chicago, IL 60611-2921; (312)787-6555

Alabama Board of Nursing, RSA Plaza, Ste. 250, 770 Washington Ave., Montgomery, AL 63130; (205)242-4060

Alaska Board of Nursing, Dept. of Commerce and Economic Development, Division of Occupational Licensing, 3601 C St., Ste. 722, Anchorage, AK 99503; (907)561-2878 — or — PO Box 110806, Juneau, AK 99811-0806; (907)465-2544

American Samoa Health Service Regulatory Board, LBJ Tropical Medical Center, Pago Pago, American Samoa 96799; (684)633-1222 x 206

Arizona State Board of Nursing, 1651 E. Morten Ave., Ste. 150, Phoenix, AZ 85020; (602)255-5092

Arkansas State Board of Nursing, University Tower Bldg., Ste. 800, 1123 S. University, Little Rock, Arkansas 72204; (501)686-2700

California Board of Registered Nursing, PO Box 944210, Sacramento, CA 94244; (916)322-3350

California Board of Vocational Nurse and Psychiatric Technician Examiners, 2535 Capital Oaks Dr., Ste. 205, Sacramento, CA 95833; (916)263-7800

Colorado Board of Nursing, 1560 Broadway, Ste. 670, Denver, CO 80202; (303)894-2430

Connecticut Board of Examiners for Nursing, 150 Washington St., Hartford, CT 06106; (203)566-1041

Delaware Board of Nursing, PO Box 1401, Dover, DE 19903; (302)739-4522

District of Columbia Board of Nursing, 614 H St., NW, Washington, DC 20001; (202)727-7468

Florida Board of Nursing, 111 Coastline Dr., E., Ste. 516, Jacksonville, FL 32202; (904)359-6331

Georgia State Board of Licensed Practical Nurses, 166 Pryor St., SW, Atlanta, GA 30303; (404)656-3921

Georgia Board of Nursing (RN), 166 Pryor St., SW, Atlanta, GA 30303; (404)656-3943

Guam Board of Nurse Examiners, PO Box 2816, Agana, Guam 96910; (671)734-7295 or 734-7304

Hawaii Board of Nursing, PO Box 3469, Honolulu, HI 96801; (808)586-2695

Idaho Board of Nursing, 280 N. 8th St., Ste. 210, Boise, ID 83720; (208)334-3110

Illinois Dept. of Professional Regulation, 100 W. Washington St., 3rd Flr., Springfield, IL 62786; (217)785-9465 or 785-0800 — or — 100 W. Randolph, Ste. 9-300, Chicago, IL 60601; (312)814-2715

Indiana State Board of Nursing, 402 W. Washington St., Rm. 41, Indianapolis, IN 46204; (317)232-2960

Iowa State Board of Nursing, State Capitol Complex, 1223 E. Court Ave., Des Moines, IA 50319; (515)281-3255

Kansas Board of Nursing, Landon State Office Bldg., 900 SW Jackson, Ste. 551-S, Topeka, KS 66612-1230; (913)296-4929

Kentucky Board of Nursing, 312 Wittington Pkwy., Ste. 300, Louisville, KY 40222-5172; (502)329-7000

Louisiana State Board of Nursing, 912 Pere Marquette Bldg., 150 Baronne St., New Orleans, LA 70112; (504)568-5464

Louisiana State Board of Practical Nurse Examiners, 3421 N. Causeway Blvd., Ste. 203, Metairie, LA 70002; (504)838-5791

Maine State Board of Nursing, State House Station, Ste. 158, Augusta, ME 04333-0158; (207)624-5275

Maryland Board of Nursing, 4140 Patterson Ave., Baltimore, MD 21215-2299; (410)764-5124

Massachusetts Board of Registration in Nursing, Leverett Slatonstall Bldg., 100 Cambridge St., Rm. 1519, Boston, MA 02202; (617)727-9962

Michigan Bureau of Occupational and Professional Regulation, Michigan Dept. of Commerce, Ottawa Towers N., 611 W. Ottawa, Lansing, MI 48933; (517)373-1600

Minnesota Board of Nursing, 2700 University Ave., W., Ste. 108, St. Paul, MN 55114; (612)642-0567

Mississippi Board of Nursing, 239 N. Lamar St., Ste. 401, Jackson, MS 39201; (601)359-6170

Missouri State Board of Nursing, PO Box 656, Jefferson City, Missouri 65102; (314)751-0681

Montana State Board of Nursing, Dept. of Commerce, Arcade Bldg., Lower Level, 111 North Jackson St. Helena, Montana 59620-0407; (406)444-4279

Nebraska Bureau of Examining Boards, Nebraska Dept. of Health, PO Box 95007, Lincoln, Nebraska 68509; (402)471-2115

Nevada State Board of Nursing, 4335 S. Industrial Rd., Ste. 430, Las Vegas, NV 89103; (702)739-1575

Nevada State Board of Nursing, 1281 Terminal Way, Ste. 116, Reno, NV 89502; (702)786-2778

New Hampshire Board of Nursing, Health & Welfare Bldg., 6 Hazen Dr., Concord, NH 03301-6527; (603)271-2323

New Jersey Board of Nursing, PO Box 45010, Newark, NJ 07101; (201)504-6493

New Mexico Board of Nursing, 4206 Louisiana Blvd., NE, Ste. A, Albuquerque, NM 87109; (505)841-8340

New York State Board for Nursing, State Education Dept., Cultural Education Center, Rm. 3023, Albany, NY 12230; (518)474-3843 or 3845

North Carolina Board of Nursing, PO Box 2129, Raleigh, NC 27602; (919)782-3211

North Dakota Board of Nursing, 919 S. 7th St., Ste. 504, Bismark, ND 58504-5881; (701)224-2974

Northern Mariana Islands, Commonwealth Board of Nurse Examiners, Public Health Center, PO Box 1458, Saipan, MP 96950; (670)234-8950

Ohio Board of Nursing, 77 S. High St., 17th Flr., Columbus, OH 43266-0316; (614)466-3947

Oklahoma Board of Nursing, 2915 N. Classen Blvd., Ste. 524, Oklahoma City, OK 73106; (405)525-2076

Oregon State Board of Nursing, 800 NE Oregon St., Ste. 465-25, Portland, OR 97232; (503)731-4745

Pennsylvania State Board of Nursing, PO Box 2649, Harrisburg, PA 17105; (717)783-7142

Puerto Rico, Commonwealth of, Board of Nurse Examiners, Call Box 10200, Santurce, Puerto Rico 00908; (809)725-8161

Rhode Island Board of Nurse Registration and Nursing Education, Cannon Health Bldg., Three Capitol Hill, Rm. 104, Providence, RI 02908-5097; (401)277-2827

South Carolina State Board of Nursing, 220 Executive Center Dr., Ste. 220, Columbia, SC 29210; (803)731-1684

South Dakota Board of Nursing, 3307 S. Lincoln Avenue, Sioux Falls, SD 57105-5224; (605)335-4973

Tennessee State Board of Nursing, 283 Plus Park Blvd., Nashville, TN 37247-1010; (615)367-6232

Texas Board of Nurse Examiners, PO Box 140466, Austin, TX 78714; (512)835-4880

Texas Board of Vocational Nurse Examiners, 9101 Burnet Rd., Ste. 105, Austin, TX 78758; (512)835-2071

Utah State Board of Nursing, Division of Occupational and Professional Licensing, PO Box 45805, Salt Lake City, UT 84145-0805; (801)530-6628

Vermont State Board of Nursing, 109 State St., Montpelier, VT 05609-1106; (802)828-2396

Virgin Islands Board of Nurse Licensure, PO Box 4247, Veterans Dr. Station, St. Thomas, US Virgin Islands 00803; (809)776-7397

Virginia Board of Nursing, 6606 W. Broad St., 4th Flr., Richmond, VA 23230-1717; (804)662-9909

Washington State Nursing Care Quality-assurance Commission, Dept. of Health, PO Box 47864, Olympia, WA 98504; (206)753-2686

West Virginia Board of Examiners for Registered Professional Nurses, 101 Dee Dr., Charleston, WV 25311-1688; (304)558-3596

West Virginia State Board of Examiners for Practical Nurses, 101 Dee Dr., Charleston, WV 25311-1688; (304)558-3572

Wisconsin Bureau of Health Service Professions, 1400 E. Washington, PO Box 8935, Madison, WI 53708-8935; (608)266-0257

Wyoming State Board of Nursing, Barrett Bldg., 2nd Flr., 2301 Central Ave., Cheyenne, WY 82002; (307)777-7601

• NUTRITION, HEALTH, AND EATING

Books:
- *Aveline Kushi's Introducing Macrobiotic Cooking,* by Wendy Esko; Japan Publishing, 1987
- *Beyond Beef: The Rise and Fall of the Cattle Industry,* by Jeremy Rifkin; Penguin Group, 1992
- *The Book of Macrobiotics,* by Michio Kushi & Alex Jack; Japan Publications, 1992
- *Jane Brody's Nutrition Book: A Lifetime Guide to Good Eating for Better Health and Weight Control;* Bantam Books, 1987
- *The Cancer Prevention Diet: Michio Kushi's Macrobiotic Blueprint For the Prevention and Relief of Disease,* by Michio Kushi; St. Martins, 1995
- *Diet for a New America: How Your Food Choices Affect Your Health, Happiness, and the Future of Life on Earth,* by John Robbins; Stillpoint Publishing (PO Box 640, Walpole, NH 03608 [800]847-4014), 1987
- *Diet for a Small Planet,* by Frances Moore Lappe; Ballantine Books, 1991
- *Doctor, What Should I Eat?,* by Dr. Isadore Rosenfeld; Random House, 1995
- *Eat More, Weigh Less,* by Dean Ornish; Harper-Collins, 1993
- *Eat Right, Live Longer,* by Neal Barnard; Harmony Books, 1995
- *Essential Fatty Acids in Health and Disease,* by Edward N. Siguel; Nutrek, 1994

- *The Facts About Fats: A Consumer's Guide to Good Oils,* by John Finnegan; Elysian Arts, 1993
- *Fats that Can Save Your Life: The Critical Role of Fats and Oils in Health and Disease,* by Robert Erdmann & Meirion Jones; Bio-Science, 1990
- *Fats that Heal, Fats that Kill,* by Udo Erasmus; 1993
- *Feeding the Whole Family: Down-to-Earth Cookbook and Whole Foods Guide,* by Cynthia Lair; Lura Media ([800] 367-5872), 1994
- *The Food Pharmacy Guide to Good Eating,* by Jean Carper; Bantam Books, 1991
- *Food — Your Miracle Medicine: How Food Can Prevent and Cure Over 100 Symptoms and Problems,* by Jean Carper; HarperCollins, 1993
- *The Healing Foods: The Ultimate Authority on the Curative Power of Nutrition,* by Patricia Hausman & Judith Benn Hurley; Rodale Press, 1989
- *In Bad Taste: The MSG Syndrome,* by George R. Schwartz; Health Press, 1988
- *The Macrobiotic Way: The Complete Macrobiotic Diet And Exercise Book,* by Michio Kushi; Avery Press, 1985
- *May All Be Fed: Diet for a New World,* by John Robbins; Avon Books, 1992
- *Nutrition Almanac: Nutrients and How They Function in the Body,* by Lavon J. Dunne; McGraw-Hill, 1990
- *Sugar Blues,* by William Dufty; Warner Books, 1976
- *Super Healing Foods: Discover the Incredible Power of Natural Foods,* by Frances Sheridan Goulart; Parker Publishing, 1995
- *You Are What You Ate: A Macrobiotic Way of Eating: An RX for the Resistant Disease of the 21st Century,* by Shelly Rodgers, MD; Prestige Publishing, 1988

African-American Natural Foods Association, 7058 S. Clyde Ave., Chicago, IL 60649; (312)363-3939

Alliance Health Products, Net: http://www.websrus.com/websrus/alliance

American Vegan Society, 501 Old Harding Hwy., Malaga, NJ 08328

The Association of Vegetarian Dietitians and Nutrition Educators is a networking and support group for vegetarian-oriented nutrition professionals. For a referral to one of these professionals, contact the
Association of Vegetarian Dietitians and Nutrition Educators, 3835 Rt. 414, Burdett, NY 14818

The Community Alliance with Family Farmers publishes the *National Organic Directory.* It lists organic farmers, wholesalers, and businesses.
Community Alliance with Family Farmers, Davis, CA; (800)852-3832

Cornell Medical Center's Garlic Information Line, (800)330-5922

Delicious! Magazine of Natural Living (subscriptions $24 a year), 1301 Spruce St., Boulder, CO 80302; (303)939-8440; E-mail: delicious@newhope.com — or — Net: http://www.newhope.com

EarthSave Foundation, PO Box 949, Felton, CA 95018-0949

Flemings Healthy Life Products, Net: http://www.ibp.com/pit/fleming

Essential Fatty Acid Information, Net: http://www.newhope.com

Food and Water is a consumer education and advocacy organization working to stop threats to food safety. The group campaigns to stop such practices as food irradiation, the use of toxic pesticides, and genetically engineered food production. They publish the *Food & Water Journal,* a quarterly magazine that features articles on the dangers of using chemicals in our food supply, the reasoning behind using organic food, the laws governing food production, and the politics of big food companies. Membership is $25 per year and includes a subscription to the journal.
Food and Water, RR1 Box 68D, Walden, VT 05873; (802)563-3300 or (800)EAT-SAFE; Fax (802)563-3310

The Human Ecology Action League focuses on the effects of chemicals on the environment and on human health. They publish a quarterly magazine called *The Human Ecologist*.
Human Ecology Action League, PO Box 49126, Atlanta, GA 30359; (404)248-1898

The Kushi Institute (macrobiotic diet information), PO Box 7, Becket, MA 01223; (413)632-5742

Macrobiotics Today, George Ohsawa Macrobiotic Foundation, 1999 Myers St., Oroville, CA 95966; (916)533-7702

The Mail Order Catalog sells books on healthy eating, vegetarian cookbooks, vegetarian diet and nutrition items, and vegetarian foods in bulk quantities.
The Mail Order Catalog, PO Box 180, Summertown, TN 38483; (800)695-2241

McBooks Press is the publisher of three books by Sharon Yntema on vegetarianism. The titles are *Vegetarian Pregnancy: The Definitive Guide to Having a Happy Baby*; *Vegetarian Baby: A Sensible Guide for Parents*; and *Vegetarian Children: A Supportive Guide for Parents*. McBooks also has a web site that provides information on vegetarian parenting.
McBooks Press, 908 Steam Mill Rd., Ithica, NY 14850; (607)272-2114; Vegetarian Parenting Site, Net: http://www.spidergraphics.com/mcb

Mothers and Others for a Livable Planet, 40 W. 20th St., New York, NY 10011; (212)242-0010

The National Coalition Against the Misuse of Pesticides seeks to focus public attention on the very serious problem of pesticide poisoning. The coalition advocates for policies that better protect the public from pesticide exposures, and assists communities and individuals with information on alternative methods of pest control. The coalition publishes brochures, booklets, and a newsletter called *Pesticides and You*.
National Coalition Against the Misuse of Pesticides, 701 E St., SE, Ste. 200, Washington, DC 20003; (202)543-5450

The National Organization to Stop Glutamates publishes the *No MSG Newsletter*. Subscriptions are $25, unless you are financially strained. For an information packet that includes a membership form, send one dollar and a self-addressed, stamped envelope to **National Organization to Stop Glutamates,** PO Box 367, Santa Fe, NM 87504; (800) BEAT-MSG

Navigator's Health and Nutrition Page, Net: http://www.nav.com/home /hnpage.html

Nutrition Action Health Letter, Center for Science in the Public Interest, 1875 Connecticut Ave., NW, Ste. 300, Washington, DC 20009; (202)332-9110

North American Vegetarian Society, PO Box 72, Dolgevill, NY 13329; (518)568-7970

Northwest Coalition for Alternatives to Pesticides, PO Box 1393, Eugene, OR 97440; (541)344-5044; E-mail: ncap@igc.apc.org — or — Net: http://www.etn.org/~ncap

Nutrition for Optimal Health Association publishes a quarterly newsletter that features nutritional information and research. Subscriptions are $8.
Nutrition for Optimal Health Association, PO Box 380, Winnetka, IL 60093; (708)786-5326

Nutritional Health Alliance, PO Box 267, Farmingdale, NY 11735

Nutrition and Health Horizons ($24 a year), 95 Brown Road, Box 1023, Ithica, NY 14850

Organic Foods Production Association of North America, PO Box 1078, Greenfield, MA 01302; (413)774-7511

Organic Trade Association, PO Box 1078, Greenfield, MA 01302; (413)774-7511

The Pesticide Action Network is an international coalition of citizens' groups who oppose the misuse of pesticides and support reliance on safe, ecologically sound alternatives. They publish a newsletter called *Global Pesticide Campaigner*.

Pesticide Action Network, 116 New Montgomery, Ste. 233, San Francisco, CA 94105; (415)541-9140; Fax (415)541-9253; E-mail: panna@igc.apc.org — or — Net: http://www.panna.org/panna/

Physicians Committee for Responsible Medicine, 5100 Wisconsin Ave., Ste. 404, Washington, DC 20016; (202)686-2210

Pure Food Campaign, 1130 — 17th St., NW, Ste. 300, Washington, DC 20036; (202)775-1132

Safe Water Foundation, 6439 Taggart Rd., Delaware, OH 43015; (614)548-5340

Seeds of Change provides 100% certified organic, open-pollinated seeds for you to grow in your garden. Their seeds have not been coated with fungicides, herbicides, fertilizers or growth hormones. For a catalog, contact
Seeds of Change, PO Box 15700, Santa Fe, NM 87506-5700; (505)438-8080; E-mail: gardener@seedsofchange.com — or — Net: http://www.seedsofchange.com

The Sproutletter is a quarterly newsletter that provides information on healthfoods, nutrition, and how to live healthier. Subscriptions are $12 a year.
The Sproutletter, PO Box 62, Ashland, OR 97520; (503)488-2326; E-mail: lolaroja@aol.com

Vegan-L Vegan Food Recipes, Net: LISTSERV@VM.TEMPLE.EDU

Vegan Outreach, 10410 Forbes Rd., Pittsburgh, PA 15235; Net: http://envirolink.org/arrs/vo/index.html

Vegan's Journal Newsletter, PO Box 2552, Madison, WI 53701-2552

The Vegetarian Resource Group is the publisher of the *Vegetarian Journal,* a bi-monthly magazine containing vegetarian recipes and news on recent scientific-based studies detailing the benefits of vegetarianism. Subjects that are also covered are animal-free products, and the interrelated issues of health, nutrition, and ecology.

VRG also publishes the *Vegetarian Journal's Guide to Natural Foods Restaurants in the US and Canada.* It is a 270-page paperback that lists over 2,500 vegetarian and natural-foods restaurants in North America. The book also lists vegetarian travel services and tours. The book is available for $14, including postage. *The Vegan Handbook: Over 200 Delicious Recipes* is available for $20, including postage.
Vegetarian Resource Group, PO Box 1463, Baltimore, MD 21203; (410)366-8343; E-mail: TheVRG@aol.com — or — Net: http://envirolink.org/arrs/VRG/home.html

Vegetarian Times is published monthly and focuses on all aspects of the vegetarian lifestyle. They also publish a cookbook that includes 600 meatless recipes. A whole section of the book is dedicated to heart disease, cancer, obesity, osteoporosis, diabetes, and pregnancy. They also sell educational videos.
The Vegetarian Times, PO Box 570, Oak Park, IL 60303; (800)435-9610; E-mail: 74651.251@compuserve.com

Vegetarian Union of North America, PO Box 9710, Washington, DC 20016

• ONLINE HEALTH INFORMATION RESOURCES

One way to obtain current medical information is by using a computer that is hooked into the Internet. The Internet allows you to converse with other people in a discussion group focused on a specific health topic. You may also access health databases at major medical schools and do a computer search for newspaper, magazine, and medical journal articles. Some Internet sites called "bulletin board services"(BBS) allow you to communicate with health professionals and medical organizations by posting a question and receiving an answer. Some libraries, medical schools and facilities are connected to a database called *Medline* that can be used to search for information on specific health concerns.

The following companies are some of the more popular online services that you can call to get your computer connected to the Internet — you will also need a modem connected to your computer that is hooked into your phone line. There also may be local online services in your town that have compatible prices and services.

AlphaOne Online, (708)827-3615
America Online, (800)827-6364
Apple Link, (800)776-2333
CompuServe , (800)848-8199
Delphi, (800)695-4005
Genie, (800)638-9636
Grateful Med, (301)496-6308 or (800)638-8480 to get Grateful Med software and hook up to the National Library of Medicine online
MCI Internet, (800)779-0949
Network USA , (516)543-0234
Prodigy, (800)776-3449

Dr. Edward Del Grosso maintains a directory of medical groups and health-related bulletin boards on the Internet.
Dr. Edward Del Grosso, E-mail: ed@blackbag.com

Electric addresses are listed throughout the research section of this book. In addition to those that are already listed, the following may provide you with information that you are looking for on certain health subjects.

Alzheimer's, Net: http://werple.mira.net.au/~dhs/ad.html

Arizona Health Sciences Center, Net: http://128.196.106.42/nutrition.html

Basic Health and Medicine Homepage, Net: http://www.nova.edu/InterLinks /medicine.html

BITNET Medical Newsgroups, Net: http://umt.umt.edu:700/1/internet/News

BONES: The Biomedically Oriented Navigator of Electronic Services, Net: http:// bones.med.ohio-state.edu

Boston University School of Public Health, Net: http://www-busph.bu.edu/

Bright Innovations, Net: http://www.Earthlink.net/~bright/

Brighton Healthcare National Health Service Trust Home Page, Net: http://www. pavilion.co.uk/HealthServices/BrightonHealthCare/

Cambridge Healthtech Institute, Net: http://id.wing.net/~chi/upcoming.html

Canadian Health Network, Net: http://hpd1.hwc.ca/

Centers for Disease Control and Prevention, Net: http://www.cdc.gov/

CGS Biomedical Information Service, Net: http://www.eskimo.com/~cgs/

Code Four Medical, Net: http://web.idirect.com/~cfm

Collaborative Hypertext of Radiology, Net: http://chorus.rad.mcw.edu/chorus.rad .mcw.edu/chorus.html

Cyberspace Hospital, Net: http://ch.nus.sg

Dept. of Health & Human Services, Net: http://www.os.dhhs.gov

The Dept. of Neurosurgery at New York University, Net: http://mcns10.med .nyu.edu/

The Dept. of Otolaryngology at Baylor College of Medicine, Net: http://www .bcm.tmc.edu/oto/page.html

The Digital Anatomist Program, Net: http://www1.biostr.washington.edu/Digital Anatomist.html

The Directory of Online Healthcare Databases, (503)471-1627

Doody Publishing Health Science Book Reviews, Net: http://www.doody.com/

Duke University Community and Family Medicine Homepage, Net: http://dmi-www.mc.duke.edu/cfm/cfmhome.html

Duke University Informatics, Net: http://dmi-www.mc.duke.edu/

Emergency Medicine, Net: http://www.njnet.com/embbs/home.html

Family Health — College of Osteopathic Medicine, Net: http://www.tcom.ohiou .edu/family-health.html

Family Medicine, Net: http://galaxy.einet.net/galaxy/Medicine.html

Family Medicine, Net: http://mir.med.ucalgary.ca:70/1/family

Fam-Med Medical References, Net: gopher://gopher.gac.edu.70/11/Librariesand Reference/MedicalReferences

Food and Drug Administration, Net: http://www.fda.gov

Gastrointestinal and Liver Pathology, Net: http://www.pds.med.umich.edu/users .greenson/

Global Emergency Medicine Archives of the Division of Emergency Medicine of the University of California at San Francisco, Net: http://herbst7.his.ucsp.edu/

Global Health Network, Net: http://www.pitt.edu/~amy/ghn/ghn.html

Global Health Network, Net: http://www.putt.edu/HOME.GHNet.GHNet.html

Global Network Navigator, Net: http://nearnet.gnn.com/wic/med.toc.html

The Good Health Web, Net: http://www.social.com/health/index.html

Good Medicine Magazine, Net: http://none.coolware.com/health/good_med /ThisIssue.html

Handicap, Net: http://handicap shel.isc-br.com

Harvard Biological Laboratories' Biosciences-Medicine, Net: http://golgi.harvard .edu/biopages/medicine.html

Health Action Network Society, Net: http://www.hans.org/

Healthcare Outlook, Net: gopher://msa1.medsearch.com:70/11/hio

The Health Connection, Net: http://www.deltnet.com/BeverlyHills/HealthConnect

Health Decisions Plus/Comprehensive Health Enhancement Support System, (800)454-4465

Health Fair Online, Net: http://www.medaccess.com

Healthline, Net: gopher://healthline.umt.edu:700

Healthnet of Canada, Net: http://debra.dgbt.doc.ca/~mike/home/html

Health Resource, Net: http://www.coolware.com/health/joel/health.html

Health Science Resources on the Internet, Net: ftp://ftp2.cc.ukans.edu/pub.hmatrix

Healthwise Health Education and Wellness Program of Columbia University Health Services, Net: http://www.columbia.edu/cu/healthwise/

Health World Online, Net: http://www.healthy.net

History of Medicine, Net: http://indy.radiology.uiowa.edu/HistOfMedHP.html

The Hospital Web, Net: http://demOnmac.mgh.harvard.edu/hospitalweb.html

Institute for Molecular Virology at the University of Wisconsin - Madison, Net: http://www.bocklabs.wisc.edu/

Interactive Body Mind Information System, Net: http://www.teleport.com/~ibis

The Interactive Patient, Net: http:medicus.marshall.edu/medicus.htm

International Health News, Net: http://vvv.com/HealthNews/

International Health News, Net: http://www.perspective.com/health/index.html

Internet-Accessible Health Science Libraries, Net: ftp://hydra.uwo.ca/libsoft .medicallibraries.txt

The Internet Medical Products Guide, Net: http://medicom.com/medicom/home
.html

Johns Hopkins University, Net: http://www.welsh.jhu.edu

Johns Hopkins University BioInformatics Web Server, Net: http://www.gdb.org/
hopkins.html

Journal of Current Clinical Trials, Net: Gopher://gopher.psi.com:2347/7?clinical

Lawson Research Institute, Net: http://Earthcube.mit.edu/uwo/lri_home/html

Lifelines Health Page, Net: http://www.rain.org/idsolute/

Mayo Medical School, Net: http://www.mayo.edu/education/rst/mms.html

MDB Information Network, Net: http://mdbinfonet.com

Medical Data Analysis of the Los Alamos National Laboratory, Net: http://www.
c3.lanl.gov/cic3/projects/Medical/main.html

The Medical Education Page, Net: http://www.primenet.com/~giva/med.ed/

The Medical Reporter, Net: http://www.dash.com/netro/nwx/tmr/tmr.html

Medical Research Council of Canada, Net: http://hpb1.hwc.ca:8100/

Medicine and Health, Net: http://nearnet.gnn.com/wic/med.toc.html

Medicine Online, Net: http://meds.com

Medicine Servers, Net: http://white.nosc.mil/med.html

Medline, Net: http://atlas.nlm.nih.gov:5700/entrezFORMSmquery.html

MedLink International, Net: http://www.medlink.com

Molecular Biology Group, Net: http://resc9.res.bbsrc.ac.uk/plantpath/molbio/

Monash University, Net: gopher://gopher.vifp.monash.edu.au

Morbidity and Mortality Report, Net: gopher://cwis.usc.edu/11/The_Health_
Sciences_Campus/Periodicals/mmwr

National Institute of Allergy and Infectious Diseases, Net: http://nearnet.gnn.com
/wic/health.03.html

National Institute of Diabetes, Digestive, and Kidney Diseases, Net: http://www
.middk.nik.gov/

National Institutes of Health, Net: http://www.nih.gov

National Institute of Health & National Library of Medicine Clinical Alerts, Net:
http://nearnet.gnn.com/wic/nutrit.02/html

National Library of Medicine, Net: http://text.nlm.nih.gov/

National Library of Medicine HyperDOC, Net: http://www.nlm.nih.gov/

To find a library near you that is connected to Medline contact the

National Network of Libraries of Medicine, (800)338-7657

Nelson Institute of Environmental Medicine of the New York University Medical
Center, Net: http://charlotte.med.nyu.edu/HomePage.html

Neuro Implant Program at Thomas Jefferson University, Net: http://he1.unstju.edu
/~doctorb.bppp.html

Neurology Dept. of the Massachusetts General Hospital, Net: http://132.183
.145.103/

Neurosciences Internal Resource Guide of the University of Michigan, Net: http:
//http2.sils.umich.edu/Publis/nirg/mirg1.html

New England Medical Center, Net: http://www.nemc.org

Online Medical Resources, Net: file://ftp2.cc.ukans.edu/pub/hmatrix

Oregon Health Sciences University, Net: http://main.ohsu.edu/

The Osteopathic Source, Net: http://www.primenet.com/~pulse/thesource.html

Palo Alto Medical Foundation Healthnews, Net: http://www.service.com/PAMF/home.html

PATHY Medical Information, Net: http://pathy.futita-hu.ac.jp/phathy.html

Physician Finder Online, Net: http://msa2.medsearch.com

Plink — The Plastic Surgery Link, Net: http://www.IAEhv.nl/users/ivheij/plink.html

Poisons Information Database, Net: http:biomed.nus.org.sg/PID/PID.html

Polio Survivors Page, Net: http://www.eskimo.com/~dempt/polio.html

Reference Library Database, Net: http://gea.lif.icnet.uk/

Repetitive Strain Injury Network, Net: ftp://sunsite.unc.edu

Rural Healthcare, Net: http://ruralnet.mu.wvnet.edu

Society for Medical Decision-making, Net: http://www.nemc.org/SMDM

Society of Critical Care Medicine, Net: http://execpc.com/sccm

Stanford University Medical Center, Net: http://med-www.Stanford.EDU/MedCenter/welcome.html

Telemedicine Glossary of the Health Science Center at Syracuse, Net: http://hellogg.cs.hscsyr.edu/Telmedicine/glossary.html

Telemedicine Information Exchange, Net: http://tie.telemed.org

Telemedicine Web Page, Net: http://naftalab.bus.utexas.edu/~mary/tmpage.html

Three-D Medical Reconstruction, Net: http://www.ge.com/crd.ive.three_dim_medical.html

Toxicology, Net: gopher://gopher.niehs.nih.gov/11/ntp

To Your Health, Net: http://www.vitamin.com

Trauma AID Project of the University of Pennsylvania, Net: http://www.cis.upenn.edu/~traumaid/home.html

Tulane University Medical Center, Net: http://www.mcl.tulane.edu/

United States Public Health Service, Net: http://phs.os.dhhs.gov/phs/

Universal Healthcare Distributors, Net: http://www.magicnet.net/UHCD

University of British Columbia Multicentre Research Network, Net: http://www.unixg.ubc.ca:780/~emerg_vh/ubc_multicentre.html

University of Chicago Health Services, Net: gopher://bio-1.bsd.uchicago.edu

University of Connecticut Health Center, Net: http://www.uchc.edu/

University of Florida Medical Informatics Home Page, Net: http://www.med.ufl.edu/medinfo/homepage.html

University of Montana Healthline, Net: gopher://healthline.umt.edu:700

University of Vermont Dept. of Neurology, Net: http://salus.uvm.edu/Neurology.html

Virtual Environments and Real-time Deformation for Surgery Simulation, Net: http://www.cc.gatech.edu/gvu/medical_informatics/research/surg_sim.html

The Virtual Hospital, Net: http://indy.radiology.uiowa.edu/VirtualHospital.html

Word on Health, Net: http://www.webcom.com/~revista/

World Health Net, Net: http://world-health.net/

World Health Organization Press Releases, Net: http://www.who.ch/press/WHOPressReleases.html

Yahoo Health Index, Net: http://www.yahoo.com/Health/

• ORGAN AND TISSUE DONATION AND TRANSPLANTS

Books:
- *Bone Marrow Transplants: A Book of Basics for Patients*, by Susan K. Stewart; BMT Newsletter ([708] 831-1913), 1995
- *Lifeguards: The Real Story Of Organ Transplants*, by Calvin Stiller; Stoddard Publishing, 1990

American Association of Tissue Banks, 1350 Beverly Rd., McLean, VA 22101; (703)827-9582

American Society for Artificial Internal Organs, PO Box C, Boca Raton, FL 33429-0468; (407)391-8589

American Society of Transplant Surgeons, Columbia University College of Physicians & Surgeons; New York, NY 10021

Brain Tissue Bank, Mailman Research Center, McLean Hospital, 115 Mill St., Belmont, MA 02178; (617)855-2400

Brain & Tissue Bank for Developmental Disorders, University of Maryland at Baltimore, Dept. of Pediatrics, 655 W. Baltimore St., Baltimore, MD 21298-2964; (800)847-1539

Brain & Tissue Bank for Developmental Disorders, University of Miami School of Medicine, Dept. of Neurology (D4-5), PO Box 016960; Miami, FL 33101; (800)59BRAIN

Canadian Transplant Society, Toronto General Hospital, Gerrard Wing 3-538, 200 Elizabeth St., Toronto, Ontario, Canada M5G 2C4; (416)595-3111

Center for Organ Recovery and Education, 204 Sigma Dr., Pittsburgh, PA 15238; (412)963-3550 or (800)366-6777

Children's Organ Transplant Association, 2501 Cota Dr., Bloomington, IN 47403; (812)336-8872 or (800)366-2682

Division of Organ Transplantation, Health Resources and Services Administration, 5600 Fishers Lane, Rm. 11A-22, Rockville, MD 20857; (301)443-7557

Eye Donation Hotline, (800)638-1818 in Maryland phone (301)269-4031

Heart of America Bone Marrow Donor Registry, 2124 E. Mayer Blvd., Kansas City, MO 64132; (800)366-6710

High Techsplantations, Net: http://www.ht.com

Human Neurospecimen Bank, Veterans Administration Medical Center, 11301 Wilshire Blvd., Los Angeles, CA 90073; (310)824-4307

International Society for Heart & Lung Transplantation, 435 N. Michigan Ave., Ste. 1717, Chicago, IL 60611-4067; (312)644-0828

Living Bank, PO Box 6725, Houston, TX 77265; (713)961-9431 or (800)528-2971

Marrow Foundation, 400 Seventh St., NW, Ste. 306, Washington, DC 20004

National Bone Marrow Donor Program, 3433 Broadway St., NE, Ste. 400, Minneapolis, MN 55413-1763; (800)654-1247

National Bone Marrow Transplant Link, 29209 Northwestern Hwy., Southfield, MI 48034; (313)932-8483

North American Transplant Coordinators Organization, PO Box 15384, Lenexa, KS 66285-5384; (913)492-3600; Fax (913)541-0156

Organ Donors of Canada, 5326 Ada Blvd., Edmonton, Alberta, T5W 4N7 Canada; (403)474-9363

Organ Transplant Fund, 1027 S. Yates Rd., Memphis, TN 38119; (901)684-1697 or (800)489-3863

People interested in becoming a tissue donor can get information or a donor card from the
Red Cross Tissue Donation Services, (800)272-5287

United Network for Organ Sharing, 1100 Boulders Pkwy., Ste. 500, PO Box 13770 , Richmond, VA 23225-8770; Organ Donor Card Hotline (800)243-6667; Net: http:// www.ew3.att.net/unos

Transplant Recipients International Organization, 1000 Sixteenth St., NW, Ste. 602, Washington, DC 20036-5705; (202)293-0980 or (800) TRIO-386

Bill Young Marrow Donor Program, 7910 Woodmont Ave., Ste. 1410, Bethesda, MD 20814; (800)MARROW-3

- **ORIENTAL MEDICINE** (Also see *Alternative and Holistic Healthcare*, and *Herbs and Plant-Based Medicines/Therapies*)

Books:
- *Between Heaven and Earth: A Guide to Chinese Medicine*, by Harriet Beinfield, Lac and Efram Korngold, LAc, OMD; Ballentine, 1991
- *Chinese Herbal Medicine*, by Daniel P. Reid; Shamhala Publications, 1987
- *Complete Book of Chinese Health & Healing*, by Daniel Ried; Shambhala, 1995
- *Macrobiotics and Oriental Medicine*, by Muchio Kushi and Phillip Jannetta; Japan Publications, 1991
- *Shang Han Lun: Wellspring of Chinese Medicine*, Oriental Healing Arts Institute; Keats Publishing, 1981
- *Shiatsu: Japanese Finger Pressure Therapy*, by Toklujiro Namikoshi; Japan Publications, 1995

Chinese medicine identifies disease as disorders of relationship, not as a singular, unvarying entity. Problems recognized early on can be dealt with before they develop into complex, deep-seated, chronic sickness.
— from the book Between Heaven and Earth: A Guide to Chinese Medicine, by Harriett Beinfield and Efram Korngold; Ballantine Books, 1991

Academy of Chinese Culture and Health Sciences, 1601 Clay St., Oakland, CA 94612

Acupuncture, Net: http://www.acupuncture.com/acupuncture/

Acupuncture Homepage, Net: http://www.demon.co.uk/acupuncture/index.html

The American Academy of Medical Acupuncture members are physicians, MDs and DOs, who include the use of acupuncture in their practice. The Academy offers a physician referral program for consumers. They publish a *Journal of Medical Acupuncture* twice a year. To obtain a pamphlet that explains acupuncture in general terms to patients, write to the
American Academy of Medical Acupuncture, 5820 Wilshire Blvd., Ste. 500, Los Angeles, CA 90036; (213)937-5514 or (800)521-2262

American Acupuncture Association, 4626 Kissena Blvd., Flushing, NY 11355; (718)886-4431

American Association of Acupuncture and Oriental Medicine, 433 Front St., Catasauqua, PA 18032; (610)266-1433

American Center for Chinese Medical Sciences, 12921 Forest View Dr., Beltsview, MD 20705

American College of Traditional Chinese Medicine, 455 Arkansas St., San Francisco, CA 94107

American Foundation of Traditional Chinese Medicine, 505 Beach St., San Francisco, CA 94133; (415)776-0502

American Oriental Bodywork Therapy Association, 6801 Jericho Turnpike, Syosset, NY 11791; (516)364-5533

Blue Poppy Press publishes books on Chinese medicine and conducts seminars on Chinese medicine.
Blue Poppy Press, 1775 Linden Ave., Boulder, CO 80304; (303)447-8372 or (800)487-9296; E-mail: 102151.1614@compuserve.com — or for seminar information (800)448-8372; E-mail: bpsem@aol.com

Chinese Medicine Works Clinic, 1201 Noe St., San Francisco, CA 94114; (415)285-0931

East West Academy of Healing Arts, 450 Sutter, Ste. 916, San Francisco, CA 94108; (415)788-2227

Institute of Traditional Medicine, 2017 Southeast Hawthorne, Portland, OR 97214; (503)233-4907

International Foundation of Oriental Medicine, PO Box 625, Oakland Gardens, NY 11364; (718)886-4431

International Institute of Chinese Medicine, PO Box 4991, Santa Fe, NM 87502; (800)377-4561

Jin Shin Do Foundation for Bodymind Acupressure, PO Box 1097, Palo Alto, CA 95018; (415)328-1811

National Acupuncture Detox Association, 3115 Broadway, Ste. 51, New York, NY 10027; (212)993-3100 or (212) 579-5183

National Commission for the Certification of Acupuncturists, 1424 — 16th St., NW, Ste. 501, Washington, DC 20036; (202)232-1404

One Peaceful World, Box 10, Becket, MA 01223; (413)623-2322

Oregon College of Oriental Medicine, 10525 SE Cherry Blossom Dr., Portland, OR 97216; (503)253-3443; E-mail: 103226.164@CompuServe.com

Oriental Healing Arts Institute, 1945 Palo Verde Ave., Ste. 208, Long Beach, CA 90815

Oriental Medical Institute of Hawaii, 181 S. Kukui St., Ste. 206, Honolulu, HI 96813; (808)536-3611

Pacific College of Oriental Medicine, 702 W. Washington St., San Diego, CA 92103

Traditional Acupuncture Institute, 10227 Wincopin Cr., American City Bldg., Ste. 100, Columbia, MD 21044; (301)596-6006

Welcome to Acupuncture, Net: http://www.acupuncture.com/acupuncture/

World Natural Medicine Foundation and World Congress of Medical Acupuncture and Natural Medicine, 9904 — 106th St., Edmonton, Alberta, T5K 1C4 Canada; (403)424-2231; Fax (403)424-8520; E-mail: steven@hippocrates.family.med.ualberta.ca

Yo Sun University of Traditional Chinese Medicine, 600 Wilshire Blvd., Santa Monica, CA 90401; (310)917-2202

• OSTEOPATHIC ORGANIZATIONS

According to the American Osteopathic Association, all DOs (Doctors of Osteopathic medicine) are trained in family practice. Many receive additional training in a specialty area, such as psychiatry, pediatrics, obstetrics, surgery, ophthalmology, and cardiology. Before entering into an osteopathic medical school, applicants typically have a bachelor's degree, with undergraduate studies that include one year each of English, biology, physics, general chemistry, and psychology. Applicants must also take the Medical College Admissions Test (MCAT).

The first two years of osteopathic medical school focus on the basic sciences. The third and fourth years concentrate on clinical work. Most of the clinical work teaching is in community hospitals, major medical centers, and other medical facilities. After graduating, DOs complete a 12-month internship where they gain experience in internal medicine, family practice, and surgery. After the internship, some DOs spend an additional two to six years in training to become a specialist.

DOs are licensed to practice medicine and perform surgery in all 50 states.

The American Osteopathic Association requires its members to earn a specified number of continuing medical education credits every three years in order to maintain membership.

American Osteopathic Association, 142 E. Ontario St., Chicago, IL 60611; (800)621-1773

American Academy of Osteopathy, 1127 Mt. Vernon Rd., PO Box 750, Newark, OH 43058-0750

American Osteopathic Hospital Association, 1454 Duke St., Alexandra, VA 22314; (703)684-7700

• OSTEOPOROSIS

As part of the normal life cycle of all the cells in the body, bone cells go through a natural life cycle process. Blood cells called osteoclasts destroy bone, and other cells called osteoblasts rebuild the bone. It is normal for bone density to decrease as a person ages, but in some people bone density changes dramatically. In these people bones can become so brittle that they fracture easily. This can lead to long-term disability and may become life threatening. This debilitating deterioration in bone mass is called osteoporosis, or brittle bone disease.

According to the National Osteoporosis Foundation, more than 300,000 hip fractures occur every year because of osteoporosis. Other bones that are commonly affected by osteoporosis are those of the spinal column and the wrist.

Osteoporosis is seen mostly in older women. As men are now living longer, the disease is being seen more often in them than it had been in the past. Men experience a slower decline in bone density because testosterone, a hormone that plays a role in bone mass, remains relatively constant.

Osteoporosis occurs more often in countries where people eat large amounts of meat, dairy, and egg products (such as in America). Avoiding meat, dairy, and eggs throughout life greatly reduces the risk of experiencing osteoporosis. Eating dark green vegetables, such as broccoli and turnip greens, and foods such as soybeans, tofu processed with calcium sulfate, soy milk, kale, bok choy, sesame seeds, and oranges can provide the body with bone-strengthening nutrients. Dietary supplements, such as calcium, zinc, manganese, and vitamin D can help strengthen bones. Vitamin D stimulates the absorption of calcium in the intestines. The vitamin is produced in the skin when it is exposed to light and may also be obtained by eating foods that contain vitamin D.

Diets that are very high in meat, egg, and dairy protein, sodium, and caffeine are not good for calcium absorption because they increase the excretion of calcium by the kidneys. Over-the-counter antacids that contain aluminum and some prescription medications, such as the anti-inflammatory steroid glucocorticoid, can also weaken or damage the bones and interfere with calcium absorption. Other ways to preserve bone health are to avoid smoking and excessive alcohol consumption.

> *Habitual inactivity results in a downward spiral in all physiologic functions. . . .*
> *Fortunately, it appears that strength and overall fitness can be improved at any age through a carefully planned exercise program.*
> — From the American College of Sports Medicine Position Stand on Osteoporosis and Exercise, 1995

Regular exercise, especially with weights, or exercises that make you work against gravity, help counteract the aging process and build stronger bones. A study done at Tufts University in Boston showed that post-menopausal women who trained on exercise machines twice weekly for a year strengthened their bones and muscles and improved their balance.

Calcium supplements may be good for the bones, but a vegetarian-based eating plan and plenty of exercise are most important of all.

American College of Sports Medicine, National Center, PO Box 1440, Indianapolis, IN 46206-1440; (317)637-9200

National Osteoporosis Foundation, 1150 — 17th St., NW, Ste. 500, Washington, DC 20036-4603; (202)223-2226

• OTHER ORGANIZATIONS NOT LISTED IN THIS BOOK

Book:
• *Medical and Health Information Directory,* Gale Research Inc. (835 Penobscot Bldg., Detroit, MI 48226-4094), (in three volumes and available in many libraries)

Centers for Disease Control and Prevention National Center for Chronic Disease Prevention and Health Promotion Technical Information Service Branch, 4770 Buford Hwy., MS K13, Atlanta, GA 30341-3724; (404)488-5080

Consumer Information Center, Pueblo, CO 81009; (719)948-4000

To find organizations doing grant research about certain diseases, call **National Health Information Center,** PO Box 1133, Washington, DC 20013-1133; (301)565-4167 or (800)336-4797

National Library of Medicine, National Institutes of Health, Bethesda, MD 20894; (800)638-8480

National Organization for Rare Disorders, 100 Rte. 37, PO Box 8923, New Fairfield, CT 06812-1783; (203)746-6518 or (800)999-NORD; E-mail: 76703,3014@compuserve.com

National Self-Help Clearinghouse, Graduate School and University Center of the City University of New York, 25 W. 43rd St., Rm. 620, New York, NY 10036; (212)642-2944

Office of Disease Prevention and Health Promotion, National Health Information Center, PO Box 1133, Washington, DC 20013; (800)336-4797

For information on groups specializing in practically any health concern, call the master toll-free number at the United States Public Health Service. If you send them $1, the National Health Information Center will supply you with a list of toll-free numbers to health-related organizations that deal with specific medical concerns. **United States Public Health Service, National Health Information Center, Dept. of Health and Human Services,** PO Box 1133, Washington, DC 20013-1133; (800)336-4797 or from Maryland call (301)565-4167

Wheaton Regional Library Health Information Center, 11701 Georgia Ave., Wheaton, MD 20902; (301)929-5520 or the Senior Health Information Line (301)929-5485

Woodward/White publishes a list titled *The Best Doctors in America.* This list contains more than 7,200 doctors nationwide in more than 350 specialties. It is available for $95. **Woodward/White, Inc.,** 129 First Ave., Aiken, SC 29801; (803)648-0300

• PAIN AND HEADACHES

Books:
• *How To Stay Well Without Pain,* by Robert and Raye Yaller; Woodland Publishing ([800]777-2665), 1994
• *Living Well: A Twelve Step Response to Chronic Illness and Disability,* by Martha Cleveland, PhD; Ballatine Books, 1993

Various non-invasive techniques and procedures used to manage pain (surgery should only be considered as a last resort when no medical emergency exists):
• Acupuncture.
• Acupressure.
• Aikido.
• Aromatherapy.
• Assertiveness training.
• Avoid sugar, caffeine, and artificial food additives.

- Biofeedback.
- Chiropractic adjustments.
- Cognitive psychological therapy (teaching the patient to think differently about the issue).
- Cold compresses.
- Electric stimulation (transcutaneous electric nerve stimulation).
- Exercise.
- Group therapy.
- Hanging from a chin-up bar (for back problems to relieve tension and stretch the back).
- Herbal treatments, such as the Chinese herb feverfew for migraines, cayenne-ginger tea for joint pain, or white willow bark for pain and fever.
- Hypnosis.
- Improved diet.
- Increased water intake.
- Learning not to feel guilty about the pain.
- Meditation, visualization, and relaxation exercises.
- Massage with oils of chamomile, clary sage, lavender, or marjoram.
- Movement, breathing, and vocal expression classes.
- Music or sound therapy to relieve stress.
- Nutritional therapy.
- Staying active.
- Stretching exercises that are controlled and mild, and performed every day.
- Swimming, water massage/hydrotherapy.
- T'ai Chi.
- Yoga to condition muscles, ligaments, and joints.

American Academy of Head, Facial and Neck Pain and TMJ Orthopedics, Atlantic Bldg., Ste. 1310, 260 S. Broad St., Philadelphia, PA 19102; (215)545-2100

The American Chronic Pain Association offers training in skills and attitudes that have proven effective in helping people deal with chronic pain. The Association publishes a quarterly newsletter, *ACPA Chronicle,* that is available for $10. They also offer books, audio tapes, and video tapes that teach pain management and helpful exercises. The ACPA can connect teenagers with chronic pain to a group called *Teen Network.*
American Chronic Pain Association, PO Box 850, Rocklin, CA 95677; (916)632-0922

American Pain Society/American Academy of Pain Medicine, 5700 Old Orchard Rd., First Flr., Skokie, IL 60077-1057; (708)966-5595

Biofeedback uses special equipment to measures skin temperature, pulse, and the frequency of the brain waves. A computer shows the results of the measurements. The patient uses his mind to change the readings and this teaches the patient to use his mind to control bodily functions. Sometimes visualizations techniques are taught and hypnosis is used in combination with biofeedback.
Biofeedback Institute of America, 10200 W. 44th Ave., Ste. 304, Wheat Ridge, CO 80033-2840; (303)420-2902

The City of Hope National Medical Center publishes two pamphlets that deal with cancer pain. *Patient Handbook for Cancer Pain Management,* and *Your Child's Comfort: A Team Approach to Managing Your Child's Cancer Pain* are available free when you request them from the
City of Hope National Medical Center, 1500 E. Duarte Rd., Duarte, CA 91010-3000

Fibromyalgia Network, PO Box 31750, Tucson, AZ 85751; (520)290-5508

Headlines Newsletter, Migraine Foundation, 120 Carlton St., Ste. 210, Toronto, M5A 4K2 Canada; (416)920-4916

For information on herbal remedies for pain relief, contact the
Herb Research Foundation, 1007 Pearl St., Ste. 200, Boulder, CO 80302; (303)449-2265 or (800)748-2617; Net: http://sunsite.unc.edu/herbs

Milwaukee Pain Clinic, 6529 W. Fond du Lac Ave., Milwaukee, WI 53218; (414)464-7246

National Chronic Pain Outreach Association, 7979 Old Georgetown Rd., Ste. 100, Bethesda, MD 20814-2429; (301)652-4948

National Headache Foundation, 5252 N. Western Ave., Chicago, IL 60625; (312)878-7715 or (800)843-2256

Roxanne Pain Institute, Net: http://www.Roxanne.com

Self-Help In Pain (SHIP), 33 Kingsdown Park, Whistable, Kent C15 2DT, England

Stress Reduction Clinic of the University of Massachusetts Medical Center, 55 Lake Ave., N. Worcester, MA 01655; (508)856-2656

- **PARALYSIS** (Also see *Back and Spine*)

American Paralysis Association, 500 Morris Ave., Springfield, NJ 07081; (800)225-0292; Net: http://www.apa.uci.edu/paralysis

American Paraplegia Society, 75-20 Astoria Blvd., Jackson Heights, NY 11370-1177; (718)803-3782

Paralyzed Veterans of America, 801 — 18th St., NW, Washington, DC 20006-3715; (202)USA-1300; TDD (202)416-7622; Fax (202)785-4452

Sigmedics manufactures and markets an electronic impulse system called Parastep that allows some people who are paralyzed below the waist to be able to have some function to their legs.
Sigmedics, Inc., Northfield, IL; (708)501-3500

- **PARKINSON'S DISEASE**

American Parkinson's Disease Association, 1250 Hyland Blvd., Staten Island, NY 10305; (800)223-2732

National Parkinson Foundation, 1501 NW 9th Ave., Bob Hope Rd., Miami, FL 33136; (305)547-6666 or (800)327-4545

Parkinson's Disease Foundation, 650 W. 168th St., New York, NY 10032; (800)457-6676

Parkinson's Speak-Out Newsletter ($24 a year), 55 Merrick St., Rumford, RI 02916-2520; (401)435-3179

Parkinson's Support Groups of America, 11376 Cherry Hill Rd., Ste. 204, Beltsville, MD 20705

Parkinson's Web, Net: http://neuro-chief-e.mgh.harvard.edu/parkinsonsweb /Main/PDmain.html

United Parkinson Foundation, 833 W. Washington, Chicago, IL 60607; (312)733-1893

- **PATHOLOGISTS**

The College of American Pathologists is the leading authority on lab testing, helps shape state and national regulations governing testing, and is responsible for how medical labs are regulated. CAP is financed by medical labs and inspects and accredits labs both in and out of hospitals. CAP does not release its records of mismanaged medical labs to the public (a true disservice to consumers). Not all labs cooperate with CAP's review and accreditation program and those labs that do participate do it on a voluntary basis.
College of American Pathologists, 325 Waukegan Rd., Northfield, IL 60093-2750; (708)446-8800

- **PATIENTS' AND CONSUMERS' RIGHTS**

Books:
- *The Consumer's Legal Guide to Today's Healthcare: Your Medical Rights and How to Assert Them,* by Stephen L. Isaacs, JD, & Ava C. Swartz, MPH; Houghton Mifflin Co., 1992

- *Ethics on Call: A Medical Ethicist Shows How to Take Charge of Life & Death Choices in Today's Healthcare System,* by Nancy Dubler & David Nimmons; Vantage Books, 1993
- *The Girl Who Died Twice: The Libby Zion Case and the Hidden Hazards of Hospitals,* by Natalie Robins; Delacorte Press, 1995
- *The Great White Lie; Dishonesty, Waste, & Incompetence in the Medical Community,* by Walt Bogdanich; Touchstone Books, 1992
- *Medicine, Money and Morals: Physicians' Conflicts of Interest,* by Marc A. Rodwin; Oxford University Press, 1993
- *Silent Violence, Silent Death: A Consumer Guide to the Medical Malpractice Epidemic,* by Harvey Rosenfield; Essential Books ([202] 387-8030), 1994
- *Smart Patient, Good Medicine: Working With Your Doctor to Get the Best Medical Care,* by Richard L. Sribnick, MD, and Wayne B. Sribnick, MD; Walker Publishing, 1994
- *Talk Back to Your Doctor: How to Demand and Recognize High Quality Healthcare,* by Arthur Levin; Doubleday, 1975
- *Wrongful Death: A Medical Tragedy,* by Sandra M. Gilbert; W.W. Norton & Company, 1995

The Agency for Healthcare Policy and Research is part of the United States Department of Health and Human Services. Copies of the agency's practice guidelines and patient guides are free.
The Agency for Healthcare Policy and Research, (800)358-9295

American Association of Dental Victims, 3316 E. 7th St., Long Beach, CA 90804

Call for Action, 3400 Idaho Ave., NW, Ste. 101, Washington, DC 20016; (202)537-1551

The Center for Medical Consumers is a health education organization and operates a library in New York City. CMC publishes a monthly newsletter called *Health Facts* that is available for $21 a year.
The Center for Medical Consumers, 237 Thompson St., New York, NY 10012-1090; (212)674-7105

Center for Public Representation, 121 S. Pinckney St., Madison, WI 53703; (800)369-0338

Champaign County Healthcare Consumers, 44 E. Main St., Ste. 208, Champaign, IL 61820; (217)352-6533

The Network Project is a citizen-supported consumer research and protection organization. It was founded in 1985 and works closely with consumer advocacy organizations in Washington and throughout the nation to educate the public about the various reform proposals. It is funded by public grants and donations.
Citizen Empowerment Project/Consumers for Quality Care/The Network Project, 1750 Ocean Park Blvd., Ste. 200, Santa Monica, CA 90405; (310)392-0522; E-mail: Network @Primenet.com. — or — Net: http://www.primenet.com/~network

Citizens for Health is a nationwide, community-based, public health advocacy network. Their goal is to educate the public and to protect consumers' rights to maintain access to a wide range of healthcare products and services relating to wellness and preventive healthcare. The group lead the national grassroots effort in support of the Dietary Supplement Health and Education Act of 1994 which guarantees consumers' continued access to dietary supplements, such as vitamins, minerals, herbal products, and amino acids, but also preserves the government's right to regulate claims used to sell them. The letter-writing campaign by consumers who feared loss of access to their vitamins if the FDA had started regulating them as strictly as prescription drugs resulted in more mail being received by members of Congress than for any other single issue since the Vietnam War. The proposed rules would have reclassified amino acids as drugs and herbs as unsafe food additives, and would have limited potency levels of vitamins and minerals.
Citizens for Health, PO Box 1195, Tacoma, WA 98401; (206)922-2457 or (800)357-2211

Coalition for Consumer Rights, 225 W. Ohio St., Ste. 250, Chicago, IL 60610

Common Cause, 2030 M St., NW, Ste. 300, Washington, DC 20036-3380; (202)833-1200

Community Health Action Center of Families USA Foundation, 30 Winter St., Boston, MA 02108; (617)338-6035

The US Government Consumer Information Center distributes a *Consumer's Resource Handbook*. The book tells consumers how to complain to get results. It lists the federal agencies that are responsible for resolving particular consumer problems, and tells where help is available in state and local governments and private organizations. Single copies are free and may be obtained by writing to
Consumer Information Center, Handbook, Pueblo, CO 81009

Consumer Product Safety Commission, 5401 Westbard Ave., Bethesda, MD 20892; Product Safety Line (800)638-2772; In Maryland phone (800)492-8104

Consumers United for Food Safety, PO Box 22928, Seattle, Washington 98122; (206)747-2659

Dept. of Justice's Americans with Disabilities Helpline, (800)514-0301

Environmental Protection Agency Public Information Center, 401 M St., SW, Washington, DC 20460; (202)424-4000; Asbestos hotline (800)368-5888; Drinking Water hotline (800)426-4791; Lead hotline (800)LEAD-FYI; Indoor Air hotline (800)438-4318; Radon hotline (800) SOS-RADON

Families Advocating Injury Reduction is based in Illinois and was founded by injury victims and families interested in advocating for public policies that will reduce the number of injuries and deaths from medical malpractice, unsafe workplaces, and dangerous products.
Families Advocating Injury Reduction, 44 E. Main, Ste. 208, Champaign, IL 61820; (217)352-6533

Families USA is a national consumer advocacy organization working for comprehensive reform of America's health and long term care systems.
Families USA Foundation, 30 Winter St., 10th Flr., Boston, MA 02108; (617)338-6035 or (202)737-6340

The Food and Drug Administration has jurisdiction over the content and labeling of foods, drugs, and medical devices. The FDA has the responsibility of evaluating the safety and value of medical treatments, and certifying them as such. The FDA can take law enforcement action to seize and prohibit the sale of products that the FDA determines as being falsely labeled. The FDA is a government entity. Activities of the FDA seem to indicate that it often bows to the pressure of well-financed lobbyists who represent the allopathic medical establishment or companies whose interests are in the process of making money — as opposed to protecting the general public. The FDA has often been strongly criticized for taking actions that support the financial interests of allopathic doctors and chemical drug manufacturers.
Food and Drug Administration, Consumer Affairs and Information, 5600 Fishers Lane, HFC—110, Rockville, MD 20857; (301)443-1544; FDA Center for Drugs (301)594-1012; Net: http://www.fda,gov/fdahomepage.html

The Federal Trade Commission has jurisdiction over the advertising and marketing of foods, non-prescription drugs, medical devices, and healthcare services. The FTC can seek federal court injunctions to halt what the FDA considers to be fraudulent claims, and may obtain redress for injured consumers.
The Federal Trade Commission, Correspondence Branch, 6th St. and Pennsylvania Ave., NW, Washington, DC 20580; (202)326-2180

Health Care for All, 30 Winter St., Boston, MA 02108; (617)350-7279

Medical device Reporting Program, (301)881-0256 or (800)638-6725

The National Center for Patients Rights is a non-profit consumer and victim of malpractice advocacy group. They can answer questions about medical misconduct, negligence, and malpractice. They do not give lawyer referrals.
National Center for Patients Rights, 666 Broadway, Ste. 520, New York, NY 10012; (212)979-6670

National Citizens' Coalition for Nursing Home Reform, 1424 — 16th St., NW, Washington, DC 20036; (202)332-2275

National Council on Patient Information and Education, 666 — 11th St., NW, Ste. 810, Washington, DC 20001; (202)347-6711

National Consumers League, 815 — 15th St., NW, Washington, DC 20005

National Headquarters — Council of Better Business Bureaus, Inc., 4200 Wilson Blvd., Arlington, VA 22203; (703)276-0100

National Women's Health Network, 514 — 10th St., NW, Washington, DC 20004; (202)347-1140

New England Patients' Rights Group, PO Box 141, Norwood, MA 02062-0002; (617)769-5720

The People's Medical Society is a nonprofit consumer education organization dedicated to the principles of better, more responsive, and less expensive medical care. The Society works to put previously unavailable medical information into the hands of consumers so consumers can make informed decisions about their own healthcare. The Society keeps records of bad doctors and inadequate health treatment. They can provide you with information on how to get copies of your medical records from uncooperative doctors. Subscriptions to their newsletter for consumers is included in their yearly $20 membership fee. They also publish books on various health subjects. **People's Medical Society,** 462 Walnut St., Allentown, PA 18102; (215)770-1670 or (800)624-8773

Public Citizen, an investigative watchdog group, was founded in 1971 by consumer advocate Ralph Nader. The group fights for a more open and democratic government, safer consumer products, quality healthcare, and a clean environment. The group includes five divisions. The Health Research Group is the country's leading consumer awareness group focused on healthcare issues. HRG has long been active in efforts to reform the nation's healthcare system, and to improve the quality of medical care. A donation of $35 or more includes a subscription to their monthly *Health Letter*.

Public Citizen's Health Research Group has compiled a list called "*10,289 Questionable Doctors*." It contains some of the names and locations of doctors who have been disciplined by their state medical boards, or by the federal government for such things as incompetence, negligence, sexual offenses, or drug and alcohol abuse. The complete list is available for $200, or a list of doctors in one state is available for $15, plus $2 shipping.

Public Citizen's recommendations to Congressional subcommittee hearings on issues relating to medical malpractice:

Rather than limit victims' rights, Public Citizen urges that the following reforms be implemented on the state and national levels to reduce medical malpractice and improve the quality of healthcare in this country:

1. Better doctor discipline is essential to reducing the incidence of medical negligence. Because a small number of doctors cause the most malpractice, removing incompetent providers from practice will lower needless injuries and deaths resulting from negligent care.

• States should give licensing boards more power to discipline physicians, including emergency suspensions pending formal hearings in cases where a doctor poses a potential danger. In addition, medical board decisions should take effect while being appealed through the court system.

• State boards should be restructured to ensure strong consumer representation and loosen ties with medical societies.

• Adequate resources should be provided to the boards to ensure timely and thorough investigations of complaints. One hundred percent of license fees should go to funding the boards. In addition, Congress should create a small program of grants-in-aid to state medical boards. The grants should be tied to the boards' agreements to meet certain performance standards.

- Consumers must have increased access to information on physicians' medical malpractice history. The National Practitioner Data Bank that holds information about actions taken against doctors should be open to the public.

   In addition, the Drug Enforcement Agency should release a monthly list of all practitioners whose controlled substances prescription licenses have been suspended.
- Insurance companies should forward all claiming and settlement information on physicians to state licensing boards.

2. Insurance should ensure sensible underwriting and thereby lower costs in the healthcare system.

- Insurance companies should be required to better spread risk by placing all physicians in a unified pool. Currently, the sub-categories used by insurance companies result in sky-high premiums for certain specialties.
- In order to differentiate "high-risk" doctors, insurance companies should charge rates based on a physician's experience. This would ensure that doctors with histories of negligent behavior would pay more.

3. Improved physician training and oversight would limit negligent behavior, and the resulting costly injuries.

- Risk management programs should be implemented to decrease medical negligence.
- Physician recertification should be implemented, requiring written examinations, and audits of medical performance through a review of patient records.
- Practice guidelines should be developed for certain procedures. A 1989 Harvard Medical School study found that practice guidelines for anesthesia have drastically reduced the incidence of death or brain damage to patients. The study also found a dramatic drop in the cost of medical malpractice premiums for anesthesiologists.
- Physicians who are aware of other doctors' incompetence should be encouraged through confidentiality and immunity to report negligence to the appropriate disciplinary body.

4. Voluntary alternative dispute resolution mechanisms should be established to enable medical malpractice victims with small claims to seek compensation through a streamlined system.

Finally, the US should adopt a single-payer national health program modeled on the Canadian system. This sensible step could provide our country's residents with universal and adequate healthcare at the same cost as the current system, which has failed a large segment of society. A universal health program would also have the effect of reducing the numbers of malpractice lawsuits, because injured victims would not need to turn to the legal system to be compensated for their healthcare expenses. Those expenses would simply be paid for through the public plan.

Public Citizen will continue to work towards the goal of universal healthcare. Likewise, we are committed to working strenuously to defeat any measures that would make it even more difficult for victims of medical malpractice to recover from wrongdoings.

> — Taken from testimony of Pamela Gilbert of Public Citizen's Congress Watch, presented to Congressional subcommittee hearing on issues relating to medical malpractice, May 20, 1993

Public Citizen's Health Research Group, 2000 P St., Washington, DC 20036; (202)833-3000

Know Your Medical Rights
1. You have the right to have complete information regarding your condition, its diagnosis, prognosis, and planned treatment, along with pros and cons of treatment.
2. You have the right to honest and competent medical care.
3. You have the right not to be kept against your will or forced to settle your bill before your discharge.
4. You have the right to pursue a second opinion.

5. You have the right to know everything about the medication or treatment you are given — its primary use, its advantages, and its disadvantages as compared to other drugs or treatment.
   — the Safe Medicine for Consumers' newsletter

Safe Medicine for Consumers is an advocacy group for patient's rights and for survivors and family members of victims of medical negligence. Although SMC concentrates its efforts in the state of California, and on the Medical Board of California, the group will send information to people outside of California to help establish chapters in other states. On request, SMC will supply information on how to successfully file complaints with state medical boards and other agencies.

SMC follows and participates in pending legislation that is in the interest of consumers' medical rights, safety, and care. It also works to protect existing public policy issues that promote quality healthcare. SMC helps to educate the public by sending out press releases to the media when there is medical patient legislation that the public should be made aware of. The group also provides consumers with education and information of their rights while obtaining medical care. As a way to help expose the tragedy of malpractice, the group regularly connects journalists and news shows with victims of malpractice. The group encourages consumers to get involved with changing the government of the medical industry, and to pressure government agencies to react faster and more responsibly to consumer demands for protection from substandard medical care.

Safe Medicine for Consumers, PO Box 878, San Andreas, CA 95249; (209)754-4408; Fax (209)736-2402

The Society of Patient Representatives is associated with the American Hospital Association and advises hospitals on how to set up patient relations programs. Not all hospitals participate.

Society of Patient Representatives and Consumer Affairs of the American Hospital Association, 840 N. Lake Shore Dr., Chicago, IL 60611; (312)280-6424

The US Government Manual is the official handbook of the federal government. Published by the National Archives and Records Administration, it describes the programs in each federal agency and lists the names of top personnel, the agency's mailing address, and a general information telephone number. It is available in most public libraries, or can be purchased for $23 by sending a check or money order along with a letter requesting the manual to the

Superintendent of Documents, US Government Printing Office, Washington, DC 20402

The United States Consumer Product Safety Commission was activated in 1973 and is headed by a chairperson and two commissioners appointed by the President with the advice and consent of the Senate. The CPSC's function is to protect the public from unreasonable risks of injury and death associated with consumer products. The Commission's objective is to reduce the estimated 28.5 million injuries and 21,600 deaths associated each year with the 15,000 different types of consumer products within the CPSC's jurisdiction. As with other government agencies that are set up to protect consumers, the CPSC has been strongly criticized for working in the interests of big business, while disregarding the safety of consumers.

The CPSC publishes booklets that describe some of the common hazards associated with the use of consumer products and recommended ways to avoid these hazards. For a list of the booklets, contact the CPSC.

To report a hazardous product or product-related injury, call the toll-free hotline at 1-800-638-2772. The phone number for the hearing impaired is: 1-800-638-8270. The Maryland TTY number is 1-800-492-8104.

United States Consumer Product Safety Commission, (301)504-0580

Created in 1980, the Center for Public Interest Law is a public interest research and advocacy organization affiliated with the University of San Diego School of Law. CPIL's goal is to make the regulatory functions of state government more efficient and more visible by serving as a public monitor of state regulatory agencies. CPIL has been

involved in studies on legislation regarding the California State Medical Board's practices of disciplining doctors. Through its law student interns, CPIL monitors the activities of 50 state agencies that regulate businesses, professions, trades, and the environment. CPIL publishes the *California Regulatory Law Reporter*.
University of San Diego's Center for Public Interest Law, c/o USD School of Law, 5998 Alcala Park, San Diego, CA 92110; (619)260-4806

The US Public Interest Research Group investigates problems having to do with the health and safety of the public and the environment, educates the public about solutions, and lobbies for reforms that preserve the environment and protect consumers. The group has a variety of publications, including reports that cover a variety of subjects of concern to the public. Among the publications are those covering pesticides in the food chain, the hazards of tanning salons, dangerous drugs, and medical devices. For a list of the publications, send a self-addressed, stamped envelope to
US Public Interest Research Group, 215 Pennsylvania Ave., SE, Washington, DC 20003; (202)546-9707

Washington Citizen Action is Washington's largest consumer group, focused primarily on health related issues, including healthcare reform, and long-term care reform. WCA is affiliated with major state church, senior, labor, and community groups concerned with consumer issues. WCA publishes a quarterly newsletter called *Outreach*.
WCA has joined with the Boston-based Families USA Foundation to publish a book titled *Seattle-Tacoma Health Care Choices*. The book is a consumer guide to healthcare in the Seattle-Tacoma area and costs $10.95. To obtain a copy of the book, contact
Washington Citizen Action Education and Research Fund, 100 S. King St., Ste. 240, Seattle, WA 98104; (206)389-0050; E-mail: wca@eskimo.com — or — Net: http://www .eskimo.com/~wca

White House Comment Office, (202)456-1111

• **PHYSICAL THERAPY** (Also see *Rehabilitation*)

Adventures in Movement for the Handicapped, 945 Danbury Rd., Dayton, OH 45420; (513)294-4611

The Internal Capsule, Net: http://www.voicenet.com/1/voicenet/homepages /levinson/

Marquette University Program in Physical Therapy, Net: http://www.mu.edu/ dept.pt

National Rehabilitation Association, 11250 Roger Bacon Dr., Ste. 8, Reston, VA 22090; (703)437-4377

The Physical Therapy World Wide Web Page, Net: http://www.mindspring.com/~ wbrock/pt.html

• **PRESCRIPTION DRUGS**

Books:
• *Beyond Antibiotics: 50 Ways to Boost Immunity and Avoid Antibiotics*, by Michael A. Schmidt; North Atlantic Press/Staying Well ([800]622-6309), 1995
• *The Complete Drug Reference*; Consumer Reports Books, 1993
• *Deadly Medicine: Why Tens of Thousands of Heart Patients Died in America's Worst Drug Disaster*, by Thomas J. Moore; Simon and Schuster, 1995
• *The Essential Guide to Prescription Drugs*, by James Long; HarperCollins, 1994
• *The Primary Source*, by Norman Myers; WW Norton & Co., 1992
• *Worst Pills, Best Pills*; published by Public Citizen's Health Research Group ([202]833-3000), regularly revised

Parsons Technology ([800]223-6925)sells a computer program titled *Medical Drug Reference*. It lists important information on over 7,000 prescription and non prescription drugs.

Alliance for the Prudent Use of Antibiotics, PO Box 1372, Boston, MA 02117; (617)956-6765

American College of Apothecaries, 205 Daingerfield Rd., Alexandria, VA 22314; (703)684-8603

American Pharmaceutical Association, 2215 Constitution Ave., NW, Washington, DC 20037; (202)628-4410

Canadian Society for Clinical Pharmacology, 33 Russell St., Toronto, Ontario, M5S 2S1 Canada; (416)595-6119

Consumer Pharmacist Newsletter (subscriptions $48 a year), ELBA Medical Foundation, PO Box 1403, Melairie, LA 70001; (504)833-3600

To report a doctor, pharmacist, or other health professional, who is abusing his Drug Enforcement Administration controlled substance (narcotics) license by selling drugs illegally, or abusing drugs, contact a diversion investigator at the diversion unit of the nearest field office of the DEA. If you cannot locate the nearest DEA office, contact the national headquarters of the DEA in Washington, DC. The DEA might conduct an investigation into the doctors' handling of controlled substances, or the doctor may be called to present evidence at a DEA administrative hearing to explain his actions and show cause of why his certificate of registration to handle controlled substances should not be revoked.

Drug Enforcement Administration, US Dept. of Justice, 1405 — I St., NW, Washington, DC 20005; (202)401-7834

Fisher Pharmaceuticals Laboratories, Net: http://www.dr_fischer.com

Food and Drug Administration, Office of Consumer Affairs, 5600 Fishers Lane, HFE-50, Rockville, MD 20857; (301)443-3170; FDA Center for Drugs (301)594-1012

The Foreign Pharmacy Graduate Exam Committee evaluates the qualifications of pharmacists who have graduated from foreign medical schools. They do this by administering an exam that measures the knowledge of the pharmacist against the standards of US pharmacy schools.

Foreign Pharmacy Graduate Exam Committee, National Association of Boards of Pharmacy Foundation, 700 Busse Hwy., Park Ridge, IL 60068; (708)698-6227

Institute for Safe Medication Practices, Warminster, PA; (215)956-9181

The Medical Letter on Drugs and Therapeutics is written for medical professionals.
The Medical Letter on Drugs and Therapeutics, 1000 Main St., New Rochelle, NY 10801-7537; (914)235-0500

Medical workers can anonymously report medication errors by calling the Medication Error Reporting Program operated by the Institute for Safe Medical Practices.

Medication Error Reporting Program, 12601 Twinbrook Pkwy., Rockville, MD 20852; (800)23-ERROR

Medscript Windows Prescription Writer for Physicians, Net: http://www.rust.net /~skindell/medscrip.html

National Association of Boards of Pharmacy, 700 Busse Hwy., Park Ridge, IL 60068; (708)698-6227

National Association of Chain Drug Stores, c/o Ronald L. Ziegler, 413 N. Lee St., Alexandria, VA 22313-1417; (703)549-3001

National Association of Retail Druggists, 205 Dangerfield Rd., Alexandria, VA 22314; (703)683-8200

National Institute of General Medical Sciences, Office of Research Reports, Bldg. 31, Rm. 4A52, Bethesda, MD 20982; (301)496-7301

Nonprescription Drug Manufacturers' Association, 1150 Connecticut Ave., NW, Washington, DC 20036; (202)429-9260

Pharmaceutical Manufacturers' Association, and America's Pharmaceutical Research Companies, 1100 — 15th St., NW, Washington, DC 20005; (202)835-3400 or (800)862-4110

Pharmaceutical Research, Net: http://cipr-diva.mgh.harvard.edu/

Pharmacology Home Page, Net: http:farmr4.med.uth.tmc.edu/homepage.html

PhRMA Homepage, Net: http://www.phrma.org

PPS Online, Net: http://www2.pps.ca/pps.html

Public Citizen publishes a 562-page book called *Worst Pills Best Pills*. The book focuses on how to prevent unnecessary illness and risks including untimely death caused by mis-prescribed or over-prescribed medications. It includes easy-to-understand information about many drugs.

Public Citizen has obtained information from the DEA about doctors who have had restrictions placed on, or have had their narcotics licenses revoked.

Public Citizen/*Worst Pills Best Pills II*, 2000 P St., NW, Washington, DC 20036; (202)833-3000

The United States Pharmacopoeia is an independent regulatory agency that sets standards for the purity and potency of drugs, vitamins, and minerals. Compliance with the standards set by the USP is voluntary on the part of manufacturers of these products. Manufacturers whose products correspond to the standards set by the USP can label their product as such. The Food and Drug Administration can take action against the manufacturers of products that are USP labeled, but that do not actually correspond to USP standards.

United States Pharmacopoeia, Rockville, MD; (301)881-0666

World Wide Drugs, Net: http://community.net/~neils/new.html

• PROFESSIONAL TITLES AND SPECIALTY DEFINITIONS

Abdominal surgery specialist: Performs surgery on the abdomen and the organs within it.

ABMP: Associated Bodywork & Massage Professionals. The Association is located in Evergreen, Colorado.

ACR: Advanced Certified Rolfer. A type of massage. Certified through the Rolf Institute in Boulder, Colorado.

ACSW: Academy of Certified Social Workers. Certified through the National Association of Social Workers in Washington, DC.

Adolescent medicine specialist: Subspecialty of pediatrics. Treats older children.

Allergist: Specialist who diagnoses and treats allergic conditions.

Allergy and immunology specialist: Subspecialty of internal medicine or pediatrics. Concentrates on diagnosing and treating allergies and the immune system.

Allopath: Practices what is known as "conventional Western medicine." Allopathic doctors control the American hospital system. The largest organization that works in the interests of allopathic doctors is the American Medical Association.

AMTA: American Massage Therapy Association. Located in Evanston, Illinois.

Anesthesiology specialist (Anesthesiologist): Administers anesthetics (drugs) so a person undergoing surgery does not feel pain. This may include preventing pain in one area of the body or total unconsciousness. The anesthesiologist monitors the patient's vital signs during surgery. An anesthesiologist may also be involved in the care of patients who are experiencing chronic pain.

AR: Assistant Resident.

ARNP: Advanced Registered Nurse Practitioner.

Ayurvedic doctor: Practices Eastern Indian medical principles encompassing what is often referred to as either "alternative," "holistic," or "complimentary" treatments. Considers body type, mood, emotion, lifestyle habits, and physical coloring. Includes diet modification; herbal tonics; inhalants and baths; exercise such as yoga; meditation; and changing surroundings to rid the patients' atmosphere of toxic thoughts and substances.

BAc: Bachelor of Acupuncture.

BSN: Bachelor of Science in Nursing.

CA: Certified Acupuncturist.

CAR: Certified Advance Rolfer.

Cardiology specialist (Cardiologist): Deals with the heart and the vascular system.

Cardiovascular surgery specialist: Subspecialty of cardiology. Performs surgery on the heart and the vascular system.

CC: Board Certified Craniopath.

CCN: Certified Clinical Nutritionist.

CCSP: Certified Chiropractic Sports Physician.

CFP: Certified Feldenkrais Practitioner. The Feldenkrais Guild is located in Albany, Oregon.

Child neurology specialist: Diagnoses and treats disorders of the nervous system in children.

Child psychiatry specialist: A subspecialty of psychiatry dealing with the emotional health of children.

Chiropractor: Has a limited license that allows him to do therapies that involve physical manipulation and adjustment of the spine and skeletal system. Treatments may also include massage, traction, hot and cold compresses, and ultrasound. Chiropractors do not prescribe drugs, are often opposed to drugs, and do not perform surgery. There are 14 accredited chiropractic schools in the US.

CHt: Certified Hypnotherapist.

CISW: Certified Independent Social Worker.

CMP: Certified Massage Practitioner.

CMT: Certified Massage Therapist.

CN: Certified Nutritionist.

CNA: Certified Nurses Aid.

CNM: Certified Nurse Midwife.

CNS: Clinical Nurse Specialist.

COI: Certified Ohashiatsu Instructor.

Colon and rectal surgery specialist: Diagnoses and treats disorders and diseases of the anus, rectum, and intestinal tract.

Cosmetic Surgeon: Plastic surgeon who operates on people who want to change their appearance for vanity reasons and are willing to take the risks of surgery to obtain their goals.

CR: Certified Rolfer.

CSW: Certified Social Worker.

DAc or DiplAc: Diplomate in Acupuncture. Has passed the national certification exam.

DC: Doctor of Chiropractic.

DDS: Doctor of Dental Surgery, or a Doctor of Dental Science.

Dentist: Doctor who specializes in the care of teeth and gums.

Dermatology specialist (Dermatologist): Doctor who specializes in the care of the skin and diseases of the skin.

DHANP: Diplomate of Homeopathic Academy of Naturopathic Physicians.

DHom (Med): Diplomate of the Institute of Homeopathy.

Diagnostic radiology specialist: A subspecialty of radiology which uses medical imaging devices to diagnose health problems.

DiplAc: Diplomate of Acupuncture.

Diplomate: When a doctor is certified by a board, he then is a Diplomate of that board.

DMD: Doctor of Dental Medicine.

DPM: Podiatrist.

DO: Doctor of Osteopathy or Osteopathic Physician: A doctor who, in addition to general medical training, has studied manipulative and therapeutic treatments of the musculoskeletal and spinal systems. Osteopaths are fully licensed physicians and surgeons who have served internships, passed equivalency exams, are able to prescribe drugs, and perform surgery, and basically have the same privileges and responsibilities as an allopathic medical doctor (MD). There are nearly 30,000 osteopathic physicians in the US.

Osteopathic therapies often concentrate on what they call the "neuro-muscular-skeletal system." Osteopathic doctors approach the body as an interrelated system. They learn different therapies and have a more holistic approach to treating ailments than allopathic doctors. They are less likely to rely on drugs and surgery than allopathic doctors, and are more likely to work with the natural healing abilities of the body. There are both general and specialist osteopathic doctors.

Osteopathy was started by Dr. A.T. Still who opened a school of osteopathy in the late 1800s in Kirksville, Missouri. Many people thought of him as a quack. There are currently sixteen osteopathic medical schools in the US. Though there have been massive changes and improvements in osteopathic medicine, many allopathic doctors still do not accept osteopathic therapies. Other allopathic doctors consult with osteopathic doctors on patient care. Most hospitals in America are controlled by allopathic doctors and some do not give admitting privileges to osteopathic doctors. There are also osteopathic hospitals. The American Osteopathic Association is located in Chicago, Illinois.

DOM: Doctor of Oriental Medicine. Some state certification boards use this title.

DSc: Doctor of Science.

Emergency medicine specialist: Usually works in a hospital emergency department.

EMS: Emergency Medicine Specialist.

Endocrinology specialist (Endocrinologist): Subspecialty of internal medicine that concentrates on disorders and diseases of the endocrine system (made up of the glands that secrete hormones — the ovaries, testes, adrenals, pineal, thymus, pituitary, and thyroid glands, and the pancreas).

ENT: Otorhinolaryngologist: Doctor who specializes in treating illnesses and diseases that affect the ears, nose and throat.

FACP: Fellow of the American College of Physicians.

FACS: Fellow of the American College of Surgeons.

FICS: Fellow of the International College of Surgeons — or — Fellow of the International Craniopath Society.

FRCOG: Fellow of the Royal College of Obstetricians and Gynecologists.

FRCP: Fellow of the Royal College of Physicians.

FRCP(C): Fellow of the Royal College of Physicians of Canada.

FRCP(E): Fellow of the Royal College of Physicians of Edinburgh.

FRCP(I): Fellow of the Royal College of Physicians of Ireland.

Gastroenterology specialist (Gastroenterologist): Subspecialty of internal medicine. Treats the organs of the digestive tract.

General Practitioner: Doctor who usually treats general health problems. Refers his patients to specialists when specific symptoms indicate the need for specialized care, such as when the patient has a serious health problem. The cost controlling measures implemented by managed care insurance-companies that now dominant healthcare has placed more influence on giving patients greater access to less expensive general practitioners and less access to more expensive specialist doctors.

General surgery specialist: May or may not perform surgery on areas of the body covered by subspecialty areas.

Geneticist: Diagnoses inherited health disorders.

Geriatrics: Subspecialty of internal medicine or general practice. Deals with elderly and the health problems associated with aging individuals.

GP: see "General Practitioner."

Gynecology specialist (Gynecologist): Specialist doctor who examines and treats disorders of the female reproductive system. Also cares for pregnant women.

Hand surgery specialist: Subspecialty of orthopedic surgery, plastic surgery, or general surgery. Performs surgery to correct disorders of the joints, bones, muscles, and ligaments of the hands.

Head and neck surgery: Subspecialty of otolaryngology. Performs surgery on the structures of the head and neck, such as the bones and muscles. Does not perform surgery on the brain or eyes.

Hematology specialist (Hematologist): Doctor who specializes in the blood and the system through which it flows.

HMD: Homeopathic Medical Doctor. See the *Alternative Medicine* section of this book.

Immunology specialist (Immunologist) : Deals with the immune system and the disorders and diseases that effect it, such as AIDS and allergies.

Infectious diseases specialist: Subspecialty of internal medicine.

Intensivist: Specializes in critical care.

Intern: Someone who has graduated from medical school and is spending a year of internship in a hospital, clinic, or ambulatory center to gain experience and to learn about taking responsibility for the care of a patient in the role of a physician by interacting and working with doctors in the treatment of patients. The internship year is organized and sponsored by a single specialty department. The majority of allopathic physicians continue their training to complete a residency program to become specialists.

Internal medicine specialist (Internist): Diagnoses and treats diseases. Nonsurgical.

LAc or LicAc: Licensed Acupuncturist. Licensed by the state and has met requirements for national certification.

Laryngology (Laryngologist): Treats the larynx and nasopharynx including the vocal cords, esophagus, and trachea.

LCSW: Licensed Clinical Social Worker or Licensed Certified Social Worker.

LD: Licensed Dietitian.

LICSW: Licensed Independent Clinical Social Worker.

LMP: Licensed Massage Practitioner.

LMT: Licensed Massage Therapist.

LPN: Licensed Practical Nurse —has had less nursing education than an RN (Registered Nurse). Has taken a state license exam.

MAc: Master of Acupuncture.

MAR: Medical admitting resident. A third year resident who is in charge of approving and assigning patients who are admitted into the hospital.

Maxillofacial surgery specialist: Deals with the boney structures of the lower front part of the face including the jaw and the immediate bones and tissues around it.

MD: Allopathic Medical Doctor. Has completed a full course of medical training. Often relies on treatments that include chemical drugs and surgery to treat many health conditions. There are 126 allopathic medical schools in the US. Allopathic doctors rule the American hospital system.

ME: Medical examiner. These are the pros who sign death certificates and conduct autopsies.

Medical Artist: Usually works in cooperation with a plastic surgeon to make drawings and models that may help to recreate the facial characteristics of a person who has had facial damage caused by an injury or disease. Also work with doctors who perform plastic surgery on children who have facial deformities.

Medical Technologist: Deals with laboratory tests, procedures, and the use of clinical laboratory equipment.

MFCC: Marriage, Family, and Child Counselor.

Midwife: A nurse-midwife is a specialist nurse who works assisting women during childbirth, and may also provide prenatal and postpartum care. Most often they are involved in the care of women with low-risk pregnancies. They work in hospitals, birth centers, or in home-birthing situations. According to Public Citizen's Health Research Group, pregnant women who are assisted by midwives are much less likely to undergo cesarean delivery. Women who previously underwent a cesarean section are also less likely to undergo another cesarean if they are assisted by a midwife. Midwives may have completed a one-year certification program, or a two-year master's program. Nurse-midwives take state licensing exams and are certified nationally. The American College of Nurse-Midwives is located in

Washington, DC. See the *Childbirth* heading in this book to find more information on midwives.

MLT: Medical Lab Technologist.

MOM: Master of Oriental Medicine.

MPH: Master of Public Health.

MSN: Master of Science in Nursing.

MSW: Master of Social Work.

MT: Massage Therapist, or a Medical Technologist.

Naturopath: May practice a combination of holistic alternative approaches, such as Chinese medicine, Indian and Native American, as well as Greek and therapies such as massage, nutrition, herbal medicine, homeopathy, water therapy, and chiropractic. Places a strong influence on prevention through lifestyle changes by doing away with unhealthful behavior, diet, and thinking, and in giving positive reinforcement. The naturopathic focus is to provide the body with what it needs to heal itself. A Natureopath may also use drugs and minor surgery, but does so as a last resort when there has not been a response to natural therapies.

The most popular school for naturopathy is Bastyr University in Seattle, Washington. That school offers a four-year program, bachelor's degrees in the natural health sciences, and master's degree programs in nutrition, herbal medicine, homeopathy, physiotherapy, botanical medicine, and acupuncture. Midwifery, women's healthcare, pediatrics, and sports medicine are also taught. Other schools where naturopathic medicine is taught include the Canadian College of Naturopathic Medicine in Ontario, the National College of Naturopathic Medicine in Portland, and the Southwest College of Naturopathic Medicine in Scottsdale.

ND: Doctor of Naturopathy. See "Naturopath" above.

Neonatal-Perinatal Medicine: Subspecialty of pediatrics. Deals with the health of newborns.

Nephrology specialist (Nephrologist): Subspecialty of internal medicine. Deals with the kidneys.

Neurological surgery specialist (Neurologist): Diagnoses and treats the disorders of the nerves, spinal cord, and brain.

Neurology specialist: Diagnoses and does nonsurgical treatments of the nerves, spinal cord, and brain.

Neurosurgeon: Doctor who specializes in the surgical treatment of the brain, nerves, and spinal cord.

NP: See Nurse Practitioner.

Nuclear medicine specialist: Uses radioactive substances to diagnose and treat diseases.

Nuclear Medicine Technologist: Prepares and administers radiopharmaceuticals, operates radiation detection devices, and other machinery to trace the distribution of the radioactive material as it flows through the body systems.

Nuclear Radiology: Subspecialty of radiology. Utilizes radioactive substances to diagnose and treat diseases.

Nurse's Aide or Nurse's Assistant: Self-explanatory. Has limited training. Usually has taken a nurse training course at a community or other type of college. But their training may also be limited to a simple class in emergency training. Should not be performing such duties as dispensing medications to patients. Works under the supervision of a registered nurse.

Nurse Manager: Head nurse. A head nurse is an RN and is the one who supervises the other nurses who work in a hospital unit.

Nurse Midwife: See "Midwife" above.

Nurse Practitioner: Nurse who has received additional medical education and works in the diagnosis and treatment of health problems on a limited level. The concept of having this type of nurse with advanced training started a few decades ago at the University of Colorado.

Nurse Practitioners may conduct physical examinations, perform preventative health screenings, work to identify specific patient needs, and, under the guidelines of a doctor, prescribe medications. Some small towns that do not have a local doctor sometimes have a nurse practitioner who they rely on for their care, and who is usually supervised by a doctor in a nearby town. There is a strong demand for nurse practitioners because they can perform some of the same tasks as doctors but at a lower cost. Salaries for nurse practitioners range from $40,000 to $65,000 per year.

NPs are nationally certified and state licensed. To keep certification, they must complete 60 to 75 hours of continuing education, and be recertified every three to five years. The American Academy of Nurse Practitioners is located in Austin, Texas.

Nutritionist: Reviews a person's diet, helps him incorporate nutrition into his meals, and teaches healthy eating habits.

OB/GYN: Obstetrician Gynecologist.

Obstetrician: Specialist who deals with pregnancy and childbirth. On average, obstetricians are sued more than any other kind of doctor.

Obstetrics and Gynecology (OB/GYN): Treats disorders of the female reproductive system. Oversees the progression of pregnancy.

Occupational medicine specialist: Subspecialty of preventative medicine. Deals with the specific health concerns of various industries and how they can be prevented or treated.

OD: Doctor of Optometry.

Ombudsman: Patient representative in the hospital or nursing home area who handles the complaints and other matters related to patient satisfaction .

OMD: Oriental Medicine Doctor. Has received an educational degree. Diagnoses from an Oriental Medical Doctor may be the result of conclusions made after examining the eyes, tongue, hair, hearing, voice tone, body odor, and factoring in of diet, age, weight, body shape, posture, and capabilities of movement. The harmony of the person is considered and disbalances are treated. Treatments may include acupuncture, massage or other manipulation, exercises, diet changes, and various herbal and substance remedies (in other words, traditional Chinese medicine).

Oncology specialist (Oncologist): Subspecialty of internal medicine. Deals with cancer, its diagnosis, and treatment in all stages.

Ophthalmologist: Specialist who treats diseases and injuries of the eyes.

Ophthalmology specialist (Opthalmologist): Observes the progression of, diagnoses of, and treatment of disorders of the eyes.

Optometrist: One who examines the eyes and prescribes corrective lenses, such as eye glasses and contact lenses.

Orthodontist: Doctor who deals with irregularities of the teeth.

Orthomolecular Physician: Usually a medical doctor. Therapies include diet changes, and assisting nutritional level with dietary supplements, such as vitamins, minerals, enzymes, and amino acids.

Orthopedist: Doctor who specializes in the musculoskeletal system (bone fractures, diseases, and malformations).

Osteopathic Physician: See "DO."

Otolaryngology specialist (Otorhinolaryngologist): Diagnoses and treats disorders of the ears, nose, and throat (ENT).

Otology: Subspecialty of otolaryngology. Diagnoses and treats disorders of the ear.

PA: Physician Assistant.

P-A: Physician-anesthesiologist.

PA-C: Physician Assistant-Certified. Certification exam is administered by the National Commission on Certification of Physician Assistants located in Atlanta, Georgia.

Pathologist: Doctor who analyzes and studies body tissues and fluids to interpret and diagnose diseases and disorders. Forensic pathologists are involved with performing autopsies to distinguish the cause and estimated time of death.

PCT: Patient care technician, or a nurse extender.

Pediatric Intensivist: Cares for children in the intensive care unit of a hospital.

Pediatric Orthopedist: A children's bone doctor.

Pediatrics specialist (Pediatrician): Deals with the health of children from babies to young adults.

PhD: Doctor of Philosophy.

Phlebotomist: Obtains patients' blood specimens and may collect other clinical laboratory specimens. They are employed by hospitals, health and medical clinics, group practices, HMO's, and public health facilities. The National Phlebotomy Association is located in Hyattsville, Maryland. The organization works to educate and certify phlebotomists. The certified membership is about 20,000. According to NPA literature, there are over 200,000 persons working as phlebotomists who have not been certified. The position does not require a degree.

Physiatrist: Specialist who focuses on the rehabilitation of the body. Helps to develop rehabilitation programs for patients who have suffered strokes or experienced physical trauma. Oversees occupational and physical therapists. Not to be confused with a psychiatrist who focuses on a patients' state of mind.

Physical Therapist: A person who helps people rehabilitate from surgery or injury to alleviate pain and restore health to its optimal level. Typically holds at least a bachelor's degree and completes a state licensing exam. Most often works in hospitals, nursing homes, rehabilitation centers, doctors' offices, and private clinics. Some physical therapists also visit patients who are recovering at home, and others have their own private practices.

Physical Medicine and Rehabilitation: Diagnoses and treats physical injuries that interfere with movement. Also treats patients who have musculoskeletal or neurologic disorders and patients who may be recovering from surgery or disease.

Physician Assistant: Works under a physician's supervision. Has less training than a physician — about four to six years of college. Some small-town clinics are run by PAs. They cannot perform any kind of complicated medical procedure, and must be supervised by a doctor. They often are involved in the taking of patient histories, and may do physical exams. Some PAs plan forms of treatment, diagnose problems, help to educate patients, and order tests. They may also stitch wounds, set some types of fractures, and assist in surgical procedures. Most PAs work in the area of family medicine. Many others specialize in areas, such as surgery, pediatrics, internal medicine, gynecology, orthopedics, and emergency medicine. To maintain national certification, a PA must complete 100 hours of continuing education every two years, and pass a national recertification exam every six years. The first PAs graduated from Duke University in 1967. Dozens of other medical schools now offer PA programs. The American Academy of Physician Assistants is located in Alexandria, Virginia.

Plastic Surgeon: Doctor who specializes in treating body parts that have been damaged or that are malformed because of a disease, injury, or birth defect. Some of today's plastic surgeons sell themselves as "cosmetic surgeons" and occupy themselves with performing unnecessary surgery on people who want to change their appearance for vanity reasons and who are willing to take the risks of surgery to obtain their goals.

PNC: Psychiatric Nurse Clinician.

Podiatrist: Foot doctor, or a doctor of podiatric medicine. Their training is in a two- or three-year course of classes and not an intense training program, such as what an MD would be exposed to. Podiatrists treat such ailments as ingrown toenails, bunions, and fallen arches. A podiatrist may sometimes perform minor foot or ankle surgery in his office.

Preventive medicine specialist: Concentrates on the prevention of disease and injury by assessing occupational and environmental factors. May treat by prescribing lifestyle or dietary changes.

Proctologist: Specializes in the diagnosis and treatment of problems with the anus, colon, and rectum.

Prosthodontist: Specialist in prosthetic dentistry.

Provider: A term used to describe anyone who delivers healthcare, such as a doctor, nurse, or pharmacist. The term may also be used to describe a hospital or clinic.

Psychiatrist: An MD who specializes in the care and prevention of mental illness and emotional and behavior disorders. Has completed post-medical training, has served a residency and is able to prescribe medication. Tends to treat more severe mental illness disorders than those treated by psychologists.

Psychologist: Doctor who studies the science of mind and behavior. Has a PhD in clinical psychology and tends to work with people who are high functioning and who are usually able to carry on normal life activities but suffer from depression or other less severe disorders than those treated by psychiatrists.

Psychosomatic medicine specialist: Concentrates on how the mind and body interact in an emotional way that may lead to disease or threaten well-being.

Public health specialist: Concentrates on the health of the community and the prevention of diseases within it.

Pulmonary specialist (Pulmonologist): Subspecialty of internal medicine. Deals with disorders of the lungs.

RAc: Registered Acupuncturist.

Radiation Therapist: Applies radiation to cancer patients and keeps a record of the treatment.

Radiographer: Operates diagnostic imaging devices, such as x-ray machines.

Radiology specialist (Radiologist): Doctor who specializes in the interpretation of x-rays and other diagnostic images used to help diagnose health problems. They also may be involved with radiation treatment of cancer patients and certain testing procedures that use technology which produces diagnostic images, such as those created by ultrasound, CAT scans, MRI machines, etc.

Radiologists are typically one of the highest paid of all doctors. When they work in a hospital, they are using equipment owned and maintained by the hospital and a staff employed by the hospital. They pay nothing for the use of hospital facilities, equipment, supplies, or staff. They interpret the images, record their findings on a tape recorder, and hand the tape over to a transcriber who types the dictation into a computer.

RD: Registered Dietitian. A person who has met the educational criteria of the Commission on Dietetic Registration, the credentialing agency for The American Dietetic Association that is located in Chicago, Illinois. Dietitians hold a Bachelor of Science degree in nutrition, have served an internship, and are required to complete continuing education courses. Dietitians are employed by hospitals, schools, nursing homes, food companies, restaurant chains, and other companies and facilities that are involved in food preparation.

Reconstructive surgery specialist (Plastic Surgeon): Performs surgery to correct abnormalities caused by birth defects, injuries, or diseases with the goal of improving function and/or appearance.

Registered Nurse: Has gone on to receive two or more additional years of education beyond that of a Licensed Practical Nurse to obtain a bachelor's degree in nursing. Registered nurses must pass a state licensing exam.

Reproductive Endocrinologist: Infertility doctor.

Residency: Next step up from an internship. Period of training in a specific medical specialty; this occurs after graduation from medical school and the length varies from three to seven years, depending on the specialty. Surgical residents have to perform a certain number of specific procedures to become certified in a specialty. To fulfill this requirement they must have patients to operate on; thus they can be too quick to perform operations, or may simply perform unnecessary operations as they seek to meet the quota requirements of their specialty.

Rheumatology specialist (Rheumatologist): Subspecialty of internal medicine. Deals with inflammations of the muscles and joints, such as arthritis.

Rhinology specialist (Rhinologist): Deals with the structures of the nose and nasal passages.

RMT: Registered Massage Therapist.

RN,C: Registered Nurse, Certified. Includes certified Registered Nurses who practice in the areas of Medical-Surgical Nurse, Gerontological Nurse, Psychiatric and Mental Health Nurse, Pediatric Nurse, Perinatal Nurse, Community Health Nurse, School Nurse, General Nursing Practice, College Health Nurse, Nursing Continuing

Education/Staff Development, Home Health Nurse, and Cardiac Rehabilitation Nurse .

RN,CS: Registered Nurse, Certified Specialist. Includes certified Registered Nurses who practice in the areas of Clinical Specialist in Gerontological Nursing, Clinical Specialist in Medical-Surgical Nursing, Clinical Specialist in Community Health Nursing, Clinical Specialist in Adult Psychiatric and Mental Health Nursing, Clinical Specialist in Child and Adolescent Psychiatric and Mental Health Nursing, Gerontological Nurse Practitioner, Pediatric Nurse Practitioner, Adult Nurse Practitioner, Family Nurse Practitioner, and School Nurse Practitioner.

RN,CNA: Registered Nurse, Certified in Nursing Administration.

RN,CNAA: Registered Nurse, Certified in Nursing Administration, Advanced.

RPh: Registered Pharmacist.

RPP: Registered Polarity Practitioner. The American Polarity Therapy Association is located in Boulder, Colorado.

RRA: Registered Record Administrator. Also Accredited Record Technician. A credential given by the American Health Information Management Association.

Scrub Nurse: Works along with a surgeon as he performs an operation.

Social Worker: Social workers are on staff at most hospitals. They have gone through supervised practical training and hold a masters degree in social work. They help patients and the patients' families with emotional support, and give therapeutic assistance. They can intervene when a patient is experiencing a problem coping with a medical condition. They may act as patient advocates and can refer patients to community or hospital services that may benefit the patient. Much of their work entails nurturing the independence of the patient. A nurse or doctor can refer a patient to a social worker.

Societies: As it applies to the medical field: Organizations of physicians or medical professionals (nurses, therapists, etc.) involved in a given field of practice. Medical societies are trade groups that represent the interests of the medical professionals. In most specialty societies, it is not necessary to be board certified to be eligible for membership.

Sonographer: Uses high frequency soundwaves (ultrasound) to create images of body tissues, bones, and organs on a screen and this can be recorded on film, or videotape. Sonographers are registered by the American Registry of Diagnostic Medical Sonographers.

Speech Therapist: Works with people who have congenital deformities or injuries of the mouth area to help them speak more clearly. Also may work with stroke or cancer patients whose ailments have interfered with speaking abilities.

Surgical critical care specialist: Subspecialty of surgery. Deals with the care of patients who are critically ill, such as burn patients, and patients who are undergoing care in the emergency or intensive care settings.

Therapeutic radiology specialist: Subspecialty of radiology. Deals with the radioactive treatment of cancer patients.

Thoracic surgery specialist (Thoracic Surgeon): Deals with surgery on diseased organs and tissues between the neck and the abdomen (the chest).

UAL: Unlicensed Assistive Personnel.

Urological surgery specialist (Urologist): Subspecialty of urology. Deals with surgery of the adrenal gland and genital urinary system, including the bladder, prostate, and reproductive organs of males.

Vascular surgery specialist: Subspecialty of surgery. Performs surgery on the blood vessels that are not in the heart, lungs, or brain.

• PROSTHETICS

American Academy of Orthotics and Prosthetics, 1650 King St., Ste. 500, Alexandria, VA 22314; (703)836-7118

American Board for Certification in Orthotics and Prosthetics, 1650 King St., Ste. 500, Alexandria, VA 22314; (703)836-7114

American Orthotic and Prosthetic Association, 1650 King St., Ste. 500, Alexandria, VA 22314-1885; (703)836-7116

Association of Children's Prosthetic-Orthotic Clinics, 6300 N. River Rd., Rosemont, IL 60018; (847)698-1694

Novacare Sabolich Prosthetic & Research Center, PO Box 60509, Oklahoma City, OK 73146; (800)522-4428

National Orthotic and Prosthetic Research Institute, PO Box 491, Lenox Hill, NY 10021

The Orthotics & Prosthetics National Office provides information on athletic organizations for disabled and handicapped individuals, and publishes various materials available to healthcare workers working in the field of orthotics and prosthetics. **Orthotics & Prosthetics National Office,** 1650 King St., Ste. 500, Alexandria, VA 22314; (703)836-7114

• PUBLICATIONS

Books:
* *Becoming a Physician: Medical Education in Great Britain, France, Germany, and the United States,* by Thomas Neville Bonner; Oxford University Press, 1995
* *Confessions of a Medical Heretic,* by Robert S. Mendelsohn, MD; Contemporary Books, 1979
* *Doctors: The Biography of Medicine,* By Sherwin B. Nuland; Vintage Books, 1988
* *The Great American Medicine Show: Being an Illustrated History of Hucksters, Healers, Health Evangelists, and Heroes from Plymouth Rock to the Present,* by David Armstrong and Elizabeth Metzger Armstrong; Prentice Hall/ Simon and Schuster, 1991
* *The Lobbyists: How Influence Peddlers Work Their Way in Washington,* by Jeffrey H. Birnbaum; Times Books/Random House, 1992
* *The Medical Detective: A Classic Collection of Award Winning Medical Investigative Reporting,* by Berton Roueche; Plume, 1991
* *Plastic Surgery Hopscotch: A Reference Guide for Those Considering Cosmetic Surgery,* by John McCabe; Carmania Books, 1994
* *Politics and Money: The New Road to Corruption,* Elizabeth Drew; Macmillan, 1983
* *The Social Transformation of American Medicine,* by Paul Starr; Basic Books, 1982
* *The Strange Case of Dr. Kappler: The Doctor Who Became a Killer,* by Keith Russell Ablow, The Free Press/MacMillon, 1994
* *The Toadstool Millionaires: A Social History of Patent Medicines in America Before Federal Regulation,* by James Harvey Young; Princeton University Press, 1961

The *Reader's Guide to Periodical Literature* is available in book or computer form in many libraries. It lists articles that were written about various subjects and can be very helpful when researching health concerns.

The *Encyclopedia of Associations* is also available in many libraries. It lists thousands of organizations and is helpful when trying to find names and addresses of various groups.

Mosey Medical Encyclopedia can be helpful in familiarizing a person with medical terminology.

The Center for the Study of Services is a nonprofit organization that publishes a Hospital Guide that lists the federal mortality rates by hospital and the mortality rates of the most common operations being done. The *Hospital Guide* is available for $12 including postage and handling. Payment can be made by way of check, money order, or credit card.
Center for the Study of Services, *Hospital Guide,* 806 — 15th St., NW, Ste. 925, Washington, DC 20005; (202)347-7283

The Department of Health and Human Services prints a variety of free and low-cost booklets that deal with various health concerns. For a copy of a catalog with the complete list of government booklets for consumers, write to the

Dept. of Health and Human Services, Consumer Information Center, Dept. 100, Pueblo, CO 81002; (719)948-4000

FDA Consumer, the magazine of the US Food and Drug Administration, provides a wealth of information on FDA-related health issues, such as food safety, nutrition, drugs, medical devices, cosmetics, radiation protection, vaccines, blood products, and veterinary medicine. For a sample copy of *FDA Consumer* and a subscription order form, write to the

Food and Drug Administration, HFI—40, Rockville, MD 20857

Medical Abstracts Newsletter uses easy-to-understand wording to explain various research findings reported in medical journals used by medical professionals. All articles in *Medical Abstracts Newsletter* cite the original source of information, including the author's name, journal, volume, page, and issue date so you or your doctor can locate the full report and evaluate its contents. A one-year subscription to the newsletter costs $21. An additional year costs $18. A $4 additional charge should be added per year of subscription for people living outside of the United States.

Medical Abstracts Newsletter, Georgetown Publishing, 1101 — 30th St., NW, Ste. 130, Washington, DC 20007; (201)836-7740

Copies of Congressional hearings on health and medicine subjects can be obtained through the

United States Government Printing Office Congressional Desk, (202)512-2470

• RARE DISORDERS

Food and Drug Administration, Office of Orphan Products Development, 5600 Fisher's Lane (HF-35), Rockville, MD 20857; (800)300-7469

Lethbridge Society for Rare Disorders/Canada, 515 7th St. S., Ste. 100B, Lethbridge, Alberta T15 2G8 Canada; (403)329-0665

The National Organization for Rare Disorders was created by a group of voluntary agencies, medical researchers, and individuals concerned with orphan diseases and orphan drugs. "Orphan diseases" are rare illnesses that strike small numbers of people. "Orphan drugs" are therapies that alleviate symptoms of some rare diseases, but that have often not been developed by the pharmaceutical-industry because they are unprofitable.

Any disorder affecting fewer than 200,000 people is considered to be an orphan disease, and products developed for these illnesses are considered by the pharmaceutical-industry as "drugs of little commercial value."

NORD, a nonprofit charity, supports itself through private donations, membership dues, fundraising events, and grants. The organization manages a database of information regarding rare disorders. The NORD Medication Assistance Program provides free prescription drugs to needy patients who cannot afford to purchase them.

Not all doctors can recognize subtleties that, in the case of some rare disorders, can mean the difference between life and death when treatment is delayed. Misdiagnosis of rare disorders or a delay in diagnosis is common. One out of three individuals with a rare disease does not receive a correct diagnosis for up to five years. NORD often hears of people who have been misdiagnosed and treated psychologically for disorders that were physical. This is because symptoms that look like one ailment can in fact be symptoms of some disorder that is so rare that there are few medical specialists who would be able to diagnose the problem correctly and know of a treatment. To help alleviate such occurrences, NORD publishes the *Physicians' Guide to Rare Diseases*.

The NORD newsletter is available through subscription. For a donation of $4, NORD will send you an information packet.

National Organization for Rare Disorders, 100 Rte. 37, PO Box 8923, New Fairfield, CT 06812-1783; (203)746-6518 or (800)999-NORD; E-mail: 76703,3014@compuserve.com

• RECORDS

Most states have laws that provide patients access to their medical records. If any doctor, medical facility, or insurance company refuses to give you a copy of your medical records, contact one of the patients' rights groups listed under the *Patients' and Consumers' Rights* heading of this book and/or contact a malpractice lawyer.

To find out if your state laws address patient access to health information and what those laws are, contact your State Department of Health. For further information, send a self-addressed, stamped envelope to the American Health Information Management Association and request a copy of their booklet titled *Your Health Information Belongs to You*.

The AHIMA was founded in 1928 and conducts qualification exams of medical records personnel. Those who become credentialed carry the title of "Registered Record Administrator" or "Accredited Record Technician."
American Health Information Management Association, Professional Practice Division, 919 N. Michigan Ave., Ste. 1400, Chicago, IL 60611-1683; (312)787-2672 or (800)621-6828

To find out if the Medical Information Bureau has a medical history file on you that is used by insurance companies and other organizations, and to order a copy of this file for your own records, write or call the offices located in Boston. Give them a few variations of your name. For instance, a person named Joseph David Doe may have a file under the name of Joe Doe, Joey D. Doe, or Joseph Doe. The MIB will also need your Social Security number, birth date, and location of your birth.
Medical Information Bureau (MIB), PO Box 105, Essex Station, Boston, MA 02112; (617)426-3660

The People's Medical Society publishes a book titled *Your Medical Rights: How to Become an Empowered Consumer*. The book gives detailed information on the rights of a patient and what rights patients have to their medical records, what information doctors and hospitals must disclose before treating a patient, how to avoid unnecessary surgery, and explanations of medical charges and how to have inaccuracies in medical bills corrected. They also publish several other books.
People's Medical Society, 462 Walnut St., Allentown, PA 18102; (215)770-1670

The *Privacy Journal* is a monthly newsletter on new technology and its impact on privacy, intended for professionals and consumers. It also publishes several books related to privacy and a yearly compilation of state and federal privacy laws.
Privacy Journal, PO Box 28577, Providence, RI 02908; (401)274-7861

A book called *Medical Records: Getting Yours* gives step-by-step instructions on how to get your medical records. The book is available for $10 plus $2 for shipping from **Public Citizen Publications,** 2000 P St., NW, Ste. 600, Washington, DC 20036; (202)833-3000

The Privacy Act of 1974 gives citizens the right to see files about themselves (subject to exemptions); to request an amendment if the record is incomplete, untimely, irrelevant, or inaccurate; and to sue the government for permitting others to see their files unless specifically permitted by the Act. A complete copy of the Privacy Act can be found in section 552a of Title 5 of the US Code. Or you may order a copy of the *Privacy Act, Public Law 93-579,* stock number 022-003-90866-8, for $2.50 from the Superintendent of Documents.

The *Citizen's Guide on Using the Freedom of Information Act and the Privacy Act of 1974 to Request Government Records,* written by the Committee on Government Operations, US House of Representatives, provides a detailed explanation of the Freedom of Information Act and the Privacy Act. The booklet (stock number 052-071-00929-9) may be purchased for $2.25 from the
Superintendent of Documents, US Government Printing Office, Washington, DC 20402

• REHABILITATION

American Academy of Physical Medicine and Rehabilitation, 122 S. Michigan Ave., Ste. 1300, Chicago, IL 60603

Association of Rehabilitation Nurses, 5700 Old Orchard Rd., 1st Flr., Skokie, IL 60077-1057; (708)966-3433

Congress on Accreditation of Rehabilitation Facilities, 101 N. Wilmot Rd., Ste. 500, Tucson, AZ 85711; (602)325-1044

Craig Hospital, 3425 S. Clarkson, Englewood, CO 80110; (303)789-8000

The Kessler Institute for Rehabilitation, 1199 Pleasant Valley Wy., West Orange, NJ 07052; (201)243-6809 or (800)248-3221

National Association of Rehabilitation Agencies, 11250-8 Roger Bacon Dr., Ste. 8, Reston, VA 22090; (703)437-4377

National Association of Rehabilitation Instructors, 633 S. Washington, Alexandria, VA 22314; (703)836-0850

National Institute on Disability and Rehabilitation Research, Dept. of Education, 330 C St., SW, Rm. 3060, Washington, DC 20202-2572; (202)732-1134

National Rehabilitation Information Center, (301)588-9284 or (800)346-2742

• REPETITIVE MOTION INJURIES

Book:
- *Conquering Carpal Tunnel Syndrome and Other Repetitive Strain Injuries: A Self-Care Program,* ,by Sharon Butler (E-mail: sbutler100@aol.com); Advanced Press ([800]909-9795; E-mail: advpr@aol.com), 1996

Carpal Tunnel Syndrome/Repetitive Strain Injury Association, PO Box 514, Santa Rosa, CA 95402-0514

National Institute for Occupational Safety and Health, 4676 Columbia Pkwy., Cincinnati, OH 45226; (800)35-NIOSH

• SECOND OPINIONS

Second Surgical Opinion Program, Dept. of Health and Human Services, 330 Independence Ave., SW, Washington, DC 20201; (202)690-8056 or (800)638-6833 or in Maryland call (800)492-6603

• SEXUAL ISSUES

American Association of Sex Educators, Counselors & Therapists, 435 N. Michigan Ave., Ste. 1717, Chicago, IL 60611; (312)644-0828

American Board of Sexology, 1929 — 18th St., NW, Ste. 1166, Washington, DC 20009; (202)462-2122 or (800)533-3521; E-mail: pp002379@interramp.com — or — Net: http://www.mentalhealth.com/PsychScapes

Intersex society of North America, PO Box 31791, San Francisco, CA 94131

National Institute of Relationship Enhancement, 4400 East-West Hwy., Ste. 28, Bethesda, MD 20814; (301)986-1479

• SEXUALLY TRANSMITTED DISEASES (Also see *AIDS*)

American Social Health Association, Herpes Resource Center, PO Box 13827, Research Triangle Park, NC 27709; Herpes Resource Center Hot Line (800)230-6039; Sexually Transmitted Disease Hot Line (800)227-8922

Citizens Alliance for VD Awareness, PO Box 31915, Chicago, IL 60631-0915; (847)398-3378

Safe Sex at the University of Canberra, Australia, Net: gopher://services.canberra .edu.au:70/11/Services/Student/Women/SAFE_SEX

Safer Sex Page, Net: http://www.cmpharm.ucsf.edu/~troyer/safesex.html

Student Health Issues, Net: gopher://nuinfo.nwu.edu:70/11/service/health

• SHOULDER AND ELBOW

American Shoulder and Elbow Surgeons/Council of Musculo-Skeletal Specialty Societies, 6300 N. River Rd., Ste. 727, Rosemont, IL 60018-4226; (708)698-1629

• SKIN

For a free pamphlet about skin cancer, write the
American Academy of Dermatology, Communications Dept., PO Box 681069, Schaumburg, IL 60168; 930 N. Meacham Rd., Schaumburg, IL 60168-4014; (708)330-0230

American Board of Dermatology, Henry Ford Hospital, Detroit, MI 48202; (313)871-8739

American College of Mohs Micrographic Surgery and Cutaneous Oncology, PO Box 4014, Schaumburg, IL 60168; (708)330-0230

American Dermatological Association, Dept. of Dermatology, University Hospital, BT 2045-1, Iowa City, IA 52242; (319)356-2274

American Osteopathic Board of Dermatology, 25510 Plymouth Rd., Redford, MI 48239; (313)937-1200

American Society for Dermatologic Surgery, 930 N. Meacham Rd., Schaumburg, IL 60173; (708)330-0230 or 9830

Dermatology, Net: http://netaxis.com/rdrugge/jan95.html

Dermatology Nurses' Association, PO Box 56, N. Woodbury Rd., Pitman, NJ 08071; (609)582-1915

Foundation for Ichthyosis and Related Skin Types, PO Box 20921, Raleigh, NC 27619; (919)782-5728 or (800)545-3286

National Arthritis and Musculoskeletal and Skin Diseases, Information Clearinghouse, PO Box AMS, Bethesda, MD 20892; (301)468-3235

National Organization for Albinism and Hypopigmentation, 1500 Loust St., Ste. 2405, Philadelphia, PA 19102; (800)473-2310

National Psoriasis Foundation, 6600 SW 92nd, Ste. 300, Portland, OR 97223; (503)244-7404; E-mail: 76135.2746@compuserve.com — or — Net: http://www.webwillow.com/npf/npf.shtml

National Rosacea Society, 220 S. Cook St., Ste. 201, Barrington, IL 60010; (708)382-8971

National Vitiligo Foundation, PO Box 6337, Tyler, TX 75711; (903)534-2925

Nevoid Basal Cell Carcinoma Syndrome Support Network, 162 Clover Hill St., Marlboro, MA 01752; (508)485-4873 or (800)815-4447; Fax (508)481-4072; E-mail: Souldansur@aol.com

The Psoriasis Research Institute runs a psoriasis medical treatment clinic and conducts drug studies to evaluate new therapies for psoriasis and other inflammatory skin diseases. The Institute is affiliated with several departments in the Stanford University School of Medicine. They publish the *Psoriasis Newsletter.*
Psoriasis Research Institute, 600 Town & Country Village, Palo Alto, CA 94301; (415)326-1848

Scleroderma Federation, Peabody Office Bldg., One Newbury St., Peabody, MA 01960; (800)422-1113

Sun Precautions - Sun Protective Clothing, 2815 Wetmore Ave., Everett, WA 98201; (206)303-8585 or (800)882-7860

United Scleroderma Foundation, PO Box 399, Watsonville, CA 95077; (800)722-4673

• SLEEP

Books:
• *Melatonin: Nature's Sleeping Pill,* by Ray Sahelian, MD; Be Happier Press, 1995

- *67 Ways to Good Sleep*, by Charles Inlander & Cynthia Moran; Walker & Company, 1995

Sleep apnea is a condition where the soft tissues at the back of the mouth and the top of the throat relax and sag during sleep. This may cause the person to choke or gasp for breath. The condition is more common among overweight and older persons. The word "apnea" is a Greek work which means "want of breath." A person who experiences sleep apnea may awake many times during one night as they gasp for breath. The American Sleep Apnea Association makes referrals to sleep study centers and self-help groups for apnea sufferers. The Association also publishes a newsletter called *Wake-Up Call*. It is published six times yearly and subscriptions are $19.95.
American Sleep Apnea Association, PO Box 66, Belmont, MA 02178-0001; (617)489-4441

The American Sleep Disorders Association is made up of physicians and scientists who are involved in the diagnosis, treatment, and basic research of sleep mechanisms and illnesses. Members of the Association include neurologists, pulmonologists, psychiatrists, psychologists, pediatrics, otolaryngologists, and other specialists. The Association develops and produces educational materials, such as patient-educations brochures, and serves as a referral source for the general public.
American Sleep Disorders Association, Rochester, MN 55901; (507)287-6006; Fax (507)287-6008; E-mail: asda@millcomm.com

Association for the Study of Dreams, PO Box 1600, Vienna, VA 22183; (703)242-0062; E-mail: ASDreams@aol.com — or — Net: http://fred.outreach.org/gmcc.asd /homepage.htm

Association of Professional Sleep Societies and the Association of Polysomnographic Technologists, 1610 — 14th St., NW, Ste. 300, Rochester, Minnesota 55901; (507)287-6006

Better Sleep Council, 333 Commerce St., Alexandria, VA 22314; (703)683-8371

Community Dreamsharing Network, PO Box 8032, Hicksville, NY 11802; (516)796-9455

Electric Dreams, E-mail: RCWilk@aol.com — or — Net: http://www.phys.unsw .edu.au/~mettw/edreams/home.html

IIDC DreamGate Projects, E-mail: iidcc-info@igc.apc.org — or — Net: gopher:// gopher.igc.apc.org:70/11/orgs/iidc

Melatonin Update Newsletter is published four times a year. Subscriptions are $16. *Melatonin Update Newsletter*, Be Happier Press, PO Box 12619, Marina Del Rey, CA 90295

Narcolepsy Network, PO Box 1365, FDR Station, New York, NY 10150

National Sleep Foundation, 1367 Connecticut Ave., NW, Ste. 200, Washington, DC 20036-1801; (202)785-2300; E-mail: natsleep@haven.ios.com

Sleep and Psychology, Net: http://web.sjsu.edu/c/s/howkins/public_html/index .html

Sleep Disorders Dental Society, 11676 Perry Hwy., Bldg. 1, Wexford, PA 15090

Sleep-SnoreCentral, Net: http://www.access.digex.net/~faust/s/dord

• SMELL AND TASTE

Book:
- *The Scent of Eros: Mysteries of Odor in Human Sexuality*, by James Vaughn Kohl and Robert T. Francoeur; Continuum Publishing, 1995

Chemical Senses Clinic at the University of California at Irvine, (714)856-5011

Monell Chemical Sense Center, Philadelphia, PA; (215)898-6666

Smell and Taste Treatment and Research Foundation, 845 N. Michigan Ave., Ste. 930 W., Chicago, IL; (312)938-1047

• SMOKING CESSATION

Books:
- *Ashes to Ashes: America's Hundred-Year Cigarette War, the Public Health, and the Unabashed Triumph of Phillip Morris,* by Richard Kluger; Alfred A. Knopf, 1996
- *The Cigarette Papers,* by Stanton A. Glantz, John Slade, Lisa A. Bero, Peter Hanauer, and Deborah E. Barnes; University of California Press, 1996
- *Smokescreen: the Truth Behind the Tobacco Industry Cover-Up,* by Phillip J. Hilts; Addison-Wesley, 1996

According to the American Cancer Society, tobacco products play a major role in about 90% of all lung cancer deaths. In addition to lung cancer, smoking is also a major cause of cancers of the mouth, larynx, and esophagus. Smoking also increases the risk of cancer of the bladder, kidney, pancreas, colon, and the uterine cervix. Smoking doubles the risk of heart disease. A smoker who has a heart attack has a greater risk of dying than a nonsmoker who suffers a heart attack.

Pregnant women who smoke increase their babies' chances of birth defects, low birth weight, premature birth, sudden infant death syndrome, and developmental setbacks. Pregnant women who do not smoke but are exposed to cigarette smoke at home and work, are also exposing their unborn babies to the cigarette smoke. A research study published in the February 23, 1994, issue of the *Journal of the American Medical Association* showed that nicotine and cotinine are present in the hair of babies newly born to nonsmoking women. The Harvard School of Public Health reports that babies born to women who smoked during their pregnancy have reduced lung function. When a nursing woman smokes, she not only subjects her baby to smoke inhalation and dramatically increases her baby's chances of experiencing lower respiratory tract infections, she also passes nicotine to her baby through the breast milk.

Children who are exposed to cigarette smoke are more susceptible to asthma, pneumonia, abnormally fast heartbeats, and are susceptible to artery damage from fatty buildups associated with heart disease. A study released by the Children's Hospital of Boston reported that children who are exposed to cigarette smoke at home have lower levels of good cholesterol than children who live in homes with nonsmokers, and this can increase a child's risk of developing heart disease.

> *Nicotine is addicting for three main reasons. First, when taken in small amounts, nicotine produces pleasurable feelings which make the smoker want to smoke more. Second, smokers can become dependent on nicotine. They suffer both physical and psychological withdrawal symptoms when they stop smoking, such as nervousness, headaches, and difficulty sleeping. Third, nicotine affects the chemistry of the brain and central nervous system, which explains how smoking affects one's mood and feelings. The addictive nature of smoking is the reason why so many people who want to stop smoking have trouble quitting.*
>
> *. . . nicotine is a poison. Taken in large amounts, nicotine can kill by paralyzing breathing muscles. In fact, taking an amount of nicotine equal to one-fifth of an aspirin tablet can be as deadly as cyanide.*
>
> — From American Cancer Society booklet *The Most Often Asked Questions About Smoking, Tobacco, and Health and The Answers*

Nicotine is a drug and thought to be more addictive than both cocaine and heroin. Certainly there are more people addicted to tobacco than both of the others. Nicotine reaches the brain only seven seconds after a person takes a puff (faster than it takes heroin to reach the brain).

The chemicals, tar, and gases in cigarette smoke literally dissolve lung tissue. This results in emphysema wherein holes are created in the lungs. A person with emphysema loses breath easily, may become unable to talk, eventually is disabled and tethered to an oxygen machine, and has a greatly reduced life expectancy. Some emphysema patients undergo lung transplants. But this is major surgery, donor organs are scarce, the procedure costs about $150,000, and the mortality rate is thirty percent. Lung reduction surgery may provide some improvement, but this surgery also carries major risks, has questionable success rates, costs $30,000, and is controversial.

Lung cancer is one of the most treatment-resistant cancers. Because lung cancer is rarely found in its early stages, only 13% of people diagnosed with lung cancer survive five years.

More than 420,000 Americans die every year from diseases caused by smoking cigarettes. This is more people than die from AIDS, automobile accidents, homicides, suicides, and alcohol abuse combined.

The medical expenses that are caused by smoking amount to billions of dollars every year.

American Cancer Society, 1599 Clifton Rd., NE, Atlanta, GA 30329; (800) ACS-2345

Americans for Nonsmokers Rights, 2530 San Pablo Ave., Ste. J, Berkeley, CA 94702; (510)841-3032; Net: http://www.sirius.com/~anr

American Heart Association, 7320 Greenville Ave., Dallas, TX 75231; (214)750-5300

American Lung Association, 1740 Broadway, New York, NY 10019-4374; (212)315-8700

The February 23, 1994 issue of the *Journal of the American Medical Association* was devoted exclusively to the health effects of tobacco. For a copy of this issue check with the periodicals desk of your local library, or contact the
American Medical Association, 515 N. State St., Chicago, IL 60610; (312)464-5000 or 2000 or (800)621-8335

Nicotine Anonymous is a fellowship of people helping each other to quit smoking and stay nicotine free. They publish a newsletter called *Fresh Air*.
California Nicotine Anonymous, PO Box 25335, Los Angeles, CA 90025; (800)642-0666

Centers For Disease Control & Prevention, Office of Smoking and Health, 5600 Fishers Lane, Rockville, MD 20857; (301)443-5287

Coalition on Smoking or Health, Washington, DC; (202)452-1184

Groups Against Smokers' Pollution (GASP), PO Box 632, College Park, MD 20741-0632; (301)459-4791

Nicotine Anonymous publishes a quarterly newsletter called Seven Minutes. Subscriptions are $7.
Nicotine Anonymous, PO Box 59177, San Francisco, CA 941590-1777; (415)750-0328; Net: http://slip.net/~billh/nicahome.html

Women and Girls Against Tobacco, 2001 Addison St., Ste. 200, Berkeley, CA 94704

• SOCIAL WORKERS

National Association of Social Workers, 750 — 1st, NW, Ste. 700, Washington, DC 20002; (202)408-8600 or (800)638-8799

• SPEECH

Book:
• *Help Me Talk Right: How to Correct a Child's Lisp in 15 Easy Lessons*, by Mirla G. Raz (E-mail: MirlaG@aol.com); Communication Skills Center (PO Box 5599, Scottsdale, AZ 85261-5599), 1996

American Speech, Language, and Hearing Association, (800)638-8255

Orton Dyslexia Society, Chester Bldg., Ste. 382, 8600 LaSalle Rd., Baltimore, MD 21286-2044; (410)296-0232 or (800) 222-3123

Compulsive Stutterers Anonymous, PO Box 1406, Park Ridge, IL 60068; (815)895-9848

Stuttering Foundation of America, 3100 Walnut Grove, Ste. 603, PO Box 11749, Memphis, TN 38111-0749; (901)452-7343 or (800)992-9392; E-mail: stuttersfa@aol.com

• STATE MEDICAL BOARDS

American Association of Dental Examiners, 211 E. Chicago Ave., Ste. 844, Chicago, IL 60611; (708)699-7900

American Association of Osteopathic Examiners, 300 — 5th St., NE, Washington, DC 20002; (202)544-5060

Association of State and Territorial Health Officials, 415 Second St., NE, Washington, DC 20002; (202)546-5400

Federation of Associations of Regulatory Boards, 400 S. Union St., Ste. 295, PO Box 4389, Montgomery, AL 36103-4389; (205)834-2415

Federation of State Medical Boards of the United States, 6000 Western Place, Ste. 707, Fort Worth, TX 76107-4618; (817)735-8445

National Board of Medical Examiners, 3930 Chestnut St., Philadelphia, PA 19104; (215)590-9500

Following is a list of the state medical boards that license, monitor, and discipline doctors in each state. To find out whether a doctor is licensed to practice in your state, contact your state's board. Additionally, there are state and county boards that license and supervise dentists, nurses, pharmacies, hospitals, and other medical professionals and facilities. Phone numbers of these other boards are available through your state medical board or state capital information operator.

To file a grievance against a medical professional, hospital, or medical center, get in contact with the proper authorities and find out what specific steps to follow. You may need to fill out forms that are supplied by the authority. (To make sure you follow the correct and most effective procedure for filing a complaint, contact the People's Medical Society, or the Public Citizen's Health Research Group, as they are listed in the *Research Resource* section of this book under the heading *Patients' and Consumers' Rights.* You may also want to obtain legal advice from an attorney before you sign your name to any letters or forms that question someone's professional skill, especially if there is the possibility of a malpractice lawsuit.)

If you are seeking to notify authorities of the illegal actions of a medical professional, you may also want to contact your state attorney general, who is the chief law enforcement officer in the state.

To successfully file a complaint that results in actions taken against a doctor, you may need to let the authorities review your medical records.

It is wise to keep records and a journal of all actions you take in the process of registering a complaint. Keep copies of all forms you sign, records of what office you called, who you spoke with, and what the main points of the conversations were.

Alabama State Board of Medical Examiners, 848 Washington Ave., Montgomery, AL 36101-0946; (205)242-4116; Fax (205)242-4155

Alaska State Medical Board, 3601 C St., Ste. 722, Anchorage, AK 99503; (907)561-2878; Fax (907)562-5781

Alaska Dept. of Commerce & Economic Development, Division of Occupational Licensing, State Office Bldg., 9th Flr., 333 Willoughby, Juneau, AK 99801; (907)465-2541; Fax (907)465-2974

Arizona State Board of Medical Examiners, 1651 E. Morten Ave., Ste. 210, Phoenix, AZ 85020; (602)255-3751; Fax (602)255-1848

Arizona Board of Osteopathic Examiners in Medicine & Surgery, 1830 W. Colter, Ste. 104, Phoenix, AZ 85015; (602)255-1747; Fax (602)255-1756

Arkansas State Medical Board, 2100 Riverfront Dr., Ste. 200, Little Rock, Arkansas 72202; (501)324-9410; Fax (501)324-9413

California State Medical Board, 1426 Howe Ave., Ste. 54, Sacramento, CA 95825; (916)263-2388 or 263-2382; Fax (916)263-2387

California, Osteopathic Medical Board of, 444 N. Third St., Ste. A-200, Sacramento, CA 95814; (916)322-4306; Fax (916)327-6119

Colorado State Board of Medical Examiners, 1560 Broadway, Ste. 1300, Denver, CO 80202-5140; (303)894-7690; Fax (303)894-7692

Connecticut Division of Medical Quality-assurance, Connecticut Dept. of Public Health & Addiction Services, Division of Medical Quality-assurance, 150 Washington St., Hartford, CT 06106; (203)566-7398; Fax (203)566-6606

Delaware Board of Medical Practice, Margaret O'Neil Bldg., 2nd Flr., Federal & Court Streets, Dover, DE 19903; (302)739-4522; Fax (302)739-2711

District of Columbia Board of Medicine, 605 G St., NW, Rm. 202, Lower Level, 20001, Washington, DC 20013-7200; (202)727-9794; Fax (202)727-4087

District of Columbia Dept. of Consumer and Regulatory Affairs, 614 H St., NW, Ste. 904, Washington, DC 20001; (202)727-7823 or (202)727-7102

Florida Board of Medicine, Northwood Centre, Ste. 60, 1940 N. Monroe St., Tallahassee, FL 32399-0750; (904)488-0595; Fax (904)487-9622

Florida Board of Osteopathic Medical Examiners, Northwood Centre, Ste. 60, Tallahassee, FL 32399-0775; (904)922-6725; Fax (904)922-3040

Georgia Composite State Board of Medical Examiners, 166 Pryor St., SW, Atlanta, GA 30303-3465; (404)656-3913; Fax (404)656-9723

Guam Board of Medical Examiners, Dept. of Public Health & Social Services, Rte. 10, Mangilao, Agana, Guam 96910; 011 (671)734-7296; Fax 011 (671)734-2066

Hawaii Board of Medical Examiners, Dept. of Commerce & Consumer Affairs, 1010 Richards St., Honolulu, HI 96801; (808)586-2704; Fax (808)586-2689

Idaho State Board of Medicine, State House Mail, 280 N. 8th, Ste. 202, Boise, ID 83720; (208)334-2822; Fax (208)334-2801

Illinois Dept. of Professional Regulation, State of Illinois Center, 100 W. Randolph St., #9-300, Chicago, IL 60601; (312)814-4934; Fax (312)814-1837 — or — 320 W. Washington St., Springfield, IL 62786; (217)524-2169; Medical Licensing Unit Fax (217)782-7645

Indiana Consumer Protection , Health Professional Bureau, One American Square, Ste. 1020, Indianapolis, Indiana 46282; (317)232-2386

Indiana Health Professions Service Bureau, 402 W. Washington St., Rm. 041, Indianapolis, Indiana 46204; (317)232-2960; Fax (317)233-4236

Iowa State Board of Medical Examiners, State Capitol Complex, Executive Hills W., 1209 E. Court Ave., Des Moines, IA 50319-0180; (515)281-5171; Fax (515)242-5908

Kansas State Board of Healing Arts, 235 SW Topeka Blvd., Topeka, KS 66603; (913)296-7413; Fax (913)296-0852

Kentucky Board of Medical Licensure, The Hurstbourne Office Park, 310 Whittington Pkwy., Ste. 1B, Louisville, KY 40222; (502)429-8046; Fax (502)429-9923

Louisiana State Board of Medical Examiners, 830 Union St., Ste. 100, New Orleans, LA; (504)524-6763; Fax (504)568-8893

Maine Board of Registration in Medicine, State House Station, Ste. 317, Two Bangor St., Augusta, ME 04333; (207)287-2480

Maine Board of Osteopathic Examination & Registration, State House Station, Ste. 142, Augusta, ME 04333; (207)287-2480

Maryland Board of Physician Quality-assurance, 4201 Patterson Ave., 3rd Flr., 21215-0095, Baltimore, MD 21215; (410)764-4777 or (800)492-6836; Fax: (410)764-2478

Massachusetts Board of Registration in Medicine, Ten W. St., 3rd Flr., Boston, MA 02111; (617)727-3086; Fax (617)451-9568

Michigan Board of Medicine, 611 W. Ottawa St., 4th Flr., 48933, Lansing, MI 48909; (517)373-6873; Fax (517)373-2179

Michigan Board of Osteopathic Medicine and Surgery, 611 W. Ottawa St., 4th Flr. 48933, Lansing, MI 48909; (517)373-6837; Fax (517)373-2179

Minnesota Board of Medical Practice, 2700 University Ave. W., Ste. 106, St. Paul, MN 55114-1080; (612)642-0538; Fax (612)642-0393

Mississippi State Board of Medical Licensure, 2688-D Insurance Center Dr., Jackson, MS 39216; (601)354-6654; Fax (601)987-4159

Missouri State Board of Registration for the Healing Arts, 3605 Missouri Blvd., Jefferson City, MO 65109; (314)751-0098; Fax (314)751-3166

Montana Board of Medical Examiners, Arcade Bldg., Lower Level, 111 N. Jackson, Helena, MT 59620-0513; (406)444-4284/4276; Fax (406)444-1667

Nebraska State Board of Examiners in Medicine and Surgery, 301 Centennial Mall S., Lincoln, NB 68509-5007; (402)471-2115; Fax (402)471-0383

Nevada State Board of Medical Examiners, 1105 Terminal Way, Ste. 301, 89502, Reno, NV 89510; (702)688-2559; Fax (702)688-2321

Nevada State Board of Osteopathic Medicine, 2950 E. Flamingo Rd., Ste. E-3, Las Vegas, NV 89121; (702)732-2147

New Hampshire Board of Registration in Medicine, Health & Welfare Bldg., 6 Hazen Dr., Concord, NH 03301; (603)271-4501

New Hampshire Licensing Board Office, 2 Industrial Park Dr., Ste. 8, Concord, NH 03301-8520; (603)2711-1203

New Jersey State Board of Medical Examiners, 140 E. Front St., 2nd Flr., Trenton, NJ 08608; (609)826-7100; Fax (609)984-3930

New Mexico State Board of Medical Examiners, Leamy Bldg., Second Flr., 491 Old Santa Fe Trail, Santa Fe, NM 87501; (505)827-7317; Fax 505 827-7377

New Mexico Board of Osteopathic Medical Examiners, 725 St. Michaels Dr., 87501, Santa Fe, NM 87504; (505)827-7171; Fax (505)827-7095

New York State Board of Medicine, Cultural Education Center, Rm. 3023, Empire State Plaza, Albany, NY 12230; (518)474-3841; Fax (518)473-0578

New York Board of Professional Medical Conduct, New York State Dept. of Health, Rm. 438, Corning Tower Bldg., Empire State Plaza, Albany, NY 12237-0614; (518)474-8357; Fax (518)474-4471

North Carolina Board of Medical Examiners, 1203 Front St., 27609, Raleigh, NC 27611-6808; (919)828-1212; Fax (919)828-1295

North Dakota State Board of Medical Examiners, City Center Plaza, 418 E. Broadway, Ste. 12, Bismark, ND 58501; (701)223-9485; Fax (701)223-9756

Ohio State Medical Board, 77 S. High St., 17th Flr., Columbus, OH 43266-0315; (614)466-3934

Oklahoma State Board of Medicine Licensure and Supervision, 5104 N. Francis, Ste. C, Oklahoma City, OK 73154-0256; (405)848-2189; Fax (405)848-8240

Oklahoma Board of Osteopathic Examiners, 4848 N. Lincoln Blvd., Ste. 100, Oklahoma City, OK 73105-3321; (405)528-8625; Fax (405)528-6102

Oregon Board of Medical Examiners, 620 Crown Plaza, 1500 SW First Ave., Portland, OR 97201-5826; (503)229-5770; Fax (503)229-6543

Pennsylvania State Board of Medicine, Transportation & Safety Bldg., Rm. 612, Commonwealth Ave. & Foster St., Harrisburg, PA 17105-2649; (717)787-2381; Fax (717)787-7769

Pennsylvania State Board of Osteopathic Medicine, Transportation & Safety Bldg., Rm. 612, Commonwealth Ave. & Foster St., Harrisburg, PA 17105-249; (717)783-4858; Fax (717)787-7769

Puerto Rico Board of Medical Examiners, Call Box 13969, San Juan, Puerto Rico 00908; (809)782-8989; Fax (809)782-8733

Rhode Island Board of Licensure and Discipline, Dept. of Health, 3 Capitol Hill, Cannon Bldg., Rm. 205, Providence, RI 02908-5097; (401)277-3855 or 56; Fax (401)277-2158

South Carolina, State Board of Medical Examiners of, 101 Executive Center Dr., Saluda Bldg., Ste. 120, 29210, Columbia, SC 29221-2269; (803)731-1650; Fax (803)731-1660

South Dakota State Board of Medical and Osteo Examiners, 1323 S. Minnesota Ave., Sioux Falls, SD 57105; (605)336-1965

Tennessee State Board of Medical Examiners, 287 Plus Park Blvd., Nashville, TN 37247-1010; (615)367-6231; Fax (615)367-6210

Tennessee State Board of Osteopathic Examiners, 287 Plus Park Blvd., Nashville, TN 37247-1010; (615)367-6281

Texas State Board of Medical Examiners, 1812 Centre Creek Dr., 78754, Austin, TX 78714-9134; (512)834-7728; Fax (512)834-4597

Utah Physicians Licensing Board, Division of Occupational & Professional Licensing, Heber M Wells Bldg., 4th Flr., 160 E. 300 S., 84145, Salt Lake City, UT 84145-0805; (801)530-6628; Fax (801)530-6511

Vermont Board of Medical Practice, 109 State St., Montpelier, VT 05609-1106; (802)828-2673; Fax (802)828-2496

Vermont Board of Medicine, 6606 W. Broad St., 4th Flr., Richmond, VA 23230-1717; (804)662-9908; Fax (804)662-9943

Virgin Islands Board of Medical Examiners, Virgin Islands Dept. of Health, 48 Sugar Estate, St. Thomas, Virgin Islands 00802; (809)776-8311; Fax (809)777-4001

Washington Dept. of Health, BME/MDB Medical Boards, 1300 SE Quince St., MS: EY-25, Olympia, WA 98504; (206)753-2287; Fax (206)586-4573

Washington Board of Osteopathic Medicine & Surgery, Dept. of Health, 1300 SE Quince St., Olympia, WA 98504-7868; (206)586-8438

West Virginia State Board of Medicine, 101 Dee Dr., Charleston, WV 25311; (304)558-2921; Fax (304)558-2084

West Virginia Board of Osteopathy, 334 Penco Rd., Weirton, WV 26062; (304)723-4638

Wisconisn Medical Examiners Board, 1400 E. Washington Ave., Madison, WI 53708; (608)266-2811; Fax (608) 267-0644

Wyoming Board of Medicine, 2301 Central Ave., 2nd Flr., Barrett Bldg., Rm. 208, Cheyenne, WY 82002; (307)777-6463; Fax (307)777-6478

• STROKE

Strokes are the third-leading cause of death among Americans and the main cause of disability, such as damaged memory, loss of speech, and paralysis among older adults. Strokes occur when a burst artery or blood clot interrupts the blood supply to the brain. The interrupted blood flow deprives the brain tissue of oxygen and damages the tissue.

Approximately 150,000 deaths are caused by stroke each year. A $20 million study funded by the National Institutes of Health found that surgery (endarterectomy) that removes fatty deposits from the two main arteries of the neck, the jugular vein and the carotid artery, can dramatically reduce the risk of stroke. The surgery also carries the risk of causing a stroke and can have a fatal outcome. (see the December, 1989, issue of the *American Journal of Public Health,* and the October 25, 1990, issue of the *New England Journal of Medicine*)

People with a diet that is low in fat and particularly low in animal content, but high in plant content, and who do not smoke, are not overweight, and who exercise daily to decrease and help manage stress, experience a significantly lower incidence of stroke.

American Paralysis Association, 500 Morris Ave., Springfield, NJ 07081; (800)225-0292

The Stroke Connection of the American Heart Association maintains a listing of over 1000 stroke support groups across the nation for referral to stroke survivors, their families, caregivers, and interested professionals. They publish a magazine called *Stroke Connection,* and sell books, videos, and literature.

The Stroke Connection of the American Heart Association, 7272 Greenville Ave., Dallas, TX 75231; (800)553-6321; E-mail: strokaha@amhrt.org.

National Institute of Neurological Disorders and Stroke, PO Box 5801, Bethesda, MD 20824; (301)496-5751 or (800)352-9424; E-mail: NINDSwebmaster@nih.gov — or — Net: http://www.nih.gov/ninds/

National Stroke Association, Englewood, CO 80110-2622; (800)787-6537 or (800) STROKES

Stroke Clubs International, 805 — 12th St., Galveston, TX 77550; (409)762-1022

• SUBSTANCE ABUSE

Al-Anon, Box 862, Midtown Station, New York, NY 10018; (800)344-2666

Alateen, 1372 Broadway, New York, NY 10018; (212)302-7240

Alcoholics Anonymous (AA), 475 Riverside Dr., 11th Flr., New York, NY 10115; (212)870-3440

Adult Children of Alcoholics (ACA), 2225 Sepulveda Blvd., Ste. 200, Torrance, CA 90505; (310)534-1815

American College of Addiction Treatment Administrators, 5700 Old Orchard Rd., 1st Flr., Skokie, IL 60077; (708)966-0181

American Council on Alcoholism, (800)527-5344

American Society of Addiction Medicine, (202)244-8948

Association of Medical Education and Research in Substance Abuse, Brown University Center for Alcohol and Addiction Studies, Box G-BH, Providence, RI 02912; (401)863-7791

Association of Recovering Motorcyclists, 1503 Market St., La Cross, WI 54601; (608)784-8462

Calix Society (Catholic Alcoholics), 7601 Wazata Blvd., St. Louis Park, MN 55426; (612)546-0544 or (800)398-0524

Children of Alcoholics Foundation, PO Box 4185, Grand Central Station, New York, NY 10163-4185; (212)754-0656

Cocaine Anonymous, 3740 Overland Ave., Ste. H, Los Angeles, CA 90034-6337; (800)347-8998

Families Anonymous, Culver City, CA; (310)313-5800

Institute on Black Chemical Abuse, 2614 Nicollet Ave. S., Minneapolis, MN 55408; (612)871-7878

Minnesota Chemical Dependency Program for Deaf and Hard of Hearing Individuals, 2450 Riverside Ave. S., Minneapolis, MN 55454; (612)672-4402 or TTY (612)672-4114 or (800)282-3323: E-mail: kasandberg@aol.com

Narcotics Anonymous, 16155 Wyandotte St., Van Nuys, CA 91406; (818)780-3951

National Association of Children of Alcoholics, 11426 Rockville Park, Ste. 100, Rockville, MD 20852; (301)468-0985

National Center for Substance Abuse Treatment, (800)662-HELP (4357)

National Clearinghouse for Alcohol and Drug Information, PO Box 2345, Rockville, MD 20847-2345; (301)468-2600 or (800)729-6686; TTY (800)487-4889

National Cocaine Hotline, (800) COC-AINE

National Council on Alcoholism and Drug Dependency, (212)206-6770 or (800) NCA-CALL

National Council on Alcoholism and Drug Information, 12 W. 21st St., New York, NY 10010; (800)622-2255 or (212)206-6770

National Institute of Drug Abuse, 11426 Rockville Pike, Rockville, MD 20852; (310)443-6245 or (800)662-4357

Resource Center for Substance Abuse and Disability, 1331 F Street, NW, Ste. 800, Washington, DC 20004; (202)783-2900; TT: (202)737-0645

Substance Abuse Program for Pregnant Women, (202)574-2480

Women for Sobriety, Box 618, Quakertown, PA 18951; (215)536-8026 or (800)333-1606

• SUPPORT AND SELF-HELP GROUPS

Support groups are made up of individuals with similar concerns and problems.

The American Self-Help Clearinghouse helps people to find and form member-run self-help support groups. It publishes a directory of over 700 different types of self-help groups that cover a broad range of addictions, disabilities, illnesses, parenting concerns, bereavement, and many other stressful life situations. The book can be obtained by sending a check or money order for $11 to

The American Self-Help Clearinghouse, Northwest Covenant Medical Center, 25 Pocono Rd., Denville, NJ 07834; (201)625-7101

The Chatback Trust, Net: http://www.tcns.co.uk/chatback

Friends' Health Connection (formerly known as Long Distance Love) matches persons with the same health problems so they may give support to, and share experiences with, each another. Participants are matched based upon a number of criteria, including age, health problem, and personal background, as well as hobbies and interests. There is a $10 fee for processing applications, but they will not deny the service to those who cannot afford it.

Friends' Health Connection, PO Box 114, New Brunswick, NJ 08903; (908)418-1811 or (800)483-7436; E-mail: fhc@pilot.njin.net — or — Net: http://www.48friend.com

Friends Network, PO Box 4545, Santa Barbara, CA 93140

Komen Kids (friendship network for children of cancer patients), (800)462-9273

National Parent to Parent Support & Information System matches families whose children have special healthcare needs, rare disorders, and children who have gone through similar surgeries. The organization is funded by a grant from the Maternal & Child Health Bureau and donations.

National Parent to Parent, PO Box 907, Blue Ridge, GA 30513; (706)632-8822 or (800)651-1151; Fax (706)632-8830; E-mail: nippsis@aol.com — or — Net: Judd103W @wonder.em.cdc.gov

Supportworks helps people organize support groups and networks which meet face-to-face or by telephone conference. They publish an 8 page booklet titled *Power Tools: Ways to Build a Self-Help Group*. To obtain a copy, send a $3 check to

Support Works, 1018 E. Blvd., Ste. 5, Charlotte, NC 28203-5779; (704)331-9500 (9 AM to noon EST)

• TERMINOLOGY USED IN MEDICINE

While virtually all medical procedures and conditions can be described by using simple English words, the medical community often uses Latin and Greek terms. These medical terms are often a combination of two or three segments. For instance, an appendectomy is the removal of the appendix using the term "ectomy," which means "to cut away." For a more detailed list and definitions, a person may use one of the many medical dictionaries that are available at their local library or book store.

Common medical prefixes describing locations, relations, amounts, sizes, types, actions, and colors:

a- or **an-**: without or not

ab-: from or away from

acou-: hearing

acro-: an extremity or an extreme state

ad-: toward or near (change the *d* to *c*, *f*, *g*, *s*, or *t* when it precedes word segments that begin with those letters)

alba-: white

amphi-: both kinds or both sides
an-: duplicate, backward, or upward
andro-: associated with the male sex
antero-: placed before or in front of
anti-: against
auto-: self progressing
ap-: detached
batho- or **bathy-**: associated with depth
blasto-: associated with original development of cells
brachy-: shortness
brady-: slow
carcin-: association with cancer
cata-: downward, against, or under
contra-: counter to, or against
cry-: cold
dia-: passing or going through, apart, across, or between
dis-: reversal, separation, or removal
dys-: an adverse, difficult, or abnormal condition
ecto-: from the exterior or outside
ectro-: congenital absence or born without
endo-: within
epi-: over, on, or upon
erthr-: red
eso-: inside
ex-: out of, away from, or outside
exo-: outside of or outward
hemi-: half
hyper-: excessive, above, increased, or beyond
hypo-: deficient, under, below, or beneath
in-: not (change the n to l, m, or r when it precedes a word segment that begins with those letters)
infra-: situated or occurring below
inter-: between
intra-: within
ization-: development
juxta-: near or within proximity of
kine-: movement
latero-: toward the side or associated with the side
leio-: indicates an association with smoothness

lepto-: fragile, narrow, or thin
leuco- or **leuko-**: white
levo-: left
macro-: large
mal-: wrong, out of order, bad, or ill
medi- or **medio-**: middle
meta-: beyond, after, or changing
nano-: very small
necro-: dead
neo-: new
noso-: associated with disease
olig- or **oligo-**: not enough, insufficient, few, or little amount
ortho-: associated with normalcy or appropriateness
pachy-: thick
pan-: all
para-: beside, or beyond
peri-: around
plano-: flat
platy-: broad or flat
pluri-: more than one
poly-: multiple, or many
post-: after
pre- or **pro-**: before or in front of
pseud-: false
re-: again
retro-: backward position or motion
sapr- or **sapro-**: decay
schizo-: divided or split
scler- or **sclero-**: hardness
semi-: half
sub-: under
super-: over, beyond, or above
supra-: over, or above
syn-: together
tachi-, **tacho-** or **tachy-**: rapid, fast, or speed-related
terato-: monster or abnormality of development
therm- or **thermo-**: heat
tox-, **toxi-** or **toxo-**: poison or poisoning
trans-: through or across
uni-: one
xantho-: yellow
xeno-: foreign or strange
xer- or **xero-**: dryness

Common medical terms indicating an association with an area or part of the body:
abdomen or **abdomin**: belly
aden-: gland
adipo-: fat
adreno-: adrenal glands
angio-: blood vessels or lymph vessels
arterio-: arteries
arthro-: joints
atrio-: atrium of the heart or within

aur-: ears
blenn-: mucus
blephar-: eye lids
brachi-: arms
bronch-: bronchial tube or windpipe
cephal-: head
cerebr-: brain
cervic-: neck area

cheil-: lip
cheir-: hand
chole-: bile ducts or bile
cholecyst-: gallbladder
chondr-: cartilage
colo-: colon
colpo-: vagina
cost-: rib
cranio-: cranium or skull
cut-: cutaneous or skin
cystido-: bladder
cyto-: cell
dent-: teeth
derm-: skin
entero-: intestines
feto-: fetus
gastro-: stomach
gnath-: jaw
hema- or hemo-: blood
hepat-: liver
hist-: tissue
hyster-: uterus
ile- or ili-: intestines
ileo- or ilio-: ilium
jejuno-: the jejunum portion of the small intestine
kerat-: cornea
labi-: lip
lact-: milk ducts
lapar-: abdomen, loin, or flank
laryng-: larynx
leuko-: white blood cells
lieno-: spleen
lipo-: fat or lipids
lumbar or lumbo: lower back or portion of spinal column in small of back
lymph- or lympho-: lymph fluids
mamm- or mammo-: breasts or milk-secreting glands
mast-: breast
maxillo-: maxilla or upper jaw
meningo-: meninges or meninx membranes of the brain and spinal chord
mento-: chin
myelo-: spinal chord
my- or myo-: muscle
myx- or myxo-: mucus
naso-: nose or nasal cavity
nephr: kidneys
neur: nerves or nervous system
occipito-: back of head
ocul- or oculo-: eyes
odont-: teeth
omo-: shoulder
omphal- or omphalo-: naval
onych- or onycho-: nails
oo-: ovum or egg
oophor-: ovary

ophthalm-: eyes
orbito-: eye socket or orbit
orchii-: testicles
oro-: mouth
os-: mouth or opening
osseo- or osteo-: bone
ot- or oto-: ear
ov-: ovaries
palato-: palate
parieto-: parietal bones of the roof of the head
pelvi- or pelvo-: pelvis
pharyng-: pharynx or throat
phallo-: penis
phleb-: veins
pilo-: hair
plasmo-: plasma
pod-: feet
ponto-: pons of the brain
procto-: rectum or anus
ptyalo-: saliva
pulmo-: lungs
pupillo-: pupil
rachi- or rachio-: spine
recto-: rectum
ren-: kidneys
retino-: retina
rhin- or rhino-: nose
sacro-: sacrum
salping-: fallopian tubes
sagui- or sanguino-: blood
sarco-: flesh
scato-: feces
sero-: serum
sial- or sialo-: saliva or salivary glands
spheno-: sphenoid bone
splen- or spleno-: spleen
spondyl- or spondylo-: vertebra or spinal column
stea-: fat
stern- or sterno-: sternum
stomato-: mouth
sudo-: sweat
talp-: ankle
temporo-: temple
teno-: tendons
thorac- or thoraco-: chest
thromb-: clot
thymo-: thymus
thyro-: thyroid gland
tibio-: tibia
tracheo-: trachea or windpipe
tricho-: hair
urano-: roof of the mouth or palate
uretero-: ureter tube
utero-: uterus
vagino-: vagina
vago-: vagus nerve

vaso-: duct or vessel
veno: vein
ventriculo-: ventricle of the heart or brain

vertebro-: vertebra of the spinal column
vesec: bladder
viscero-: internal organs
vulvo-: vulva

Common medical suffixes describing what is being done surgically:

-centesis: puncture with a needle to take or "draw" fluid
-cryo: freeze
-desis: bind or fuse together
-ectomy: excise, cut away or out
-lysis: freeing of
-nyxis: puncture
-ostomy: artificially open or create an opening

-pexy: fixate, stabilize
-plasty: repair or reform
-rhaphy: sew or bind
-rhexis: break or fracture on purpose to realign or restructure
-scopy: look at or examine internally with an instrument
-tomy: surgical incision into an organ
-stomy: surgical opening

Common medical suffixes describing the state or what is happening or being experienced:

-agra: seizure or sharp pain
-alge or **-algia:** associated with pain
-asis: taking place
-blast: the initial development or original growth
-cele: a swelling, tumor, protrusion, or hernia
-cide: destruction
-dynamo: strength or a force
-esis: a condition or action
-ferous: bearing or yielding
-genesis: production of something
-glycemia: sugar in the blood
-hydr: having to do with liquid
-iasis: produced by disease or disease producing characteristics
-itis: inflammation
-lepsia, -lepsis, or **-lepsy:** associated with seizures

-megaly: enlarged or very large
-oid: resembling
-oma or **-ome:** a mass, tumor, or swelling
-osis: indicating a diseased or abnormal condition
-pathy: indicates disease or abnormal state
-penia: deficient or less than what is considered normal
-plegia: paralysis
-pnea: associated with breathing
-poiesis: production of
-ptosis: drooping or sagging
-rhage: abnormal discharge, bursting, or flow
-rrhea or **-rhea:** flow or discharge
-scler: hardening
-uria: characteristic or constituent of urine

• THERAPY THROUGH ART, DANCE, MUSIC, AND WRITING

American Art Therapy Association, 1202 Allanson Rd., Mundelein, IL 60060; (708)949-6064

American Association for Music Therapy, PO Box 50012, Valley Forge, PA 19484-0012; (215)265-4006

American Dance Therapy Association, 2000 Century Plaza, Ste. 108, Columbia, MD 21044

American Society of Psychopathology of Expression, 74 Lawton St., Brookline, MA 02146; (617)738-9821

Association for Applied Poetry, 60 N. Main St., Johnstown, OH 43031; (614)967-6060

Association of Youth Museums, 1775 K St., NW, Ste. 595, Washington, DC 20006; (202)466-4144

Certification Board for Music Therapists, 6336 N. Oracle Rd., Ste. 326, PO Box 345, Tucson, AZ 85704-5457

National Association of Music Therapy, 8455 Colesville Rd., Ste. 930, Silver Spring, MD 20910; (301)589-3300

• THYROID

National Graves' Disease Foundation, 320 Arlington Rd., Jacksonville, FL 32211; (904)724-0770

Thyroid Foundation of America, Massachusetts General Hospital, Ruth Sleeper Hall 350, Boston, MA 02114; (617)726-8500

• TRAVEL FOR MEDICAL REASONS — LODGING FOR FAMILIES — SPECIAL AIRPLANES

Book:
• *The Travel Health Clinic Pocket Guide to Healthy Travel*; by Lawrence Bryson; Silvercat Publications, 1994

Air Life Line is a voluntary association of pilots who fly medical missions to transport patients or supplies.
Air Life Line, 1716 X St., Sacramento, CA 95818; (916)446-0995

Airline Medical Directors Association, American Airlines Medical Dept., PO Box 66033, AAMF Ohare, IL 60666; (312)686-4192

The Angel Planes, 2756 N. Green Valley Pkwy., Ste 115, Green Valley, NV 89014-2100; (702)261-0494 or (800)Fly-1711; Fax (702)261-0497

Association of Air Medical Services, 35 S. Raymond, Ste. 205, Pasadena, CA 91105; (818)793-1232; Fax (818)793-1039; E-mail: NatlOffice@aol.com

Corporate Angel Network, Westchester County Airport, Bldg. One, White Plains, NY 10604; (914)328-1313

Flying Doctors of America, 1951 Airport Rd., DeKalb-Peachtree Airport, Atlanta, GA 30341; (404)451-3068; Fax (404)457-6302

International Association for Medical Assistance to Travelers, 417 Center St., Lewiston, NY 14092; (716)754-4883

The National Association of Hospital Hospitality Houses promotes the creation and development of hospitality houses, offering lodging and other support to families traveling to receive medical care away from home. The Association is affiliated, as members, with the American Hospital Association, and Independent Charities of America.
National Association of Hospital Hospitality Houses, 4013 W. Jackson St., Muncie, IN 47304; (800)542-9730

National Emergency Medical Service Pilot's Association, 5810 Hornwood, Houston, TX 77081

National Flight Nurses Association, 6900 Grove Rd., Thorofare, NJ 08086; (609) 384-6725

National Flight Paramedics Association, 35 S. Raymond Ave., Ste. 205, Pasadena, CA 91105; (818) 405-9851; Fax (818)793-1039

The National Patient Air Transport Hotline is operated by Mercy Medical Airlift on behalf of the Air Care Alliance. They are associated with the Association of Air Medical Services, the National Air Transport Association, and the Air Care Alliance. The hotline is answered 24 hours-a-day. They make referrals to all known appropriate charitable, charitably assisted, and special patient discount commercial flight services based on the evaluation of the patient's condition, type of transport required, and departure/destination locations.

NPATH provides information on referral as follows:

1. For patients and patient families who must find a way to move a loved one or themselves to distant locations for specialized treatment or recovery after illness or accident.
2. For health care industry personnel (doctors, nurses, social workers, and discharge planners) and travel industry personnel who must find the most cost-effective means to move a patient and/or patient family member long-distance by air.
3. For volunteer pilots and/or medical personnel who want to serve with one of the many volunteer pilot organizations that fly for the public benefit, or with other charitable agencies that serve needy patients with charitably-assisted transport.

National Patient Air Transport Hotline, PO Box 1940, Manassas, VA 22110; (800)296-1217

Ronald McDonald House, One McDonald's Plaza, Oakbrook, IL 60521; (708)575-7048

World Health Organization Travel & Health Information, Net: http://www.who .ch/TravelAndHealth/TravelAndHealth_Home.html

• WEIGHT AND EATING PROBLEMS

To lose weight:
* Be aware of how many fat grams and calories you are consuming.
* Do not eat fried foods.
* Avoid white rice, white bread, white sugar, soda pop, and other empty calorie items.
* Avoid refined sugars, artificial sweeteners, and foods that contain them.
* Do not add salt to your foods and do not use salt substitutes. When you must add salt to a recipe, use sea salt (available at healthfood stores).
* Do not eat at fast food restaurants.
* Do not purchase fattening foods.
* Never eat cheese.
* Take your lunch to work so that you can control what you eat and avoid the temptation of fattening restaurant or snack foods.
* If you do eat meat, do not make it the main item of your meal.
* Use small plates, bowls, and utensils instead of large ones.
* Drink larger glasses of water.
* Snack on fruit or vegetables instead of other foods that may be packed with fat, cholesterol, salt, sugar, or empty calories.
* Do not eat desert. Eat a fruit in place of fatty desert items.
* Drink water or herb tea instead of snacking or drinking sodas or coffee.
* Exercise daily and do a variety of little exercises throughout the day.
* Admit that you have an eating problem or a weight problem when one or both exists.
* Get rid of your cookbooks that contain fattening recipes.
* Read a variety of books about fitness and nutrition.
* Consult with a nutritionist to find ways to improve your diet.
* Take high-quality vitamin supplements to help you get rid of cravings to overeat.
* Avoid dwelling on what you consider to be your failures and disappointments in life.
* Change what you can, confront what you should, and do not take your aggravations out on your stomach.
* Attend a support group, such as Overeaters Anonymous.
* Start each day with the goal of eating only healthy foods, and stick with the goal.

For a referral to a certified fitness trainer call the
Aerobics and Fitness Association of America, 15250 Ventura Blvd., Ste. 310, Sherman Oaks, CA 91403; (818)905-0040 or (800)446-2322

American Anorexia and Bulimia Association, 418 E. 76th St., New York, NY 10021; (212)734-1114

American Dietetic Association, PO Box 39101, Chicago, IL 60639; (800)366-1655

American Society of Bariatric Physicians, 5600 S. Quebec, Ste. 160, Englewood, CO 80111; (303)779-4833

Anorexia Nervosa and Related Eating Disorders, Inc., PO Box 5102, Eugene, OR 97405; (541)344-1144

Association for Glycogen Storage Disease, PO Box 896, Durant, IA 52747; (319)785-6038

Center for Child and Adolescent Obesity, UC San Francisco School of Medicine, Dept. of Family & Community Medicine and Pediatrics, Box 0900, San Francisco, CA 94143-0900; (415)476-4575

Center for the Study of Anorexia and Bulimia, 1 W. 91st St., New York, NY 10024; (212)595-3449; Fax (202)265-4954

Cooper Clinic, 12200 Preston Rd., Dallas, TX 75230; (800)444-5764

Exercise — Abdominal Training, Net: http://clix.aarnet.edu.au/misc.fitness .abdominaltraining.html

Fitness, Net: http://www.fanzine.se/fitness/

Formula One, Net: http://www.wondernet.com/alliance/formula1.html

Hippocrates Health Institute, 1443 Palmdale Crt., W. Palm Beach, FL 33411

Mankato State University Athletic Training, Net: http://vax1.mankato.msus.edu /~k061252/MSUATC.html

The McDougall Newsletter includes information on improving health through diet and exercise. It is published by Dr. John McDougall and his wife Mary who are also the authors of the books *The McDougall Plan,* and *The McDougall Program.* John McDougall has a weekly syndicated radio show and conducts seminars. The newsletter is published six times per year and subscriptions are $20.
McDougall Newsletter, PO Box 14039, Santa Rosa, CA 95402; (707)576-1654 or (800)570-1654; Fax (707)576-3313

National Anorexic Aid Society, 1925 E. Dublin Granville Rd., Columbus, OH 43229; (614)436-1112

National Association of Anorexia Nervosa and Associated Disorders, PO Box 7, Highland Park, IL 60035; (708)831-3438

National Digestive Diseases Education & Information Clearinghouse, 1555 Wilson Blvd., Ste. 600, Rosslyn, VA 22209

National Health Video, Net: http://www.frp.com/healthvid

National Institute of Fitness, PO Box 938, Ivins, UT 84738; (801)673-4905

Nutrition Action Healthletter ($20 a year), 1875 Connecticut Ave., NW, Washington, DC 20009; (800)237-4874

Overeaters Anonymous, PO Box 92870, Los Angeles, CA 90009; (310)618-8835 or (800)743-8703

The Pritikin Longevity Centers are preventative health education hotels. Guests undergo a physical exam, take classes in exercise, and learn to prepare lowfat/low-cholesterol meals. The book *Pritikin Program for Diet and Exercise* is available in many book stores.
Pritikin Longevity Center, 1910 Ocean Front Walk, Santa Monica, CA 90405; (310)450-5433 or (800)421-9911 — or — 5875 Collins Ave., Miami Beach, FL 33140; (305)866-2237 or (800)327-4914

Rancho La Puerta, PO Box 69, Tecate, CA 91980; (619)744-4222

Tufts University *Diet & Nutrition Letter,* 203 Harrison Ave., Boston, MA 02111; (617)482-3530 or (800)274-7581

Theodore B. VanItallie Center for Nutrition and Weight Management at St. Luke's— Roosevelt Hospital Center, New York, NY; (212)523-8440

• WISHES FOR TERMINALLY ILL CHILDREN

Sunshine Foundation, 2001 Bridge St., Philadelphia, PA 19124; (215)535-1413 or (800)767-1976

Make-A-Wish Foundation, 100 W. Clarendon, Ste. 2200, Phoenix, AZ 85013-3518; (800)332-9474

• WOMEN'S HEALTH

Books: (Many of the books listed here may be purchased with a credit card over the phone by calling Medea Books of Santa Cruz, California; (408)425-0913

- *Black Women's Health Book: Speaking for Ourselves*, edited by Evelyn White; Seal Press, 1994
- *Body and Soul: The Black Women's Guide to Physical-health and Emotional Well Being*, edited by Linda Villarosa; Harper-Perennial, 1994
- *The Endometriosis Sourcebook*, by Mary Lou Ballweg and the Endometriosis Association; Contemporary Books, 1995
- *The Estrogen Decision*, by Susan M. Larke, MD; Westchester Publishing, 1995
- *The Female Heart: The Truth about Women and Heart Disease*, by Marianne J. Legato MD and Carol Colman; Avon, 1993
- *A Gynecologist's Second Opinion: The Questions and Answers Your Need to Take Charge of Your Health*, by William H. Parker, with Rachel L. Parker; Plume, 1995
- *The Hysterectomy Hoax: A leading surgeon explains why 90 percent of all hysterectomies are unnecessary, and describes all the treatment options available to every woman, no matter what age*, by Stanley West MD with Paula Dranov; Doubleday, 1994
- *Male Practice: How Doctors Manipulate Women*, by Robert S. Mendelsohn, MD; Contemporary Books, 1981
- *Men Who Control Women's Health*, by Diana Scully; Houghton Mifflin, 1980
- *Menopause Without Medicine*, by Linda Ojeda, PhD; Hunter House Publishers ([510]838-6652), 1995
- *The Menopause Self-Help Book: A Women's Guide to Feeling Wonderful for the Second Half of Her Life*, by Susan M. Lark; Celestial Arts (PO Box 7327, Berkeley, CA 94707), 1990
- *The New Our Bodies, Ourselves*, by the Boston Women's Health Book Collective; Simon & Schuster, 1992
- *Our Health, Our Lives*, by Eileen Hoffman; Pocket Books 1995
- *Outrageous Practices: The Alarming Truth About How Medicine Mistreats Women*, by Leslie Laurence and Beth Weinhouse; Fawcett Columbine, 1994
- *Unequal Treatment*, by Nechas and Foley; Simon and Schuster, 1994
- *Women and Doctors: A Physician's Explosive Account of Women's Medical Treatment — and Mistreatment — in America Today and What You Can Do About It*, by John M. Smith, MD; Atlantic Monthly Press, 1992
- *Women's Bodies, Women's Wisdom: Creating Physical and Emotional Health and Healing*, by Christine Northrup, MD; Bantam Books, 1994
- *The Women's Guide to Hysterectomy: Expectations and Options*, by Adelaide Haas & Susan L. Puretz Berkeley; Celestial Arts, 1995
- *Women's Health Alert: What Most Doctors Won't Tell You About*, by Sidney M. Wolfe and Rhoda Donkin Jones; Addison-Wesley Publishing, 1991
- *Women Under the Knife: A Gynecologist's Report on Hazardous Medicine*, by Herbert H. Keyser, MD; George F. Stickley Company, 1984

According to the United States Department of Health and Human Services, two out of every three healthcare dollars are spent on women. Women visit doctors more often than men, take the majority of medications, and undergo a large majority of the surgeries. As a result, women are subject to the greater amount of negligent care, questionable procedures, and so-called cures. Though the majority of money spent on healthcare is spent on women, they have not been included in most health research studies of diseases, drug therapies, surgical procedures, and lifestyle effects on health.

Studies have shown that women are more likely to have the proper testing done if they go to an obstetrician/gynecologist who is female because they follow screening guidelines for mammograms and pap smears better than male doctors. A woman should be forewarned that unnecessary mastectomies and hysterectomies are more common than any other type of surgery.

"We were making rounds in the hospital," she recalls. "I was the only woman, and we were discussing the case of a woman who had checked into the hospital for a hysterectomy. 'She doesn't really need it,' said the physician who was leading the rounds, 'but let's do it anyway, because you can all use the practice.'" Outraged, the young doctor couldn't stop herself from blurting out, "And while we're at it, why don't we remove your testicles for practice, too!" She nearly got kicked out of the training program.
— From the book *Outrageous Practices: The Alarming Truth About How Medicine Mistreats Women*, by Leslie Laurence and Beth Weinhouse; Fawcett Columbine, 1994

About 4,500 women in America die every year from cervical cancer. It is one of the most common cancers in women and, according to researchers at Johns Hopkins School of Hygiene and Public Health, the human papilloma viruses may play a part in over 90% of all cervical cancers. Women who smoke, who had intercourse early in life, who have had multiple sexual partners, or who have been infected with the sexually transmitted human papilloma virus are at a higher risk of developing cervical cancer.

Developed in the 1940s by Dr. George Papanicolaou and made widely available in the 1950s, a Pap smear can detect cervical cancer in its earliest stages. The test is done by taking a small sample of tissue cells from the cervix and examining them for abnormalities.

Before undergoing a Pap smear, be sure not to have intercourse or put anything in the vagina for at least 48 hours before the test. Also, because menstrual flow may interfere with the accuracy of a Pap smear, women are advised to undergo the test at mid-cycle.

When Pap tests results are abnormal, an exam of the cervix with a microscope called a colposcope can be done. A tissue biopsy can be performed if further testing is needed.

Modern medicine, women, and mishaps:

- The synthetic female hormone diethylstilbestrol (DES): Used between 1938 and the early 1970s, it was prescribed to several million pregnant women to prevent miscarriages. It was available in pill form, as well as by injection and suppositories, and was sold by over 200 drug companies under different brand names. Women who were exposed to DES have a slightly increased risk of breast cancer.

  Daughters of women who took DES have an increased risk of a rare form of vaginal and cervical cancer called clear-cell adenocarcinoma. Sons of women who took DES have an increased risk of having undescended testicles, cysts on the epididymis, and infertility.

- The Copper-7 and Dalkon Shield IUDs: These intrauterine birth-control devices (IUD) caused infections that left many women sterile, perforated the uteruses of some women, and caused the death of others. Additionally, intimidating tactics were practiced against the women who subsequently sued the manufacturers when the lawyers claimed the women's problems were caused by their sexual practices and not by the faulty devices doctors had placed in their uterus.

- Strictly cosmetic operations done to the breasts: Starting in the early 1960s, millions of silicone gel-filled implants were surgically placed in women's breasts. Only after many of these women complained about the health problems these devices caused and the mutilations done to women at the hands of plastic surgeons did the government stand up to the medical lobbies and limit the use of the implants. The ongoing legal battles between implant recipients and manufacturers reflect that of those carried out between recipients of the Dalkon Shield and the A.H. Robins Company.

- Cesarean sections: America has the highest cesarean section rate in the world. In contrast, the Netherlands has one of the lowest cesarean birth rates and one of the lowest maternal and neonatal mortality rates in the world. A doctor makes more money if he performs a cesarean section instead of working with the woman to have the baby naturally. According to the Atlanta-based Centers for Disease Control and Prevention, there were 349,000 unnecessary Cesarean birth deliveries performed in America in 1991 at a combined cost of more than $1 billion. A report released in May of 1994 by Public Citizen's Health Research Group estimated that half the 421,000 cesarean sections performed in 1992 were unnecessary and added $1.3 billion to America's healthcare bill. These types of doctor-assisted births, where the abdomen and uterus are cut open to deliver the baby, are finally on the decrease as women are becoming more educated in this area of their health.
- Hysterectomies: More than 550,000 hysterectomies are performed in the US each year at an approximate cost of $2 billion. US women undergo twice as many hysterectomies as women in Britain, and four times as many hysterectomies as women in France. This figure is much lower than 20 years ago, but still is much higher than many professionals believe it should be. According to a study conducted by the Santa Monica based think tank, Rand Corporation, about 16% of hysterectomies performed in a study group of 642 people in five states were clearly unnecessary. Forty-one percent of the hysterectomies were unneeded or of questionable necessity. Another 25% were of questionable value.
- Norplant: This birth-control device consists of six matchstick-size silicone rods containing the synthetic hormone progestin, an ingredient in many birth control pills, that are implanted into the skin of the upper left arm and then left in place for up to five years. More than one million American women have received this product. The product literature lists side effects that include rare instances of stroke, phlebitis, and birth defects. Available in America since 1990, the device is now the subject of lawsuits filed by hundreds of women across the country who claim the product has caused severe side effects, such as heavy bleeding, headaches, depression, and, when the implanted rods are removed, heavy scarring and other complications. The company that distributes the product in America, Wyeth-Ayerst Laboratories of Philadelphia, has said the complication rate remains low and many of the problems may be attributed to the medical professionals inserting the devices, and lack of consumer preparation.

Action for Cancer Prevention Campaign, Women's Environment & Development Organization, 845 Third Ave., 15th Flr., New York, NY, 10022; (212)759-7982; E-mail: wedo@igc.apc.org

American Association of Gynecological Laparoscopists, 1301 E. Florence Ave., Santa Fe Springs, CA 60670; (310)946-8774

American Board of Obstetrics and Gynecology, 2915 Vine St., Ste. 300, Dallas, TX 75204-1069

American Gynecological and Obstetrical Society, University of Utah, 50 N. Medical Dr., Salt Lake City, UT 84132; (801)581-5501

American Medical Women's Association, 801 N. Fairfax St., Alexandria, VA 22314; (703)838-0500

American Society for Colposcopy and Cervical Pathology, c/o American College of OBGYN, 409 — 12th St., SW, Washington, DC 20024; (800)787-7227

American Urogynecologic Society, 401 N. Michigan Ave., Chicago, IL 60611; (312)644-6610

Association of Women's Health, Obstetric, and Neonatal Nurses, 700 — 14th St., NW, Washington, DC 20005; (202)662-1600

Breast Lump & Cervical Cancer Information Hotline, (800)4-CANCER; In Alaska call (800)638-6070

The Boston Women's Health Book Collective operates on the belief that women's health issues must be addressed in an economic, political, and social context, and that women should have a much greater role in health policy decisions. The Collective provides a feminist critique of health care systems and information on women's health through publications, advocacy, and media work. Their Health Information Center collects material from around the world in the area of women's health, and the impact of various social systems on the health of women. Books that the Collective sells cover such subjects as Norplant; hormone replacement therapy risks and benefits; alternatives to allopathic healthcare; the economic and political issues of women's health; reproductive rights; the RU 486 abortion pill; AIDS; the global health issues of women; diagnostic health tests; and childbearing. To obtain a current literature list, send a self-addressed, stamped envelope to the
Boston Women's Health Book Collective, 240 A Elm St., PO Box 192, W. Somerville, MA 02144; (617)625-0271; Fax (617)625-0294; E-mail: bwhbc@lgc.apc.org

Canadian Pelvic Inflammatory Disease Society, PO box 33804, Station D, Vancouver, BC V6J 4L6, Canada

Candida and Dysbiosis Information Foundation, PO Box JF, College Station, TX 77841-5146; (409)694-8687

Center for Research on Women with Disabilities, 6910 Fannin, Ste. 310-South, Houston, TX 77030; (713)797-6282; Fax (713)797-6445; E-mail: mnosek@bcm.tmc.edu

Center for Women Policy Studies, 2000 P St., NW, Ste. 508, Washington, DC 20036; (202)872-1770

Conversations: The Newsletter for Women Fighting Ovarian Cancer is published monthly and subscriptions are free. Donations toward expenses are very welcome. A pen pal/phone pal list called *Voices* is available to subscribers of the newsletter. These are support services to any woman who is in any phase of fighting ovarian cancer.
Conversations, PO Box 7948, Amarillo, TX 79114-7948; (806)359-0111

The *DES Action Voice* newsletter is published quarterly. It contains information about the health risks of the synthetic form of the female hormone estrogen (Diethylstilbestrol).
DES Action, USA, 1615 Broadway, Ste. 510, Oakland, CA 94612; (510)465-4011 or (800)DES-9288; E-mail: desact@well.com

DES Cancer Network, PO Box 10185, Rochester, NY 14610; (716)473-6119; E-mail: desnetwrk@aol.com

Endometriosis Alliance of Greater New York, PO Box 326, Cooper Station, New York, NY 10276; (212)533-3636

The Endometriosis Association is a self-help organization of women with endometriosis and others interested in exchanging information on endometriosis. EA offers mutual support and help, educates the public and medical community, and promotes related research. The EA also publishes a newsletter and other materials.
Endometriosis Association, 8585 N. 76th Place, Milwaukee, WI 53223; (414)355-2200 or (800)992-3636; Fax (414)355-6065

Feminist Bookstore News is published six times per year. It carries articles, letters, and news items relating to women, and also includes book reviews. Though it is a communications vehicle for feminist bookstores in America and other countries, it is a very informative publication in general. Nor for the closed-minded. Subscriptions are $70 per year.
Feminist Bookstore News, 2358 Market St., PO Box 882554, San Francisco, CA 94188; (415)626-1556; Fax (415)626-8970

A Friend Indeed newsletter focuses on issues relating to women in mid-life. Subjects covered include the risks of hysterectomy, estrogen therapy, osteoporosis, and menopause. Ten issues are published each year. Subscriptions are $30.

A Friend Indeed Publications, Inc., Box 515, Place du Parc Station, Montreal, Quebec, Canada H2W2P1 — Or — Box 1710, Champlain, NY 12919-1710; (514)843-5730; E-mail: janine@odyssee.net — or — Net: http://www.odyssee.net/~janine

Harvard Women's Health Watch ($24 a year), Harvard Health Publications, 164 Longwood Ave., Boston, MA 02115; (617)432-1485

The Hysterectomy Educational Resources and Services Foundation is a non-profit foundation which provides information about the alternatives to hysterectomy, the risks of the alternatives, and the potentially dangerous consequences of the surgery. The Foundation maintains a free lending library of books, videos, and audio tapes which circulate via the mail. The *HERS Newsletter* is available for $20 a year. HERS also sells scientific journal articles that cover various aspects of hysterectomy and women's health.

Hysterectomy Educational Resources and Services Foundation, 422 Bryn Mawr Ave., Bala Cynwyd, PA 19004; (610)667-7757; Fax (610)667-8096

International Dalkon Shield Victims Education Association, 212 Pioneer Bldg., Seattle, WA 98104; (206)624-4961

Medea Books is a bookstore in Santa Cruz, California. They specialize in books and other items for women. They publish a catalog, accept credit card orders by phone, and ship anywhere in the US. The store is named after Medea, the ancient Goddess of female healing wisdom.

Medea Books, 849 Almar Ave., Ste. C-285, Santa Cruz, CA 95060; (408)425-0913

Menopause News is an independent publication that contains research results, and medical and psychological opinions, as well as letters and book reviews. It is published six times a year and subscriptions are $23.

Menopause News, 2074 Union St., San Francisco, CA 94123; (800)241-6366

The National Asian Women's Health Organization develops and implements a broad agenda for Asian women's and girls' health, addressing the numerous factors that impact the physical, emotional, mental, social, and spiritual well-being of Asian women and girls.

National Asian Women's Health Organization, 250 Montgomery, Ste. 410, San Francisco, CA 94104; (415)989-9747; Fax (415)989-9758; E-mail: Nawho@aol.com

National Association of Women's Health Professionals, 175 W. Jackson Blvd., Ste. A 1711, Chicago, IL 60604; (708)869-0195

National Black Women's Health Project, 1237 Ralph D. Abernathy Rd., Atlanta, GA 30310; (404)758-9590

National Ovarian Cancer Coalition, PO Box 4472, Boca Raton, FL 33429-4472; (407)393-3220 or 392-6188

National Vulvar Pain Foundation, PO Drawer 177, Graham, NC 27253; (910)226-0704

National Vulvodynia Association, PO Box 19283, Sarasota, FL 34276-2288; (813)927-8503

National Women's Health Network, 514 — 10th St., NW, Ste. 400, Washington, DC 20004 (202)628-7814

National Women's Health Resource Center, 2440 M St., NW, Ste. 325, Washington, DC 20037; (202)293-6045

The Older Women's League is a national membership organization that focuses on the economic, political and social equality of mid-life and older women. The League sells publications, videos, and audio tapes that cover such issues as women and heart disease; menopause; osteoporosis; retirement income and financing; pensions; elder abuse; and divorce. For an information packet, send a self-addressed, stamped envelope to the

Older Women's League, 666 — 11th St., NW, Ste. 700, Washington, DC 20001; (202)783-6686 or (800)825-3695

Ovarian Plus is an independent quarterly newsletter. The editor and publisher is an investigative journalist. The newsletter covers such topics as risk reduction, screening, early detection, psychosocial issues, and political awareness. Subscriptions are $50 per year.
Ovarian Plus: Gynecologic Cancer Prevention Newsletter, PO Box 498, Paauilo, HI 96776-0498; (808)766-1696; Fax (808)776-1266; Net: http://www.monitor.com/ovarian/

PMS Access, PO Box 9326, Madison, WI 53715; (608)833-4PMS or (800)222-4767

Public Citizen's Health Research Group publishes two books on women's health — *Women's Health Alert: What Most Doctor's Won't Tell You About* ($7.95), and *Unnecessary Cesarean Sections: Halting A National Epidemic* ($10). Include $2 for shipping.
Public Citizen, 2000 P St., NW, Ste. 600, Washington, DC 20036; (202)833-3000

Rhonda Flemming Mann Resource Center for Women With Cancer, 200 UCLA Medical Plaza, Ste. 502, Los Angeles, CA 90024; (310)794-6644

Somali Association for Relief and Development/Female Circumcision Information, Research, and Support Institute, 95 W. 95th St., Ste. 25, New York, NY 10025

Toronto Women's Health Network, 1884 Davenport Rd., Toronto, Ontario M6N 4Y2 Canada; (416)392-0898

Vulvar Pain Foundation, PO Drawer 177, Graham, NC 27253; (910)226-0704; Fax (910)226-8518; Net: http://www.lifeplay.net/health/vpFoundation

Women's Cancer Research Center, 3023 Shattuck Ave., Berkeley, CA 94705; (510)548-9272

Women's Health Advocate Newsletter ($24 per year), Aurora Publications, 3918 Prosperity Ave., Fairfax, VA 22031

Women's International Pharmacy, (800)279-5708

Women Wise is a quarterly publication of the Concord Feminist Health Center of Concord, New Hampshire. The newspaper-type publication covers women's health issues and includes book reviews, information on feminist issues, reproductive rights, and gay & lesbian rights. Subscriptions are $10 per year.
Women Wise, Concord Feminist Health Center, 38 S. Main St., Concord, NH 03301; (603)225-2739

Yeast Consulting Services, PO Box 11157, Torrance, CA; (310)375-1073

Final Notes

If you have information that you believe should be included in future updates of this book, or have comments about this book, please write to John McCabe in care of the publisher: **Carmania Books, PO Box 1272 , Santa Monica, CA 90406-1272. E-mail to TheJMcCabe@aol.com — or — CarmaniaBk@aol.com.**

About Carmania Books

Carmania Books is a source of health reference information for consumers. So that we may keep our health research database current, we encourage health organizations to keep our address on file and notify us whenever there is a change in address, phone number, fax number, or electric address.

Because we provide health organizations with valuable exposure, many organizations keep us updated on their activities by providing us with complimentary subscriptions to their newsletters and magazines. Book publishers also regularly send us review copies of their newest health titles.

If you are a health organization sending information for inclusion in the Research Resources section of this book, include (where applicable):

- The full name of the organization.
- The mailing address.
- Phone number.
- Fax number.
- E-mail address.
- Net address.
- Name and title of a contact person.
- Information on the history of the organization.
- Information on the activities or function of the group.
- If the organization deals with a particular disease or condition, please provide a definition.
- Include information on how the organization is funded, particularly if it receives money from any pharmaceutical company, medical supply company, or professional organization.
- Information on professional associations or affiliations.
- Amount of yearly membership fee.
- Number of members and information on how to become a member.
- Name of newsletter or other publications and literature along with sample copies. Also, include information on how your newsletter is funded — through subscriptions and membership fees, or if funding is provided by a pharmaceutical company or other business that could benefit financially from the readers of the newsletter (disclosure information on funding sources should be included in every issue of the newsletter).
- Review copies of books (damaged copies are okay).

Ordering a copy of this book

Additional copies of this book are available from Carmania Books for $19.95. Shipping charges include $3 for the first book and $1 for each additional book. California residents must include sales tax. Send to: Carmania Books, PO Box 1272, Santa Monica, CA 90406-1272.

YES! We do offer quantity discounts on this book. Contact Carmania Books at the address above for more information, or send e-mail to CarmaniaBk@aol.com.